Dual Disorder Heroin Addicts

Icro Maremmani • Matteo Pacini
Angelo G. I. Maremmani

Dual Disorder Heroin Addicts

Clinical and Therapeutical Aspects

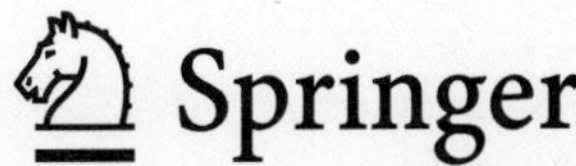 Springer

Icro Maremmani
Addiction Research Methods Institute
World Federation for the Treatment of
Opioid Dependence
New York, NY, USA

Matteo Pacini
V.P. Dole Research Group
G. De Lisio Institute of Behavioural
Sciences
Pisa, Italy

Angelo G. I. Maremmani
Association for the Application of
Neuroscientific Knowledge to Social Aims
(AU-CNS)
Pietrasanta, Italy

ISBN 978-3-031-30095-0   ISBN 978-3-031-30093-6   (eBook)
https://doi.org/10.1007/978-3-031-30093-6

This Springer imprint is published by the registered company Springer Nature Switzerland AG
The registered company address is: Gewerbestrasse 11, 6330 Cham, Switzerland

Foreword

Although substance use disorders are defined as mental disorders in international classifications (DSM-5 TR and ICD-11), their consideration as such is not common in the field. The persistent difficulty in conceptualizing the relationship between addictive and other mental disorders stands out among the many challenges faced by the field of Psychiatry.

Icro Maremanni is one of the European and international opinion leaders who quickly understood that substance addictions are inseparable from the presence of other mental disorders, a clinical condition known as Dual Disorders (DDs) [1].

This book contains a comprehensive review of the evidence and draws from Prof. Maremanni's extensive experience in the field of heroin dual disorders.

Multiple epidemiological studies have established that DDs are an expectation rather than an exception: a substantial fraction of patients suffering from a mental disorder, at some point in their lives, will also experience an addictive disorder, and vice versa. In fact, more than 75% of severe psychiatric disorders occur with other mental disorders, such as substance use disorders and other addictions [2].

From a neuroscience perspective, addiction involves a set of brain interconnected processes, rather than being a disorder defined principally by a single behavior (such as uncontrollable excessive drug use) [3].

For these epidemiological and neuroscientific reasons, people with addictions always present other mental symptoms, pathological personality traits or disorders, that is, Dual Disorders, which are explored in this guide.

An important point to consider when discussing DDs is that only a small proportion of individuals exposed to licit and illicit drugs will ultimately develop addictions. Genetic factors have been strongly implicated in the development of substance use disorders, but the role of this pre-existing vulnerability is still poorly understood and is an area that requires more research [4].

Finally, diagnostics remains a challenge in the field of DDs. Due to the lack of sensitivity and reliability of current diagnostic criteria of psychiatric disorders, clinical scientists seek to identify transdiagnostic processes that may help explain symptom expressions in mental disorders [5]. Dual Disorders, the main topic of this book, is a good example of this approach. Adopting a transdiagnostic perspective to define specific phenotypes can allow the identification of vulnerability or resilience factors to developing different addictions and other mental disorders.

Based on Prof. Maremanni's research background, this book allows one to consider, in particular, the role of the opioid system in mental disorders. Recent studies have investigated certain mental states/personality traits that are linked to addiction and the opioid system of healthy subjects [6]. As a result of genetic or acquired factors, the opioid system may be disrupted and then produce specific functional deficits or excesses in perception, cognition, emotion, and behavior with overlapping phenotypic expressions across psychiatric domains, including addictions and other mental disorders.

This academic and clinical book is an important step towards integrating mental health care, which, until now, has been separated into different treatment concepts, one for addictions and another for other mental disorders. We are advancing towards a future of personalized and precision psychiatry in the field of Dual Disorders, an important aspiration of clinical neuroscience.

References

1. Szerman N, Torrens M, Maldonado R, Balhara YPS, Salom C, Maremmani I, Sher L, Didia-Attas J, Chen J, Baler R; World Association on Dual Disorders (WADD). Addictive and other mental disorders: a call for a standardized definition of dual disorders. Transl Psychiatry. 2022;12(1):446. doi: https://doi.org/10.1038/s41398-022-02212-5. PMID: 36229453; PMCID: PMC9562408.
2. Alsuhaibani R, Smith DC, Lowrie R, Aljhani S, Paudyal V. Scope, quality and inclusivity of international clinical guidelines on mental health and substance abuse in relation to dual diagnosis, social and community outcomes: a systematic review. BMC Psychiatry. 2021;21:209.
3. Nora D. Volkow. Personalizing the treatment of substance use disorders. Am J Psychiatry 2020;177:2.
4. Belin D, Belin-Rauscent A, Everitt BJ, Dalley JW. In search of predictive endophenotypes in addiction: insights from preclinical research. Genes Brain Behav. 2016;15(1):74–88. doi: https://doi.org/10.1111/gbb.12265. Epub 2015 Nov 13. PMID: 26482647.
5. Yücel M, Oldenhof E, Ahmed SH, Belin D, Billieux J, et al. A transdiagnostic dimensional approach towards a neuropsychological assessment for addiction: an international Delphi consensus study. Addiction. 2019;114(6):1095–109.
6. Alan F. Schatzberg. Opioids in psychiatric disorders: back to the future? Am J Psychiatry 2016;173(6):564–5

Institute of Psychiatry and Mental Health,   Nestor Szerman
Gregorio Marañón University Hospital
Madrid, Spain

Contents

Guiding Principles for the Treatment of Dual Disorder Patients

1

1.1 Terminology

1.1.1 Habit

If a substance is used 'habitually', that means it is consumed frequently, either continuously or intermittently. The habit of resorting to a substance depends on the subject's proneness to its use for various reasons, the most frequent of which is self-stimulation and reward. Habitual use, or habit of using a substance, never looms as a disorder, though it may be of medical interest due to its toxic effects. Although the habit of using a drug may be influenced by pharmacological means, an intervention of that kind would not have a medical meaning or goal [1, 2].

1.1.2 Abuse or Non-medical Use

The term 'abuse' (or, more precisely, 'non-medical use') indicates recurrent substance use despite known harmful effects and consequences. In other words, a subject decides to engage in substance non-medical use beyond the threshold of unwanted consequences but does so while experiencing a pleasurable or desirable state. Non-medical use may forerun addiction but is not the addiction itself; the relationship with the substance and the reward mechanism is physiological, whereas the capacity to limit pleasure to avoid unwanted consequences is impaired. When control is lost over the ability to interrupt a habit of consumption that no longer brings pleasure, independently of its increasingly negative effects, we will use the term 'addiction' [3].

Recently, many parties have disputed the term 'abuse' because it is judgmental. It is, in fact, ambiguous because it implies intentional misconduct; if this term is used, therefore, it could be denied that substance use disorders (SUDs) are a medical condition. The correct terms would be 'non-medical use' or, simply, 'use'. To

© The Author(s), under exclusive license to Springer Nature
Switzerland AG 2023
I. Maremmani et al., *Dual Disorder Heroin Addicts*,
https://doi.org/10.1007/978-3-031-30093-6_1

avoid too much repetition in a text, at first mention, 'non-medical use' can be chosen, followed by 'use' at further occurrences. Note that 'harmful use', 'hazardous use', 'recreational use', and 'compulsory use' are overlapping with non-medical use but are not identical to the latter. They can only be alternatives under specific circumstances. If used, these words should be used in a non-moralizing manner and be well defined, e.g. the context should make clear to whom the use is harmful and what type of harm is done. In the case of using 'recreational use', this cannot be put on par with 'non-medically' automatically, as it depends on the substance and can be different for each user and even differ from one occasion of use to another [4].

1.1.3 Addiction

Addiction is a non-medical substance use characterized by losing control before substance use. For addicted subjects, the only chance of holding back from substance use is the absolute unavailability of the substance. In this case, the subject abstains with varying degrees of discomfort. In any other case, the addicted subject will produce stereotyped behaviour with a high level of impulsiveness, which increases when obstacles challenge the subject's search for the substance. The only obstacle that would extinguish the subject's desire to use the substance is unavailability. Such uncontrolled appetition is called craving and is the core symptom of addiction [3, 5–9].

The concept of 'control' usually refers to a possible inability to prevent negative consequences in social and productive terms. On medical grounds, control is maintained if subjects are rewarded by substance use and can organize their resources to keep themselves supplied with the substance, although negative social consequences may develop, and involvement in substance use may leave no room for other life activities. The amount or frequency of substance consumption does not permit discrimination between a habit and a disease, nor do the toxic effects, the exclusiveness and intensity of engagement in substance use, or the level of social adjustment. The addicted subject loses the ability to handle his/her habit, and that is when the disease is born. Several substance users apply for treatment when driven by legal issues, social impairment, or lack of money and succeed in stopping the habit when strongly challenged by its negative consequences. Others stop when the substance no longer gives them the desired effects so that it is no longer worth the effort. Unlike simple users, addicted subjects may seek help even in the absence of psychosocial impairment or a history of adverse events. For example, heroin use disorder (HUD) patients can be classified in a variety of psychosocial categories, which comprise the 'stable' mode, i.e. with no course towards social disruption, but with a stable, though not satisfactory, level of working activity and significant relationships. Besides this, the 'two worlders' mode has been described; that term is used to evoke the condition of a subject who leads an everyday life except for a recurrent involvement in clandestine, drug-related activities, crime included.

An individual who is thoroughly and exclusively dedicated to a substance which, in his/her intentions, will give him pleasure, without ever being able to attain this aim and despite the loss of available resources and a deterioration in the quality of life, is, by definition, addicted to that substance. A subject who complains about having no control over a habit (which implies a chronic discrepancy between the drive to use a substance and the intention to use it in a controlled way) is, by definition, addicted to that substance. However, even when a subject does not complain about an irreversible loss of control, a complaint about dissatisfaction or unhappiness from an expected source of pleasure, without a physiological evolution towards the extinction of appetitive behaviour, is enough to justify a diagnosis of addiction.

Addiction suits a variety of situations, some featuring a chemical substance as the object of craving, others featuring a situation or a gateway towards possible pleasure (such as pathological gambling).

1.1.3.1 Dependence Versus Addiction

Dependence is that pharmacological state in which someone is susceptible to emerging discomfort if deprived of a substance, but recovers a state of well-being when the same, or a cross-reactive, substance is reintroduced. Dependence may be spontaneous or result from an acquired condition: insulin dependence is a spontaneous state in a diabetic person who has lost his/her endogenous resources. A person with diabetes will develop significant metabolic disturbances due to insulin deficiency, but the provision of exogenous insulin supplies will restore his/her metabolism. Also, a person with a chronic self-immune disorder may depend on cortisone drugs, which do not replace any lost function, but counteract a harmful pathophysiological process. Secondary addictive features include dependence on beta-blockers in a person with chronic high blood pressure or the dependence on barbiturates of a person with epilepsy. In this case, any abrupt interruption of exposure to the substance will be followed by a rebound syndrome featuring symptoms opposite those induced by the substance. Rebound symptoms are also the opposite of the symptoms that the substance is meant to counterbalance. The pharmacological basis for this phenomenon is tolerance, which consists of a progressive lowering of the sensitivity threshold in response to exposure to stable dosages. Tolerance is an elastic phenomenon; one result of this is that the interruption of exposure drives a tolerant subject into a sudden state of imbalance due to a relative deficiency of the substance; the outcome is that the system 'rebounds' by progressively lowering the sensitivity threshold until the original level is restored. Before the swing back is complete, the transient imbalance is expressed by rebound symptoms.

Rebound symptoms (commonly referred to as withdrawal symptoms) are usually transient. After the withdrawal has stopped, the eventual state will depend on why the substance was started. If there was a therapeutic reason, and the disease is chronic, the original disease symptoms will strike back. If the disease has been extinguished in the meantime, the subject will just be well. If the disease is a chronic-relapsing one, subjects may stay symptom-free for a period of variable length before they relapse [2].

For addicts receiving treatment, methadone dependence is a consequence of therapy. Its interruption means going back to the natural course of the addictive disease, which implies a perspective of relapse.

Addiction is a radically different condition. Addiction is a cerebral state consisting of a behavioural drive towards consuming an object in response to a subjective feeling called craving, which is intense, self-syntonic, and spontaneous. It is associated with an incapacity to control the urgency or exclusiveness of this drive through one's intentions. Addiction may be compatible with a social life, intellectual and productive functioning, and an ability to keep the law, although it usually leads in the opposite direction. Anyway, by definition, it is incompatible with a happy life and a satisfactory level of reward.

As noted above, on subjective grounds, addiction is coupled with an intense feeling of desire, which cannot be handled (i.e., craving). In a condition of abstinence, the craving will emerge sooner or later, regardless of withdrawal-related discomfort and relapsing behaviour. The old word for addiction was 'toxicomania', which will later be replaced by the term 'drug addiction' or 'drug-dependence'. The first word is more precise and less ambiguous, whereas 'drug-dependence' should be avoided. In fact, 'toxicomania' suggested a 'toxic' effect coupled with an irresistible drive to use the substance and recalled the concept of 'mania' as the psychopathological model to describe the syndrome. Dependence on a toxic substance sounds meaningless: in a condition of dependence, that person is uncomfortable in the absence, not in the presence, of the substance. Even assuming that a toxic effect can be viewed as the price to be paid for gaining benefit from substance use, the cost/benefit ratio must favour the benefit e.g. as happens in the treatment of epilepsy). The toxic aspect of dependence cannot be attributed to withdrawal, which does not develop if someone is constantly exposed to the substance. It can be overcome by gradual tapering [6, 10, 11].

On the other hand, saying that someone is 'addicted to a toxic substance' provides an accurate idea of the tragic tie between that person and the substance. Some addictive diseases also correspond to a state of dependence, but, if so, only for limited periods. Withdrawal is just incidental in an addictive syndrome and does not add anything substantial in terms of diagnosis or prognosis, though it may change presentation symptoms. Stabilization dosages, too, are similar in non-tolerant subjects.

On clinical grounds, the course of addiction follows a course divergent from that taken by dependence:

- The re-emergence of craving is not gradual; craving becomes intense even without tolerance.
- When narcotic dependence sets in, it is complained about since it makes substance use more awkward and interferes with the original reasons for using narcotics (those reasons were forms of reward).
- During attempts to 'detoxify', the addicted person can buffer withdrawal symptoms by using a cross-reacting substance or, possibly, by reacting in a 'cold turkey' way, i.e. without getting any chemical help. Nevertheless, addicts continue to be incapable of preventing the development of relapses after detoxification.
- To handle withdrawal, i.e. dependence, the addict must learn to be able to live without dealing with the substance, over which he/she has no control. That

explains why addicts can go through a 'cold turkey' experience but remain incapable of comfortably detoxifying by tapering narcotics.

The term 'addict' can be defined as undesirable. It is not a person-first use of language (as it reduces the person to one characteristic); it is pejorative and stigmatizing under various circumstances. 'Addiction' comes from Latin'addicere': making someone the slave of someone else, and it has the trait of being pejorative and stigmatizing. In this book, the term 'addiction' will refer to a SUD of high severity [4].

1.1.3.2 Addictive Ambivalence

In addicted people, thoughts, affects, and behaviours are all displayed ambivalently. This observable ambivalence mirrors a psychopathological one, which is itself an expression of a neurobiological 'conflict'. Addicted patients behave in a contradictory way: they apply for treatment intending to persist with their inclination to continue their substance use. Such behaviour corresponds to their intention, or 'will', misleadingly called. A 'will' to stop addiction is usually claimed when help is being asked for, but the drive to reproduce addictive behaviours overpowers that 'will'. The diagnosis is 'addiction', a term that allows identifying a category of 'difficult patients' who apply for therapeutic intervention against reckless behaviour that pulls in the opposite direction; these features provide the dynamics of 'making allowance for disease'. To make the point more simply, addicted patients cannot counteract the symptoms of their disease. Since addiction is centred upon craving, its course will drag the patient away from a therapeutic setting in imposing a self-perpetuating search for the substance. Many develop a wrong idea of addiction, mistaking it for a strong habit and interpreting a request for treatment as a tricky attempt to escape the consequences of one's illicit and disruptive behaviours.

On clinical grounds, it is possible to discriminate between the hope of remission, which corresponds to intention and not to will, i.e. an elaborate kind of thought inspired by personal experience, which can be translated into a series of graduated actions tending towards treatment adherence and is based on the activity of the cortical brain. Addictive behaviour, on the other hand, is produced by an instinctual drive that moves forward side by side with an affective state, remains self-syntonic, and becomes ever more pertinent (an urgent priority). The instinct is directly reinforced by exposure to substances and eventually becomes self-perpetuating by long-lasting substance-produced imprinting. Because it is related to subcortical brain activity, an instinctual drive takes the form of a rapid, one-step process.

Addictive behaviour results from a more robust, 'addictive' component, induced by substances and finding expression as an instinct, possibly reinforced by the substance itself, and a weaker, more rational component, which develops gradually, following the negative consequences of substance use. The two dynamics, the addictive instinct and the anti-addictive intention, are challenged in different ways by the substance: in fact, the substance first impacts the instinctual component and soon afterwards on the intention, through the main features of substance-related experiences. The honeymoon phase, in which the person develops addiction, always precedes the later stage in which an intention to quit will develop and overlap with the earlier intention. The same sequence is reproduced before and during relapses. Even if the intention to stay abstinent remains prominent after detoxification, a single episode of consumption is enough to trigger relapse; apparently, sound intentions are quickly overwhelmed by quick instinctual dynamics that had been extinguished [9, 12]. It is a misconception to expect that continuous abstinence, possibly reinforced by environmental rewards, should restore an addict's capacity to avoid substance use. As time passes, the intention to stay abstinent does not become sounder but usually weakens and loses the urgency initially displayed at the time of detoxification treatment when it was related to heavy global impairment. As conditions improve, time does not heal but brings on relapse. The addictive instinct, though without any reinforcement due to enduring abstinence, rapidly comes back to drive a person towards the substance against their intentions.

In moving from relapse to relapse, a process of sensitization seems to take place: relapsing takes place more and more rapidly, and the period of latency between the first slip and full involvement in substance use becomes shorter. In the struggle between the intention to abstain and the drive to use, the odds are always loaded against the gambler, and the match lasts for shorter times.

On psychopathological grounds, the ambivalence of addicts is founded on the core of addiction, i.e. the instinctual drive and its affective correlate (craving); these are self-syntonic. Some authors fail to recognize craving as self-syntonic and refer to it as compulsive (sometimes this term is used to indicate very intense craving with short-loop usage). The discrepancy between the intention to abstain from and the drive to use a substance may be mistaken for a compulsion, if the intention is misunderstood for a drive. The two components struggling in the addict's mind are not of the same kind and do not come into conflict on the same level; the drive itself is not ambivalent and is directed towards the substance. Craving drive and behaviour are all oriented towards the substance, making the whole complex a self-syntonic phenomenon. The intention pulling in the opposite direction cannot be referred to as self-dystonic (compulsive) since it acts on a different brain level, rational vs. instinctual. Resorting to the substance despite the intention to stop addiction is not a matter of compulsion; it is a conflict between a pursued and unwanted behaviour. The conflict takes place both during and after the behavioural output [3].

Ambivalence does characterize addiction at different degrees of severity. Higher severity corresponds to a more significant discrepancy between intention and drive; the latter turns out to be even stronger. In a severely ill addict with years of substance use and a history of repeated treatment failures, the intention to stop addiction may be sound and structured. However, the drive is always 'sounder' in the addict's brain. Therefore, since the drive is becoming more rapid and can count on reinforcement, the intention to abstain is always weaker. In proportion, severely ill addicts become more willing to stop but less capable of doing so.

A severely ill addict is usually pessimistic about acquiring the capability of stopping addiction and staying detached from the substance. Because of this factor, along with more significant psychosocial impairment and independent complications (e.g. infective diseases), the intention to abstain eventually weakens, leaving further room for addiction. A hard-core addict will ultimately think that the only realistic chance is to acquire partial control over substance use, resulting from an addictive way of thinking and growing pessimism about a healing perspective. Addicts often need to be motivated because of such pessimism, while the addictive way of thinking becomes a target to be removed by treatment. Motivation should not be mistaken for an element of treatment. No patient can be motivated so strongly as to make his/her intention prevail over the addictive drive. On the other hand, acting on motivation increases the patient's trust and compliance with treatment, so restoring a healing perspective to their mind. When addicted patients approach treatment settings, they are characterized by a spontaneous request for help, a different motivational status, and a constant ambivalence towards compliance with treatment, which they may be aware of to a certain degree.

1.1.3.3 Addiction and Insight

When patients ask for help, they are usually aware of the severity of their current condition and realize that they have lost control over substance use. On the other hand, they have no real insight into the nature of the disease concerning its chronicity, endogenous pathophysiology, and irreversibility [13]. Addicts will think the problem is their recent past instead of their future and deny having any long-term trouble with substance use control. In this way, addicts underrate or decline the risk of relapse and aim to achieve a controlled use or spontaneous abstinence rather than understanding that this should be a relapse-prevention treatment. As soon as they reach a state of partial well-being, they will identify it with definitive healing. When relapses occur, they will think of each relapse as a separate episode, with its precursors, reasons, and treatment perspectives.

Substance users usually deny or lack any awareness of their problem. Recent neuroscientific evidence suggests that the denial of problems related to drug use may be associated with alterations in various brain networks that contribute to insight. This integrated model includes the insula, which is involved in enteroception, self-awareness, and drug craving; the anterior cingulate, which is involved in behavioural monitoring and response selection; and the frontal and dorsal striatum, which is involved in automatic habit formation and self-awareness [14, 15]. Of particular interest is the role played by the insula in processes related to conscious enteroception, emotional experience, and decision-making. Within this framework, the insula contributes to the way addicted individuals feel, remember, and decide about taking drugs— the main result being that drug addiction turns out to be like a naturally motivated behaviour, closely comparable with eating and sex [16].

As to alcohol, a close relationship has been observed between the state of patients' insight and their level of motivation to change their behaviour [17]. Some papers have pointed out the effect of insight on patients' willingness to change their lifestyle, suggesting the need for brief insight-enhancement interventions addressed to patients with alcohol dependence [18]. When a contemporary mental illness is present (in cases with dual disorder—DD), this has been hypothesized to act as a fundamental factor in impairing insight level [19].

A few studies have been dedicated to investigating the role of insight in cocaine dependence. Some authors have examined the potential association between awareness of illness and drug-seeking behaviour and have proposed, especially with cocaine subjects who are urine-negative, interventions to enhance insight to improve their longer-term clinical outcomes [20]. Active cocaine users display a diminished neural response to errors, particularly to the anterior cingulate cortex, which is closely involved in error processing. The inability to detect or adjust performance in response to mistakes has been linked with clinical symptoms, including the loss of insight and perseverative behaviour. According to this theory, behavioural deficits that probably contribute to the maintenance of drug-dependence could derive directly from a cognitive dysfunction [21].

Concerning cannabis, there has been a great deal of debate over the role of the delta-9-tetraidrocannabinol (THC) in the pathogenesis of psychotic disorders; to date, cannabis use has been one of the most critical risk factors for psychosis [22–25]. Whatever the cause, it is complicated for many subjects to bring cannabis use to a stop during the early phases of recovery, not only because of prior habits of use, but also because of the attendant psychotic symptoms, including poor insight and judgement, lack of impulse control, and, most crucially, cognitive impairment. Moreover, most of these subjects cannot grasp the fact that cannabis use relates to the onset of symptoms. Of course, patients' insight is a basic condition for understanding the need for treatment programmes and is still further damaged by ongoing substance use [26].

Lastly, it is correct to assess dependence on nicotine as a severe form of dependence; it is, consequently, distinguished by impairment of awareness and the reward system. The description of smoking as an autonomously chosen lifestyle appears to be cynical and calls for vigorous rejection. Most older smokers would like to quit smoking and have repeatedly tried to do so without ever succeeding. High-risk patients with comorbidities, who are highly motivated to quit smoking, often fail to achieve success, even if they are fully aware of the significant benefits of effective smoking cessation [20, 27].

In the field of heroin addiction, there is, in the literature, a worrying and unjustified shortage of data. This fact is even more disquieting when it is borne in mind that HUD patients often fail to comply with methadone treatment when prescribed at appropriate blocking dosages. Lack of insight is a complicated state for building the motivation for compliance or abstinence.

In our opinion, medicine and, especially, addiction medicine can no longer be considered a simple intervention whose results depend exclusively on a physician's decision. Patients have become ever more closely involved in the therapeutic process, especially on rehabilitative grounds, so they participate in their treatment, though not at a decision-making level [28]. Increasing efforts have been dedicated to informing and educating patients and significant ones about health issues, making possible the active participation of any concerned citizen [28–30]. Thus, on rehabilitation and prevention grounds, it is crucial to provide information about the nature of the disease, its features, and its course while making precise which available treatments are the most effective [28, 31, 32] and overcoming misleading thinking styles.

Table 1.1 Predictors of impaired insight in 1066 DD/BIP1-HUD patients

Predictors	OR (CI 95%)	p
Heroin intake		
Multi-weekly	0.55 (0.32–0.96)	0.036
Daily	1.57 (1.10–2.25)	0.013
Modality of use		
Junkies	0.42 (0.20–0.87)	0.020
Two worlders	0.37 (0.18–0.79)	0.010
Polysubstance use, absence	1.79 (1.33–2.42)	0.000
Household: satisfactory situation	0.56 (0.42–0.76)	0.000
Dual diagnosis, absence	1.75 (1.29–2.37)	0.000

We assume that a patient's compliance with therapy is to some degree related to his/her insight. As a result, the insight assessment is necessarily preliminary to an educational process that improves the patient's active role in the therapeutic process. Correlations between the patient's degree of insight and the history of addiction may be helpful to clinicians in identifying which patients are most in need of an educational intervention.

In one of our studies on a group of 1066 HUD patients who were seeking treatment for opioid agonist treatment, we looked for differences in historical, demographic, and clinical characteristics between patients with different levels of awareness of illness (insight) (Table 1.1).

The results showed that in the cohort studied, most subjects lacked insight into their heroin-use behaviour. Compared with the impaired-insight group, those who possessed insight into their illness showed significantly greater awareness of past social, somatic, and psychopathological impairments and had a more significant number of past treatment-seeking events for heroin addiction. In contrast with other psychiatric illnesses, awareness appears to be related to the passing of time and the worsening of the disease. Methodologies to improve the insight of patients should, therefore, be targeted more directly on patients early in their history of heroin dependence because the risk of lack of insight is greatest during this period [33].

1.2   Dual Disorders and Its Flaws

The first step in structuring an effective treatment for DD patients is the definition of a correct psychiatric diagnosis; this is not always easy because there is an overlap area between outbursts of primary psychiatric disorders and drug- or alcohol-related psychopathology.

The SUD may trigger or, on the contrary, mask the symptoms of concomitant psychiatric pathology (Table 1.2).

It can cause psychopathological symptoms, typical of almost all psychiatric pathologies, the duration and severity of which correlate with the type, dose, and duration of substance use; it can accelerate development, cause relapse, or worsen the severity of a concomitant psychiatric pathology; it may be motivated by a desire

Table 1.2 Psychiatric symptoms due to substance use disorder

Psychiatric symptoms	Primary used substance	State
Delirium	Alcohol and CNS sedatives	Intoxication and withdrawal
	CNS stimulants and cocaine	Intoxication
	Hallucinogens and PCP	Intoxication
	Inhalers	Intoxication
	Opioids	Intoxication
Psychosis	Alcohol and CNS sedatives	Intoxication and withdrawal
	CNS stimulants and cocaine	Intoxication
	Cannabinoids	Intoxication
	Hallucinogens and PCP	Intoxication and flashback intoxication
	Inhalers	Intoxication?
	Opioids	Withdrawal
Memory disorders	Alcohol and CNS sedatives	Prolonged use
Dementia	Inhalers	Prolonged use
Mood disorders	Alcohol	Intoxication
	CNS sedatives	Withdrawal
	CNS stimulants and cocaine	Intoxication and withdrawal
	Hallucinogens and PCP	Intoxication
	Inhalers	Intoxication
	Opioids	Intoxication?
Anxiety disorders	Alcohol and CNS sedatives	Intoxication and withdrawal
	CNS stimulants and cocaine	Intoxication
	Caffeine	Intoxication
	Cannabis	Intoxication
	Hallucinogens	Intoxication
	Inhalers	Intoxication
Sexual dysfunctions	Alcohol and CNS sedatives	Intoxication and withdrawal
	CNS stimulants and cocaine	Intoxication
	Opioids	Intoxication
Sleep disorders	Alcohol and CNS sedatives	Intoxication and withdrawal
	CNS stimulants and cocaine	Intoxication and withdrawal
	Caffeine	Intoxication
	Opioids	Intoxication and withdrawal

to mitigate the symptoms of a psychiatric disorder or the side effects of drugs used to combat the psychopathological picture; it can cause psychiatric symptomatology when this use is abruptly discontinued; it can induce changes in the nervous system that produce and support psychiatric syndromes that are then persistent even in the absence of use, or even posthumous onset compared with cessation of use.

Psychopathological symptoms, if residual, may cause SUD to be misinterpreted as partially 'in remission'; may interfere with the patient's aptitude and motivation to follow rehabilitation treatment. For example, anxiety disorders or phobias can compromise the result of group psychotherapy; the absence of motivation to undertake addiction treatment may depend on depression; interpersonal relationships can be limited by odd behaviours in psychotic or manic patients. Often, all these phenomena are interpreted as signs of resistance to treatment or relapse into the use of substances in patients in the phase of remission concerning addiction; they can mimic the maladaptive behaviour typical of substance users, conditioning a misdiagnosis of 'SUD'. Lastly, they can accompany the course of addiction as markers of severity and chronicity, anticipating the tendency to relapse soon after the first period of use, thus falling within the specific psychopathology of SUD but being open to a mistaken interpretation as an additional diagnosis.

It is also possible that psychiatric pathology and the use of substances coexist while remaining autonomous throughout the disease.

Dual disorder is a term applied to people who have an addictive disorder and another co-occurring mental disorder. It is related to interacting neurobiological and environmental factors involved in behaviours of substance- and non-substance-related disorders. Nobody chooses to become an addict. Addiction is not a matter of weakness of will, a consequence of self-indulgent behaviour, or a result of the mere pursuit of pleasure [34].

In the past, other terms have been used. The acronym MICA (mentally ill chemical abusers) was sometimes used for subjects with a SUD and a severe and persistent psychiatric condition, such as schizophrenia or bipolar disorder. Another definition classified a subject as being 'mentally ill and chemically affected' since the term 'affected' describes the condition better while carrying no negative connotation. Other acronyms used are MISA (mentally ill substance abusers), CAMI (chemical abuse and mental illness), and SAMI (substance abuse and mental illness). In this book, the term 'dual disorder' (DD) will be used. The most frequent associations are major depression and cocaine use, panic disorder and alcoholism, schizophrenia, alcoholism and substance non-medical use, and borderline personality disorder with polysubstance use. It is not uncommon to come across patients with more than two coexisting disorders, for which it is possible to apply the same considerations that were made concerning DD.

Nevertheless, a confounding effect was produced by the clinical and nosological overlap between comorbidity, DDs, and simple state-related symptoms. More recently, some Italian authors have pointed to the need to define addiction-related psychopathology beyond intoxication, withdrawal, and craving. A non-specific, persistent clinical picture dominated by depressed mood, anxiety, and impulsivity was described as the standard expected psychiatric profile of heroin addiction before accounting for any specific DDs [35–42]. Other than comorbidity, such a clinical picture could be said to stand as the rule for recognizing the psychiatric impairment of HUD patients. It is usually sensitive to opioid agonists [43], as well as being enhanced by antagonists or on-going chronic intoxication [44]. On the other hand, these symptoms are more than state-related abnormalities and run parallel to their activity and severity, thus looming as a helpful indicator of relapse and insufficient therapeutic coverage [45].

After 20 years of segregation, we should, instead, bring addictive diseases back to the area of general psychiatry to avoid any further misconception of behavioural diseases as being other than located in the brain and likely to express themselves also through secondary mental abnormalities. The segregation of addiction treatment to a position separate from the academic psychiatric environment has led to the thought that addictions are distinct behavioural disorders, which is correct, but disorders somehow not belonging to the field of psychiatry, as if they took place at some different level, 'in between the brain and society'. Across 20 years of studies on DDs, the data have shown a wide variability between countries. Apart from that, reports do not seem to share a single vision of what a DD is supposed to be. The diagnostic definition has not gone beyond a 'comorbidity' level, not allowing us to differentiate transient syndromes from independent disorders, which may run parallel to them and sometimes overlap. This problem mirrors the diagnostic trends of addictive diseases in general psychiatric environments. Psychiatrists usually tend not to separate addiction from non-medical use or simple physiological consumption. Whenever the precise situation is concerned with illegal drugs, any use is labelled as misuse, and any heavy use as addiction. Heroin use and misuse are seldom reported as such. Legal drug use is considered abnormal in psychiatric patients because it may be a risk factor or exert a negative influence. Overall, psychiatrists are partly blind to addiction and the physiological use of substances. Addiction is merged with non-medical use and is sometimes regarded as secondary to other disorders by applying a hypothesis of self-medication or symptomatic expression (impulsiveness). On the other hand, addictologists are hypersensitive to psychiatric symptoms and are unlikely to record them as part of the addictive picture [46].

DD patients must be evaluated in terms of case severity, chronicity, and the degree of functional impairment. A wide range of different clinical conditions calls for specific interventions. Still, there is a trend for patients to be clustered around specific treatments instead of others based on which clinical features are prominent. For instance, methadone-maintained populations include many addicts with comorbid personality disorders. Schizophrenic alcoholics tend to be treated in hospital in-patient units or local mental health services or within homecare programmes.

Mentally ill subjects run a high risk of developing SUDs, and, conversely, substance users are likely to be future psychiatric patients. Approximately one-third of all psychiatric patients use substances, a frequency twice that found among the general population. Over 50% of substance users report symptoms of psychopathology, though these are primarily interpretable as substance-induced rather than due to any independent mental disease.

In cases of DD, there is a clear trend towards greater chronicity and severity and more serious somatic, social, and psychological problems than in cases of uncomplicated addiction. Moreover, relapses into substance use are more likely; this, in turn, causes psychiatric symptoms to become exacerbated, setting up a vicious circle. DD patients take longer to complete any treatment successfully, are likely to undergo several critical phases over time, and tend to recover more slowly.

1.2.1 Relationship with a Dual Disorder Patient

When psychiatric illness and substance non-medical use coexist, the medical approach to the patient is inevitably awkward. This fact is due both to the patient's psychiatric condition and addictive behaviours and to a cultural context that does not favour a scientific approach to mental illness in general or, more emphatically, to addictive diseases. On the one hand, depression and doubts about effectiveness are unlikely to prevent patients from resorting to medical services. On the other hand, environmental issues interfere with a correct medical intervention: patients are unlikely to know what kind of treatment is provided by which service; some types of facilities are only available if paid for; and some types of service, though effective, are only available in some areas, so that addicts in some parts of a country face disadvantages.

Usually, when DD patients apply to an outpatient clinic to treat their addiction, acute psychiatric syndromes are often mistaken for substance-induced alterations, or, conversely, withdrawal or intoxication phenomena are misinterpreted as psychiatric illness. In the latter case, patients are usually referred to psychiatric services. Paradoxically, the same happens with psychiatric patients who apply for treatment at psychiatric facilities if they are also current substance users [46]. The intensity and frequency of psychiatric symptoms and substance-induced symptoms usually fluctuate. So, it may be that the need to buffer intermittent acute variations on a basis comprising a chronic psychiatric illness and an addictive condition catch the clinician's attention more than the need to control the independent aspects of the case, which will be psychiatric, addictive, and social. The result may be that the health system becomes an obstacle to patients seeking treatment rather than a way of providing them with adequate health facilities. Currently, a correct approach to DD patients requires not only attention to the specific issues of each case but also an awareness of the continuing divergence between the health system, as it is implemented now, and the needs of DD patients.

1.2.2 Dual Disorder Patient Case Management

Traditionally, the public health system has always given patients the responsibility of seeking treatment, as if that was a sign of their motivation to be cured. More recently, the same issue has been raised in connection with what is called 'case management' (CM), considering that most patients with other psychiatric illnesses are reluctant to resort to services or are not capable of taking advantage of available facilities. CM may be a crucial resource in dealing with addiction when the aim is to start patients on treatments and favour retention in treatment. CM may also be valuable in attenuating the negative results of dropping out of treatment. Conversely, programmes lacking a CM approach are more likely to be hampered by psychopathological crises and hospitalization episodes, while the most severe cases are unlikely to be successfully handled. The broad aim of CM is to encourage reluctant patients to enter treatments and limit the negative impact of treatment failures on the personal history of subjects. DD patients need to be followed up for their conditions, applying strategies devised to fit their condition. Physicians and patients should share the responsibility for the treatment. At present, patients who deny the presence or minimize the severity of their condition are treated with excessive severity by physicians. DD patients require a completely different approach to be persuaded to enter and comply with treatment programmes. It is advisable to avoid confrontation with patients whose conditions are particularly severe, such as psychotic ones, because they are unlikely to comply with the programme's rules until the severity of their condition has been at least partly improved. Too often, addictive diseases are regarded with a 'here and now' attitude by physicians themselves, who also tend to overrate the background aspects of associated psychiatric disorders. SUD tends to be interpreted as symptomatic of previous psychic trauma rather than an independent condition. Too often, treatment strategies focus on resolving some evolutional problem, in the mistaken conviction that addiction will achieve remission once its background has been readjusted. So far, the primary outcome of this attitude has been the perpetuation of the vicious circle of addictive behaviours.

Some treatment programmes require patients to be drug-free as a condition for admission. In most patients with a severe DD condition (such as people with schizophrenia), a drug-free state should only be considered a possible long-term outcome of adequate methadone maintenance. On the other hand, a drug-free condition may be helpful for patients suffering from depression or panic disorder to allow an earlier, better-defined diagnosis and, later, a proper therapeutic plan. For DD patients, the requirement of a drug-free condition as a preliminary to programmes actually functions as an obstacle [47]. We, therefore, suggest that the concept of a 'drug-free state' be redefined as a therapeutic goal to be approached step by step along a route mapped out by an adequate treatment programme. Homeless patients, who dwell in highly drug-polluted environments, cannot be expected to be brought to a drug-free condition by any deadline, especially an early one.

1.2.3   Dual Disorder Patient and Treatment Systems

Several operators work together in psychiatric services: psychiatrists, psychologists, social workers, counsellors, and others. Treatment strategies vary from one service to another and within the same service. Psychiatric patients must be provided with integrated treatments, comprising counselling, case management, hospitalization, and rehabilitative and residential programmes, to satisfy the needs arising from both acute and chronic conditions. In some cases, psychotropics are used to treat psychiatric disorders and, simultaneously, SUDs. The frequency of psychotropic use among general psychiatric patients is low, whereas DD patients tend to use otherwise innocuous agents, such as sedative tricyclic antidepressants. Therefore, trouble may follow from the incautious prescription of psychotropics to non-medical use-prone patients. This fact is why psychiatrists should broaden their knowledge of substance-related medical issues, while physicians who deal with drug addicts should also be knowledgeable about psychiatry, especially the use of psychotropics. As in the field of general psychiatry, a variety of therapeutic solutions are available for the treatment of SUDs (short- and long-term detoxification programmes, agonist maintenance, therapeutic communities, and self-help programmes), which often apply divergent basic principles and may be incompatible with each another.

Some programmes require a drug-free condition as a starting point, whereas that condition is simply the long-term result of other programmes. Some programmes, such as methadone or buprenorphine maintenance, do not invariably aim at the complete elimination of heroin use. Controlled heroin use may be acceptable when no evolution towards abstinence is feasible, if methadone maintenance treatment (MMT) ensures satisfactory personal and social readjustment. The extent of heroin-assisted treatment (HAT) in countries where it is available is modest compared to other agonist maintenance treatments for opioid dependence. Within the European Union, the role of HAT is marginal. A range of therapeutic, safety, prevention, and economic concerns about potential adverse effects of HAT for patients and the treatment system are discussed in the light of relevant research evidence. None of the concerns is justified. Positive effects for the treatment system and public order prevail. The present model of HAT has good outcomes for previously treatment-resistant HUD patients, is a safe and cost-effective therapy, and is a helpful element in a comprehensive treatment system for HUD patients [48].

As is true of treatment for psychiatric patients in general, teams working in addiction medicine units comprise physicians, psychiatrists, psychologists, and counsellors. Other operators may also be involved, offering a variety of adjuvant skills. A biopsychosocial approach, incorporating and integrating various professional skills, should lie at the core of any service for addictive diseases. Psychotropics are currently used to treat whatever complications may follow substance misuse (overdose and withdrawal), but some of them, especially disulfiram, naltrexone (NTX), and methadone, are effective on addiction too. Addiction physicians are often knowledgeable about psychotropics, but a prejudice exists that any psychotropic is quite likely to induce dependence. Therefore, many addiction physicians avoid prescribing psychotropics, whereas they should be able to decide when to resort to them and what category is required for specific psychopathological conditions. Unless DD patients are provided with effective treatment for their psychiatric illness, the risk of relapse is bound to remain high.

Self-help associations, such as Alcoholics Anonymous and Narcotics Anonymous, may have much to offer to other types of treated patients. Self-help interventions should not be viewed as alternative treatment options but be part of integrated treatment programmes. On the other hand, unfounded fears and misinformation may spread within self-help contexts, if participants only report opinions and views strictly on personal experiences. Specific self-help programmes for DD patients have been developed in the United States; these do indeed focus on improving patients' compliance with psychopharmacological therapies.

DD patients frequently get in touch with their general practitioners (GPs), but they usually win little attention. Moreover, GPs are likely to deal with cases of DD by prescribing generic psychotropics, such as antidepressants and anxiolytics, or misuse-targeting agents, such as disulfiram and NTX, which should be included in integrated treatment programmes. GPs are the category of physicians most likely to prescribe anxiolytic drugs, especially benzodiazepines (BDZs), which are those most likely to be non-medically used. GPs show they are most concerned about the side complications of addiction, such as withdrawal, overdosing, or somatic issues, rather than aiming for a specific intervention directed at the core of the addictive disease.

1.3   Dual Disorder and Treatment Models

1.3.1   Sequential Model

The sequential model is the first to have been applied and, to date, has been the most frequently employed. According to this, psychiatric disease and addictive disease are approached in two different stages. Some clinicians reckon that the addictive disease should always be approached first and that it only makes sense to treat the comorbid psychiatric illness once any misuse has been halted. Others argue that specific treatments for the psychiatric illness may be feasible even when there is on-going substance use before any intervention for addiction has been started. Another view is that the decision on treatment priority should consider the severity of each condition, the preference going to the condition most urgently calling for intervention. To exemplify all this, we could select the case of a DD depressed heroin addict who seeks treatment at a mental health service when still suffering from depression and attends a specific programme for substance use to cure recurrent alcohol binges.

1.3.2   Parallel Model

On the parallel model, the patient is enrolled in two programmes simultaneously, the first targeting the psychiatric illness and the second focusing on substance use. A 12-step programme may, for instance, be combined with psychiatric treatment under the supervision of mental health operators. As with the previous (sequential) model, this model also consists of already running programmes. Psychiatrists deal with psychiatric illness, and addiction physicians or operators manage the addiction-related issues.

1.3.3   Integrated Treatment

The integrated model pairs psychiatric treatment with intervention against substance use within a programme precisely planned for DD patients. Theoretically, two distinct categories of physicians and skills should be involved, together with a twofold CM approach, to allow patients to overcome both psychiatric and addictive relapses.

Each of these treatment models has pros and cons. Requirements for treatment adequacy vary with different states of comorbidity, symptom severity, and global functioning impairment. The sequential and parallel models may best fit severely addicted patients who also suffer from a minor form of psychiatric disease. The main drawback to these approaches is that patients may be given contradictory information in the two different settings they attend. Conversely, when a CM facility is available and is embodied in a single operator possessing two sets of skills in a specific setting, patients benefit from a homogeneous treatment approach.

1.3.4 Towards a Hierarchical Approach to Dual Disorder Treatment

When treating patients with dual disorder and DD/BIP1-HUD (DD/HUD), it is advisable to follow a hierarchical algorithm [49] (Fig. 1.1).

SUD should be dealt with first: by detoxification possibly and certainly starting most patients on anti-craving pharmacological maintenance, although aversion therapy may suit a few patients. HUD patients may have opioid antagonists administered to them if they are mildly ill, whereas agonist medications (buprenorphine and methadone) suit moderately and severely ill patients, respectively. Achieving control of mood instability or psychotic episodes is the next step, followed, eventually, by a prevention strategy to counter residual cravings and breakthrough episodes of mood disorders or psychotic episodes using long-term pharmacological maintenance with a double target. Relapse prevention must never be understood as complete extinction but as a trend towards a lower grade of severity, a reduction in frequency, and a delayed occurrence of possible relapse. HUD patients are a population in which it is possible to study and register the effects of chronic opioid injury

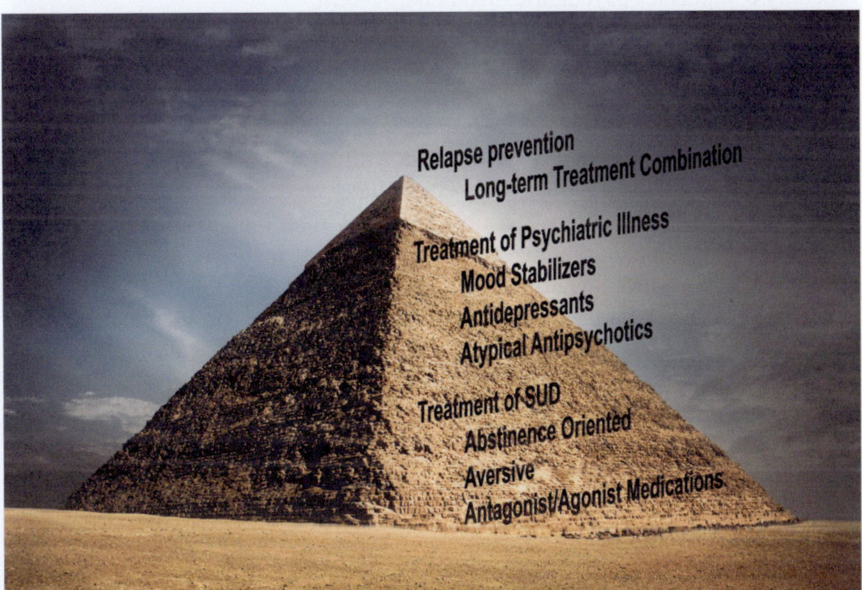

Fig. 1.1 Hierarchical approach to dual disorder treatment

and the following dysfunction. The backdating body of pharmacological knowledge about psychiatric properties of opioid agonists seems to corroborate what emerged from the description of opioid agonist-treated HUD patients suffering from DD by our research group [50–56]. On the one hand, the toxic properties of fast-acting opioids and the therapeutic properties of slow-acting opioids are crucial issues in uncomplicated and DD/HUD patients. Opioid agonists such as methadone and buprenorphine should first be thought of as psychoactive drugs, with valuable properties in the treatment of opioid addiction and a more comprehensive therapeutic potential when heroin addiction is combined with further psychiatric disturbance [49].

1.3.5 Criteria to Be Used in Treating Dual Disorders

In some isolated cases, the two professional figures involved have succeeded in working as a team. In others, a single person has possessed both professional skills. In all other cases, addicts tend to ask for help or be referred to both facilities and attend them according to the prevalence of craving or other psychiatric symptoms.

In most cases, patients have poor insight into their addiction and may have poor insight into their other disorders, too, as in the case of psychosis [33]. Several studies from the literature confirm that there is a mutual negative interaction between substance use and psychiatric disorders, in terms of both a more severe substance use history and an unfavourable treatment prognosis for DD patients. Substance use generally complicates psychiatric disorders [57–62].

Nevertheless, it should not be assumed that DD patients are destined to drop out, whatever the conditions of treatment may be. In some contexts, it has been reported that they stay the course better and continue in treatment to a greater extent than single-diagnosis addicts [52, 55, 56, 63]. Italian data on the long-term stabilization of DD patients following an MMT have shown that no poor dropout percentages need be expected, if the treatment protocol includes no dose limitation and does not encourage premature treatment termination. As a rule, bipolar spectrum patients require higher stabilization dosages, which would rule them out of effective treatment as far as dose-limiting attitudes are concerned.

As a personal hint, our recommendation would be to consider unrecognized bipolar disorder in patients who fail to taper their methadone despite recurrent attempts and possible hospitalizations because of outbursts of rage or dysphoric excitement. These patients, who are usually looked down on because they do not get satisfactory results despite sticking to 'higher doses', are likely to be the best responders when doses are further increased due to a virtuous circle between psychiatric improvement, treatment compliance, and craving suppression.

It would be unfounded to regard DDs as having a low potential for treatment adherence. A study on anonymous Internet consultation about opioid misuse-related issues showed an opposite trend. Patients were classified according to the kind of issue they came with side effects and interactions, addictive symptoms, and other psychiatric symptoms unrelated to addiction or intoxication. Clarification was possible because of an open consultation mode, with no limits to answers and rebuttals. Patients could describe their situation and history in detail, and physicians could ask for whatever information was missing for them to express an opinion. Based on these interactions, patients could be further classified as having or not having insight into three crucial aspects of addiction dynamics: the automatism of relapsing behaviour; the loss of control over substance use, when the substance is being used; and a unitary vision of relapses, instead of an incomplete interpretation of each episode. Findings reveal that independent psychiatric symptoms are related to a better understanding of addiction as a chronic disease and recognizing the impossibility of handling the substance. Coexisting psychiatric diagnosis may lead patients to an earlier and more complete perception of themselves as being impaired. Their compliance with treatment can be based on the control of psychiatric symptoms. Addiction itself implies poor insight, and the absence of significant psychiatric impairment allows patients to think they can handle each relapse separately, control environmental factors to stop relapses, or come to terms with substance use [64].

We could state that DD patients benefit most from virtuous treatment protocols for reasons that account for inadequate protocols' most severe detrimental effects. As mentioned elsewhere, the dosage is a simple exemplification of this 'biphasic' effect. Under similar conditions for the severity of addiction, DD patients (especially when the disorders and psychoses are affective) present as resistant patients when their treatment is based on an averagely ineffective dosage. Conversely, they amazingly turn into brilliant responders when treated with higher dosages. After admission into treatment, the short term seems to be when most differences between single and DDs emerge. Early attrition, in other words, is still the most significant obstacle even for higher-dose programmes. Due to the importance of dosage in the achievement of craving suppression, less potent opioid agonists and pure antagonists fail to reach out to the therapeutic needs of severely addicted and mentally ill addicts. A group of early attrition survivors in NTX maintenance showed a dropout rate related to the presence of psychotic disorders, affective disorders, and otherwise unspecified aggressiveness [44]. The same diagnoses predicted better long-term retention within a high threshold MMT [55]. A study was conducted on the so-called 'resistant patients' in Norway [65], where enhanced maintenance treatment with opioid medications is not made available. These patients, who have a poor level of retention in some standard programmes (non-therapeutic forms of intervention) and are less capable of coping well in the transient phase after detoxification, may be distinguished by a higher rate and severity of mental disorders. Surprisingly, their treatment compliance improves drastically when challenged by methadone in a low-threshold programme. At lower dosages, which are usually largely ineffective in preventing relapses and blocking the course of addiction, some rapid-onset benefits could derive from a positive impact of methadone on the independent psychiatric symptoms. Together with previous observations about the relationship between methadone dose and outcome for DD patients, we propose a scheme comprising four-dose ranges (Table 1.3).

Table 1.3 Methadone dose, retention in treatment, and positive outcome in patients with and without dual disorder

	Patients without dual disorder		Patients with dual disorder	
Medication and dosage	Retention in treatment	Outcome	Retention in treatment	Outcome
Opioid antagonists	Poor	Average	Very poor	Average to poor
No specific treatment	Poor	–	Very poor	–
Methadone, <60 mg/day	Poor	Poor	Poor to average	Mediocre
Methadone, 60–120 mg/day	Average	Poor to average	Poor to average	Mediocre
Methadone, 120–200 mg/day	Average	Average to good	Average to good	Average to good
Methadone, 200–1500 mg/day	Good	Good	Good	Good

It could be objected that, if DD patients do well at higher dosages (150 mg/day), it is contradictory that the same effect should be seen at lower dosages (60 mg/day). It should, however, be noted that the first finding comes from a high-threshold programme, in which patients who have shown a poor response to the standard Italian treatment dosage (50–60 mg/day) are enrolled. In the second case, patients are presented as resistant, but they are, in fact, simply responders to methadone while not responding to non-specific treatments [47] and are gathered within a low-threshold approach. In conclusion, DD patients are expected to do best at higher dosages within higher-threshold programmes, but they may also achieve results at lower dosages in low-threshold programmes. In non-specific programmes, despite the possible use of psychotropics, these patients are destined to have an outcome of poor retention and poor response.

Heroin addiction, considered separately in this study, is expected to improve in response to around 100 mg/day of methadone, but not below 60 mg/day (lack of narcotic blockade and a weaker direct anti-craving effect) [3, 66]. When a DD is present, a virtuous circle may be established even at low dosages (especially for anxiety disorders) or will not start to function unless higher dosages are reached (especially in cases of bipolar disorders and psychosis) [67]. Therefore, retention and positive outcome do not always run parallel in DD patients as they do in their single diagnosis peers. The early attrition rate in high threshold programmes remains a problem, and side interventions are needed to improve initial motivation to treatment and compliance with opioid medication up-titration. In low-threshold programmes, the rules are typically less strict, and doses allow ongoing opioid use, which may explain the dramatic effect on retention in the Norwegian study mentioned earlier. In the longer term, a common pathway towards dose adjustment is needed to make response and retention converge and run parallel.

The importance of treatment environment has not yet been widely studied. It can, however, be stated that the common approach to DDs is to increase the number of facilities, which may hamper the feasibility of multimodal intervention. A better outcome for DD patients may be favoured by a single physical place of treatment, with no need to be referred elsewhere or deferred to 'some other time' for psychiatric intervention. Even better, the same physician should oversee both aspects and possess both skill sets.

Psychiatrists have been involved and trained to deal with drug users. Still, sometimes their skill is limited to a basic knowledge of the potential anti-craving effects of common psychotropics or the psychiatric effects of substances. An addiction-centred skill based on general training in psychiatry seems to be the ideal profile.

Unpublished data from an outpatient care and rehabilitation service within a large urban area (Rome, Italy) describe one doctor's shopping resource model for the treatment of DD/alcohol use disorder (DD/AUD) patients. Patients were required to attend a place where different treatments could be administered to them and then be evaluated by a team of operators. After daily attendance at a day hospital facility (varying in duration according to the accomplishment of a thorough medical examination and diagnosis), patients were left free to decide whether they wished to be followed up (every second week); in addition, they were obviously welcome to do that at the same place. Substance-related diagnoses and further psychiatric evaluations were performed by a single group of professionals, and so was the follow-up. Considering the first 99 consecutive patients, dropout was significantly related to DDs. No later than 3 months after discharge from day hospital, DD patients had been followed up in treatment (about 55% vs. 25%). After that term, patients were basically followed on a 'flexible schedule' basis, which may mean they should attend 'as needed'. During the following 3 months, the rate of attendance obviously dwindled; even so, the trend was less sharp for DD patients.

In several studies, a DD status (at least of a major kind) is considered an exclusion criterion. Consequently, anti-addictive treatments cannot be said to be generally effective, even in the light of positive findings. Studies of selected psychiatric samples may enlighten us in assessing their effectiveness on DDs, but to tell the truth, such an approach has little value. A DD diagnosis should never be considered in the same way as a single, one-item diagnosis: it is therefore more reasonable to include all dual diagnoses in a general assessment of an anti-craving medication, rather than study all dual diagnoses separately. In fact, the impact of the treatment of single-diagnosis addicts may be closer to that of—for instance—addiction plus anxiety disorders, than it may ever be between the latter and another type of DD (e.g. bipolar disorder). In addition, the algorithm of DD treatment accounts for addiction as the first aspect to stabilize, to be followed by the other disorder. There may be a few exceptions, but it is more useful to first reduce or abolish substance use, and then diagnose what remains of all previous psychiatric symptoms, to clarify their course. The last stage would be to intervene on the dual syndromes [49].

Even in cases where we should plan to start with the treatment of general psychiatric impairment, and then move on to addiction, we have few instruments, which, however, prove useful even in the presence of substance use. Most psychiatric treatments are hampered by concurrent substance use, which is why most studies rule substance users out of the study sample. It may be admitted that the exclusion of addiction from studies of single psychiatric diagnoses has some justification, but it is not sensible to do things the other way around. The very notion that DDs are treatment-resistant a priori is gratuitous and is contradicted by the data discussed above. Obviously, DD patients are expected to do worse in pseudo-therapeutic programmes, which require the absence of symptoms in order to rate patients as having 'improved' or as 'doing well' or as having been 'rehabilitated', so that those with a double source of symptoms are likely to have a worse outcome. That kind of course is just the spontaneous expectancy that depends on the disease and could never be considered a treatment outcome.

A recent Italian study checked the correspondence between DD and the features of craving, some of which were found to be specific to mentally ill addicts [68]. In particular, the cueing of craving by the availability of heroin during rehabilitation attempts was rather specific (OR over 6) and resorting to any substance in the absence of heroin was more unlikely than it was among single-diagnosis peers (OR 1.75). These findings suggest the importance of craving coverage after detachment from heroin, especially after detoxification, due to the need to avoid triggering a relapse. The same subjects do not show proneness to generic substance use, but are focused on heroin and may endure the difficulties of withdrawal, rather than resorting to symptomatic medications, while struggling to eventually supply themselves with heroin. As a logical consequence, this category of patients is expected to benefit from treatment as a result of the medication of psychiatric symptoms. For 'treatment-resistant' patients, the coverage of psychiatric symptoms seems to be achieved at doses 30% higher than average effective doses for uncomplicated patients. Nevertheless, it can be hypothesized that patients with severe mental illness coupled with a mild form of addiction will benefit from opioid agonist treatment even at lower dosages.

Reference should be made here to detoxification, too. Despite its worldwide popularity, that kind of intervention is seldom required for medical purposes and is mostly employed as a result of a misunderstanding of addiction diagnosis. What is worse, since the so-called 'detoxified' patients are often still intoxicated, due to the characteristics of long-term withdrawal and are subdued by their recurrent craving, successful detoxification does pave the way for some acute complications of addiction, such as lethal overdosing at relapse. In DDs, detoxification is just a doubly missed chance of getting addicts enrolled in effective treatment. The greatest misconception that is now being applied to the treatment of DDs is to base the perspectives and outcomes of patients on basic mistakes in the treatment of addiction. Unless we get rid of these mistakes, we may continue to believe that DD patients are destined to have poor outcomes in abstinence-oriented programmes and that hardcore, resistant patients may be allowed to get methadone treatment as an ultimate harm reduction approach. A study conducted in Cyprus illustrates this upside-down view in an emblematic way. A small group of patients were observed in a 'therapeutic community'" programme, and DD diagnosis was ascertained as one main correlation with dropout/relapse. Patients were requested not to be on any opioid agonist, although some of them were addicted to heroin (a few were addicted to heroin only), whereas psychotropic drugs were allowed in the case of DD ones. After approximately 1 year, all DD patients had dropped out, whereas 20% of single-diagnosis patients were still following the programme after a year had elapsed. Authors conclude that DD patients, even if the effort has been made to set up an integrated programme, are expected to have a poorer prognosis, in line with previous data from the literature. Surprisingly, they also quote exceptional data from authors (namely us) reporting a good prognosis for diagnosis, although these data, they claim, are obtained in harm reduction methadone programmes. In other words, prognosis may be good with no perspective of true remission, while DD patients do poorly on abstinence-oriented community programmes. By contrast, we should stress and stigmatize that our study was a high-threshold, rehabilitation-oriented methadone programme with no dose or time limitations, and it showed a better 8-year retention rate for DD patients kept on an average 150 mg/day stabilization dosage [56]. In the community study, all patients had relapsed after 50 months, the DD ones being the first to drop out (as already noted, all during the first year). We may say that no abstinence-oriented programme is reasonable if it requires the absence of agonist treatment in cases of opioid addiction. Obviously, complicated patients will do worse, just because they do so in the absence of any intervention. Encouraging abstinence by omitting effective treatment for addiction offers DD patients nothing other than the spontaneous course of their 'double trouble'. On general grounds, such programmes (either for single or DDs) function as waiting lists for spontaneous relapse [69].

1.3.5.1 Dead Ends and Start Lines in Dual Disorder

Several studies or reviews have discussed the issue of the disease chronology of DDs, in other words: how can one distinguish primary psychiatric disorders from substance-induced transient or persistent disorders with similar symptoms? A *Statistical Mental Disorders Manual (DSM)*-based classification is of little help, since the exclusion of putative substance-induced pictures from a primary psychiatric category resulted in little attention being paid to these secondary disorders. In fact, substance-induced pictures are commonly regarded as difficult to handle, resistant to treatment, and without any standard treatment algorithm. We consider this issue to be a dead end, for the following reasons. First, the assumption that substance-induced pictures are basically different from spontaneous ones is gratuitous. As far as we know, certain substance-induced psychiatric disorders may just be phenocopies of spontaneous versions of the same biological disorder. Moreover, the time overlap between onset periods may also lead to overrating the effect of a substance on the development of certain psychiatric disorders, which would find a way to emerge, possibly later, or more gradually, or with a sharper profile of classic symptoms instead of a substance-filtered clinical picture. Lastly, the diagnosis of a 'secondary' disorder does not automatically imply that detachment from the substance will lead to the stable extinction of symptoms. On the other hand, the persistence of symptoms long after detachment from substance use and the accomplishment of detoxification do not necessarily indicate a primary disorder. The emergence of psychiatric symptoms after the subtraction of agonist opioid treatment (AOT) may indicate a therapeutic effect of that kind of treatment on an independent psychiatric disorder, as in the case of methadone-withdrawal psychoses. These disorders are easily disguised during agonist treatment and may be considered as transient withdrawal-related accidents instead of primary disorders that were initially masked within a picture of severe chronic intoxication, and then disappeared during anti-craving treatment.

Psychiatric disorders are heterogeneous, as they share no common source for all psychiatric symptoms. Instead of splitting a patient population into sharply defined clinical pictures (for instance, affective psychosis and methamphetamine use; or panic disorder and alcoholism), most studies deal with obscure 'all-in' categories, such as dual diagnosis, dual disorders, psychiatric comorbidity, and psychiatric symptoms. Moreover, no distinction between substance classes is made. The result is that we find ourselves having to reason over treatment approaches to methamphetamine addicts with psychotic symptoms together with opioid addicts with depression, or AUD patients with social phobia. We agree on the usefulness of a research 'field' that resorts to grouping together all such conditions, due to a common ground of clinical and biological knowledge, but research efforts would achieve more if they were based on specific targets and study populations.

SUDs are heterogeneous, too, since not all clinical pictures correspond to a chronic relapsing loss of control over use (addiction). Also, not all cases of polydrug use have the same dynamics with respect to the primary addiction and the concurrent psychiatric disorder. In greater detail, we assessed patients with alcohol–heroin polydrug use, cocaine–alcohol polydrug use and heroin–cocaine polydrug use, comparing them with exclusive users of heroin, alcohol, and again heroin, respectively, possibly with other minor substances (mostly cannabis and BDZs, which had not, however, been the original reasons for treatment). Studies agreed on indicating cocaine use as a correlate of axis I bipolar disorder, whether it is combined with alcohol or heroin. On the other hand, the heroin–alcohol polydrug use pattern is typical of highly cyclothymic subjects, but below the threshold of clinical diagnosis [70–74]. Depressive disorders are unrelated to either combination. The heroin–alcohol combination often develops because of treatment omission, premature termination, or under-medication, so that it appears to be a surrogate or enhanced form of a common opioidergic drug disorder [75, 76]. The cyclothymic profile is, in fact, the only profile that discriminates heroin- and AUD patients from healthy controls [77, 78].

Apart from addiction-centred studies, other authors have indicated stimulant use, possibly coupled with alcohol and cannabis, as peculiar to a bipolar diathesis, and proposed the concept of bipolar-stimulant spectrum disorders, going beyond the causal distinction between spontaneous, associated, and induced bipolar disorders [79].

1.3.5.2 Screening and Definition Criteria for Dual Disorder Heroin Addiction

In several studies, no psychiatric category is featured when reporting about the comorbidities of substance users; instead, authors refer to comorbid mental disturbance by drawing on syndrome names as labels, or naming series of key symptoms.

The first criterion for the screening of DDs should be the deviance of putative diagnosis from the stereotype of transient chronic intoxication, either during substance use or soon after detoxification. Such a stereotype varies according to which substance is accounted for and may not be defined during mixed polydrug use phases. Nevertheless, the stereotype of heroin addiction has been reliably defined as a depressive-anxious-hypersensitive-somatic syndrome. This clinical picture runs parallel to acute opioid impairment (susceptibility to withdrawal) and to the severity of addiction. A variant of the same syndrome can be identified as the hypophoric syndrome ('reward deficit' syndrome) [80] following detachment from opioids or agonist treatment subtraction, otherwise known as the late withdrawal syndrome. This latter condition is well known to be an indicator of relapse, is sensitive to opioid agonists, and is worsened by antagonists. Italian authors have worked to ascertain the exact reasons why the above conditions should not be labelled as DDs or at least are not enough to authorize the recognition of an independent mood or anxiety disorder.

On the other hand, psychotic states are quite unlikely during opioid maintenance, as well as substance-related excitement, even in patients who may be abusing cocaine during MMT [81].

European data on the prevalence of psychosis in AOT populations show a relatively low rate of schizophrenia or delusional disorder, regardless of the rate of global comorbidity. In the Netherlands, as many as 39% of opioid users in treatment do display psychotic symptoms, out of an 84% overall comorbidity rate, but current (acute) psychosis does not reach the 10% level. A small population Italian study on hospitalized substance users (heroin being featured as the main primary substance) described the effects of methadone dose increase and the reduction of antipsychotics and mood stabilizers at discharge, under equal conditions for the length of stay in hospital and the kind of index diagnosis at admission [82]. Overall, it may be that opioid agonist treatments have a therapeutic influence on psychotic states (an influence that is dependent on the doses being used) and that this link may mask the prevalence of psychotic disorders in populations maintained on over-standard doses.

To sum up, DDs may be present in cases of intense affective discomfort, especially when patients are free from current intoxication or are emerging after a long period of well-being after discharge from opioid agonist treatment. In all other cases, an addiction-related profile should be first considered—a profile that is likely to be improved by opioid agonist initiation, dose increase, or reintroduction. Psychotic symptoms are more likely to indicate a DD as being responsible for psychosis, unless during forced acute withdrawal or acute psychotomimetic intoxication [83].

The intermingling between substance use and psychiatric risk disposition, or primary milder disorders, may lead to full-blown syndromes which would not have developed spontaneously, but do so because of exposure to at least one substance. In such cases, it is not always possible to ascertain the course of the associated disorder, especially when anti-craving therapies are used, which may have a dual effect. Otherwise, the course of the disorder in the absence of relapse will help to bring clarification, and the latest clinical configuration should be accounted for: for instance, a bipolar 2 disorder ranking up to type 1 after substance use should be rated as bipolar 1, though the course is expected to be more favourable in a substance-free condition [84].

1.3.6   Diversion of Medications Used in the Treatment of Dual Disorder DD/BIP1-HUD Patients

1.3.6.1 Street Opioid Medication Use, Low-Threshold Programmes, and Dual Disorders

The use of medications outside a treatment programme is usually rated as 'misuse' or non-therapeutic use. Certainly, self-medication is something different from treatment, although the results in some cases may be similar. To make this point clear, when self-medication employs a medical drug without any change in the route of administration, the effects may be thoroughly therapeutic. Some patients happen to apply for treatment after they have decided to switch from street heroin to street methadone, because of the difficulty of obtaining effective treatment from local services. Such patients tend to present themselves as self-medicating from psychiatric disorders and would stick to methadone in a therapeutic way against their psychiatric disorder, incidentally, experiencing an anti-craving effect, too. Their insight into the psychotropic effects of methadone is high, even if their insight into the role of methadone in the extinction of craving is low. As a category, women seem to end up using street methadone, together with other substances, more often before entering treatment and earlier in their opioid-using history [85]. Such a finding may indicate that, at least in an early phase, the contribution of primary mental illness to self-medication dynamics is higher for women, so that their global mental balance is impaired earlier, but they instinctively use a slow-acting stable opioid, in order to cope with this loss of balance.

1.3.6.2 Impact of MMT in the Natural History of HUD Patients

Methadone treatment has been widely employed since the late 1980s for the treatment of heroin addiction. Nevertheless, Italian methadone treatments have not followed the original Dole and Nyswander standard model dating back two decades previously [86]. In that model, HUD patients were conceptualized as people with a neurological susceptibility to narcotics, who needed opioid agonists to maintain a condition of balance [10]. Methadone-induced narcotic blockade (by which the addict's brain is disabled for stimulation by heroin) is effective in leading heroin craving to extinction and prevents heroin-induced highs that reinforce craving. Once-a-day oral methadone corresponds to stable blood levels over a 24-h period. Lastly, methadone itself is inexpensive and the whole treatment setting has proved to be cost-effective [87, 88]. A number of studies have agreed on ascertaining its effectiveness as compared with an alternative of opioid addiction [89]. Evidence for this treatment effectiveness is so sound that, should there be a lack of improvement, it is usually ascribed to errors in attendant psychosocial interventions rather than true psychopharmacological refractivity [90].

In any case, methadone has intrinsic pharmacological properties that often prove to be appealing to addicts. Back in the 1950s, attempts to use methadone as a non-medical drug were reported, in some cases by adopting intravenous routes [91]. Moreover, some patients resorted to illegal methadone while in treatment, which may be related to on-going heroin use or be independent phenomena [92].

The use of 'street methadone' during MMT may either depend on addictive properties of methadone formulations or simply be due to its availability in drug-related contexts through take-home supplies delivered to addicts who are being treated [93–98]. Also, the use of illegal methadone may be a consequence of the ineffective administration of methadone treatment (due to arbitrary dose limitations below blocking values, or premature tapering and termination [86]). In order to investigate the reasons for 'street methadone' use and its clinical correlates, it is more useful to evaluate street samples (sought after by treatment-seeking addicts), rather than subjects who have been in treatment for variable periods. In one of our studies [85], we compared the clinical features and addiction histories of HUD patients who are currently using street opioids, at the time of first treatment entrance, selected according to their use of 'street methadone'. The reason for such sample selection is to limit the confounding effect of previous acknowledgement about methadone's properties in a therapeutic setting. We hypothesized that 'street methadone' may be used either as a single non-medical drug, so contributing to global impairment and worsening the patient's clinical conditions, or otherwise, as some sort of self-medication in order to combat craving and try to influence controlled heroin use. Illegal methadone use should correspond to better clinical conditions and less global impairment with respect to the general narcotic addict stereotype.

Although methadone addiction has never been reported in the literature, addicts are thought to misuse any substance they may happen to handle in the absence of medical supervision.

If this is correct, methadone is likely to have become a misused drug through diversion from take-home supplies delivered to addicts in treatment. In other words, if methadone had become a misused drug, addicts who also use methadone would have behaved in a way like others, i.e. similar to those frequently engaged in poly-drug use, with similar addiction histories and a similar degree of psychosocial impairment throughout their course of addiction.

In our study, HUD patients who also resort to 'street methadone' are less likely to use BDZs, hypnotics, speed-uppers, hallucinogenic drugs, and cannabinoids. In methadone-maintained patients, we reported how effective methadone dosages also reduce the use of depressants and speed-uppers [81]. Results suggest that such an effect is already produced out of a therapeutic setting, and below therapeutic dosage levels. Such a hypothesis is supported by the fact that 'street methadone' users are less often polydrug users; a state of opioid impairment due to heroin addiction often leads to misuse of different kinds of drugs apart from heroin itself [75].

Table 1.4 reports the most important characteristics of this kind of patients.

'Street methadone' users have a milder form of disease: they use heroin less frequently, took longer to become addicted, and spend less time before seeking

Table 1.4 Severity of addiction and concomitant substance use in street methadone users and no-users at their first AOT

	Heroin plus Methadone	Heroin		
	$N = 54$	$N = 251$		
Addiction severity	N (%)	N (%)	χ	p
Physical complications	35 (64.8)	147 (58.6)	0.72	0.395
Mental state	45 (83.3)	139 (55.4)	14.5	0.000
Workspace	26 (48.1)	167 (66.5)	6.46	0.011
Family area	18 (33.3)	155 (61.8)	14.6	0.000
Romantic area	19 (35.2)	131 (52.2)	5.14	0.023
Socialization/leisure area	28 (51.9)	146 (58.2)	0.72	0.395
Legal area	46 (85.2)	206 (82.1)	0.30	0.583
Using multiple substances (>3)	19 (35.1)	139 (55.3)	7.22	0.007
Concomitant substance use				
Alcohol	15 (27.8)	72 (29.0)	0.03	0.853
Benzodiazepines	8 (14.8)	116 (46.2)	20.77	0.000
Hypnotics	6 (11.1)	74 (29.4)	12.18	0.000
Cocaine	26 (48.1)	199 (79.2)	16.23	0.000
Amphetamines	15 (27.7)	163 (64.9)	27.32	0.000
Hallucinogens	14 (25.9)	128 (50.9)	12.38	0.000
Cannabinoids	31 (57.4)	214 (85.2)	14.05	0.000
Inhalants	5 (9.4)	16 (6.4)	0.60	0.424
Heroin use				
Daily	32 (61.5)	194 (78.5)	6.73	0.009
As stable user	39 (72.2)	188 (75.8)	0.30	0.580
Periodic abstention	42 (82.4)	197 (82.1)	0.00	0.963
	$M \pm SD$	$M \pm SD$	T	p
Age at first contact (years)	20 ± 4	19 ± 4	1.81	0.075
Age at continuous use (years)	24 ± 6	21 ± 4	2.95	0.005
Dependence duration (months)	5 ± 4	8 ± 5	−4.58	0.000

treatment. As for social adjustment, 'street methadone' users have less work, family, and partnership impairment.

One possible explanation is that the use of 'street methadone', together with heroin, results in a lower degree of consequences than heroin use alone, at least in some social spheres. 'Street methadone'" use does not loom as a multiple opioid addiction, and methadone itself does not seem to take place in an addictive way. The implications of methadone treatment delivery and take-home policies are easy to figure. Logistic regression analysis shows that female sex and dual disorder are discriminant between the two subgroups (and so are polydrug use and the frequency of heroin use, though to a shorter extent). The meaning of this gender-specific correlate remains obscure. The psychotropic properties of methadone [99] and its normalizing effect upon the hypophysis–gonadal axis [100] may concur to make it particularly useful to buffer opioid-related discomfort in female addicts rather than male ones.

In Italy, 'street methadone' use by HUD patients, who apply treatment for their first time, seems not to be addictive, but somehow symptomatic of a better capacity to cope with opioid-related discomfort caused by chronic exposure to heroin, and a prelude to their first therapeutic attempt, maybe as a simple precursor or a favouring factor. These data should be accounted for when deciding about treatment policies, about take-home limitations and the prevention of methadone diversion.

1.4   Use of Opioid Medications in Heroin Addiction

1.4.1   Agonist Opioid Treatment in DD Patients. The PISA-V. P. Dole Research Group Experience

In this section, we report clinical information about methadone treatment for DD patients, based on our personal experience in the PISA-V.P. Dole Research Group experience.

MMT took root in the 1960s and continues to be the most widespread treatment solution for opioid addiction. It starts with an induction phase, through which dosages are gradually increased to reach an optimum value. MMT then follows, consisting in the administration of a constant methadone dosage. At the same time, medical facilities, rehabilitative interventions, and counselling are available too. When this technique is properly applied, patients' conditions, which are bound to be displayed in a critical form at treatment entrance, will significantly improve as maintenance goes forward.

In patients without dual disorder (NDD), initial methadone dosages are used to soothe withdrawal symptoms (early induction). As soon as withdrawal has been buffered, proper induction can be started, with the aim of identifying a therapeutic dosage value, which is expected to vary between individuals. For NDD patients, initial dosages range between 20 and 40 mg/day, and early induction takes no longer than 24 h. Actual induction, which allows a therapeutic dosage level to be reached, lasts no longer than 5–10 days. The following stabilization phase, during which an optimum dosage is sought, and after which that dosage is stably administered as the maintenance dosage, is usually complete within a month. During the maintenance phase that follows, behavioural and psychosocial readjustments are allowed to develop, based on what has been achieved during the previous phases. At this stage, opioid receptors are stably bound by the medication, so suppressing craving and addictive behaviours, on one hand, and compensating for the conditioning due to chronic opioid intoxication, on the other. Maintenance should continue for as long as patients show they are benefiting from it and for as long as patients agree to stay in treatment. The best way of evaluating the therapeutic results is, in fact, the retention rate.

Independently of its essential target, MMT also plays an important role in social medicine. It can be crucial in limiting the spread of HIV and HCV infection among HUD patients, but it can also improve mental health among opioid-addicted patients. In fact, DD patients who are successfully treated by MMT tend to be retained in treatment longer than their uncomplicated peers.

In this section, we have reported the guidelines for the treatment of DD/HUD, as defined by the results from our decennial naturalistic follow-up experience at the PISA-V.P. Dole Research Group. Reported indexes include first-day dosage, weekly dosage during the first month, and average dosage over the first 4-month interval. Dosages are compared between DD/HUD and NDD/HUD. Moreover, stabilization dosage and the time taken to reach it are also accounted for: the term 'stabilization dosage' is used to refer to the maximum dosage administered for at least 4 months with constantly positive outcome. The outcome is evaluated as positive or negative according to two parameters: level of psychosocial adjustment and recent heroin use, as occurring more or less than twice in the previous 2 months.

Figure 1.2 displays first-day, weekly dosages for the first month of treatment, and every quarter month until 3 years. DD patients need an average of 40 mg on the first day, like their uncomplicated peers. Highest first-day dosages for dual disorder addicts, of 80–100 mg/day, are slightly lower than those for NDD peers (up to 200 mg). First-day dosages for dual disorder addicts, then, tend to be lower. During the first month of treatment, dosages were increased by 40% in the first week, by a further 20% in the second week, by 10% in the third week, and, lastly, by 5% in the fourth week. Again, dosages for uncomplicated addicts are slightly higher. Nevertheless, stabilization dosage is higher for dual disorder addicts (140 mg/day vs. 100 mg/day). In fact, the dosages required for DD patients tend to continue to rise through the second month, but then stay the same throughout the whole of the rest of the observation period. Overall, it can be said that uncomplicated addicts require higher induction dosages but become stabilized at lower dosages. The time needed to reach stabilization is longer for DD patients, an average of 7 months vs. 3 months among uncomplicated peers. This gap is not fully justified by the fact that eventual stabilization dosages are higher, so DD patients can be said to proceed

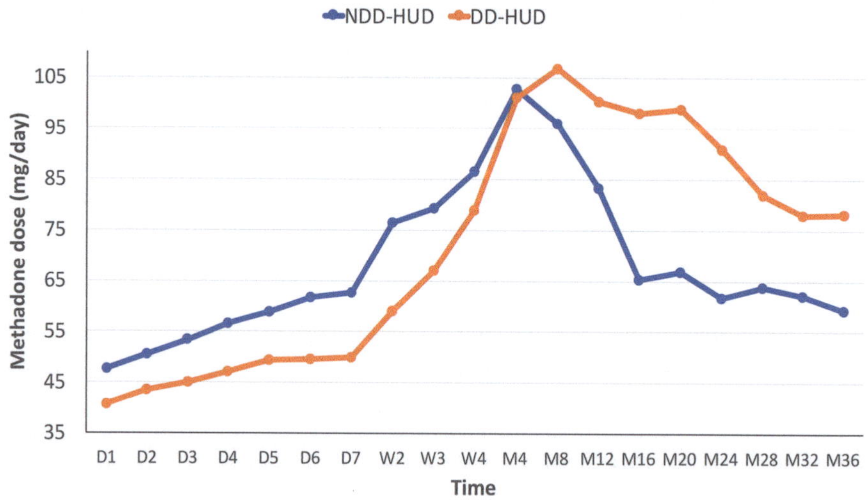

Fig. 1.2 Methadone dosage in HUD and DD/HUD patients according to the clinical experience of PISA-V.P. Dole Research Group

more slowly towards stabilization. Methadone tapering during treatment accomplishment does not proceed in divergent ways in the two groups, but it does take place more slowly in DD patients.

As for retention rates, it was noted that DD patients experience a higher early rate of attrition, but no difference is left after 8 months of treatment. In a 10-year follow-up, the rates for survival-in-treatment were about 50% for NDD patients and about 70% for DD patients. After 4 years of treatment, such rates tended to become stable onwards. DD patients showed better outcome measures than NDD patients. A significantly higher methadone dose was needed to have DD patients stabilized. Contrary to expectations, treatment-resistant patients with psychiatric comorbidity showed a better long-term outcome than treatment-resistant patients without DD [56]. Regarding bipolar 1 DD/HUD patients (DD/BIP1-HUD), the rates for survival-in-treatment were 58% as opposed to 44% for NDD/HUD patients. After 3 years of treatment, such rates tended to become progressively more stable. DD/BIP1-HUD patients showed better outcome results than NDD/HUD patients regarding Clinical Global Index (CGI) severity and *DSM-IV* Global Assessment of Functioning—GAF ($p < 0.001$). No differences were found regarding urinalyses for morphine between groups during the observational period. Bipolar 1 patients needed a higher methadone dosage in the stabilization phase, but this difference was not statistically significant [52]. The 10-years rates of endurance in the treatment of DD chronic psychotic HUD (DD/PSY-HUD) patients were 36%, compared with 34% for NDD/HUD patients ($p = 0.872$). Also, in this case, after 3 years of treatment, these rates tended to become progressively more stable. DD/PSY-HUD patients showed better outcome results than NDD/HUD patients regarding CGI severity and *DSM-IV*-GAF ($p < 0.001$). No differences were found regarding good toxicological outcomes or the methadone dosages used to achieve stabilization. The time required to stabilize DD/PSY-HUD patients was shorter. An enhanced MMTP seems to be equally effective in patients with DD/PSY-HUD and those with NDD/HUD [101].

First-day dosage is crucial for treatment retention: it is important to achieve complete control of withdrawal symptoms within 24 h, by using a cumulative dosage of 80–100 mg when necessary. If patients are left in a condition of partial withdrawal, it is quite unlikely that they will stay in treatment any longer. So, what precautions are needed when the dosage exceeds 40 mg on the first day? As a rule, when withdrawal symptoms are assessable, 20 mg should be administered, and evaluation of withdrawal repeated after a couple of hours. If withdrawal shoots up again or persists, a further 20 mg should be administered, and patients should be kept under observation for the next 2 h. This procedure can be repeated until withdrawal is complete. The eventual cumulative dosage administered on the first day will be repeated through the following days (induction phase), until a steady state is supposedly reached (normally on the third or fourth day). No differences due to the presence of absence of DD are expected in these stages of treatment. In other words, the presence of DD only seems to influence the management of the maintenance phase. From a clinical point of view, admission into MMT should not depend on DD. However, with the criteria currently being applied, DD patients are likely not to be retained in treatment, since there is a trend to administer lower rather than higher methadone dosages. In fact, it must be recalled that DD patients require higher dosages during the stabilization phase. If DD patients display resistance to standard treatment, they are likely to be considered as non-responders, whereas they are simply not receiving adequate treatment. The time required to reach stabilization is longer for DD patients, so it is important to monitor patients through quite a long period, before they can be expected to achieve stabilization. If these guidelines are applied, it is unlikely that an under-treated patient will be taken for a non-responder. Methadone tapering should only be considered after at least 1 year, given that it must be introduced very slowly with DD patients. However, if tapering results in a worsening of psychosocial adjustment or a relapse into substance use, the previously used dosage should be restored.

1.4.2 Pondering Antagonist Opioid Medication Use in DD/ BIP1-HUD Patients

Opioid antagonism in opiate dependence has been used for decades for two therapeutic purposes: to achieve abstinence within detoxification and maintenance programmes and to treat respiratory depression, which is often responsible for fatal overdoses.

With regard to detoxification treatment [102] and maintenance treatment [103] programmes, they have been based on administering NTX since the late 1970s [104], when a report issued by the US National Research Council Committee made it clear that a narcotic antagonist was an acceptable treatment for a small number of patients undergoing treatment for opiate dependence. The patients most likely to qualify and be chosen for such therapy were those who were relatively opiate-free (known as 'post-addicts') and highly motivated to seek treatment. With patients showing that kind of profile, NTX was able to slightly increase both retention in treatment and opiate-free urine tests, with respect to placebo [105]. One interesting study has investigated the predictors of successful outcome in a population of 149 current heroin users undergoing long-term NTX treatment (NTX maintenance), after their selection based on being assessed as opioid non-tolerant by a baseline naloxone test. Higher rates of retention in treatment were predicted by a higher degree of psychosocial adjustment, and by a less severe psychopathological impairment, with special reference to mood, aggressiveness, and delusions [44]. In order to face the poor compliance with NTX shown by addicts, an injectable, sustained-release formulation of NTX has been devised. A randomized, double-blind, placebo-controlled 8-week trial investigated the efficacy and safety of this formulation on 60 heroin-dependent adults, randomized to receive placebo or 192 or 384 mg of depot NTX. Doses were administered at the beginning of weeks 1 and 5. Retention in treatment was dose-related, with 39%, 60%, and 68% of patients in the placebo group, in the group taking 192 mg of NTX daily and in the group taking 384 mg of NTX daily, respectively. Mean time to dropout was 27, 36, and 48 days for those taking the placebo, for those taking 192 mg of NTX, and for those taking 384 mg of NTX, in those respective groups. It should be noted that the percentage of urine samples that turned out to be negative for opioids and other substances varied significantly as a function of dose [106]. A 1-year open label study has reported similar results in a sample of 114 heroin addicts from 13 clinical sites in Russia. With a NTX implant of 380 mg, 62.3% of patients completed the programme. Urine testing revealed that 50.9% were abstinent from opioids at all assessments during the evaluation period. Problems in liver function tests occurred in 16.7% of patients, while no severe adverse events were reported [107]. Extended-release NTX treatment is often preceded by a procedure known as rapid NTX induction, based on the administration of a buprenorphine–clonidine combination. A study carried out on 150 participants concluded that lower age and indicators of greater substance dependence severity (more current opioid use and/or other substance use) predict difficulty in completing a rapid NTX induction procedure [108]. When the level of heroin craving was monitored in patients receiving NTX on a regular basis, with meetings and interviews held twice weekly, a pattern of craving reduction was attested in most of but not all the addicts, and it usually took 3–5 weeks for this effect to occur [109]. More recently, it has become clear not only that depression frequently occurs in heroin addicts who are undergoing an NTX maintenance treatment, but also that the risk of a non-fatal heroin overdose is significantly higher after NTX treatment, as a result of reduced tolerance. In a more recent study, data from clinical trials demonstrated that the mortality rate subsequent to NTX treatment appears to be equivalent to or even greater than that for untreated heroin users [110]. Moving from the putative implication of kappa opioid receptors in opioid dependence, one study tried to determine the effectiveness of a functional kappa antagonist as a treatment for opioid dependence. This was accomplished by combining a partial mu agonist/kappa antagonist (buprenorphine, 4 mg, sublingual) with a mu antagonist (NTX, 50 mg by mouth), theoretically leaving kappa antagonism as the major medication effect. After inpatient detoxification and a naloxone-challenge test to verify that they were not physically dependent on opioids, subjects received NTX. Starting on the fourth day, patients also received liquid buprenorphine; 33% of patients completed the 3-month study. The positive response to treatment exceeded that expected from NTX alone (90% dropout), but was still less than that expected from an agonist maintenance treatment [111].

About the treatment of opiate overdoses, the drug of choice is naloxone, which can be administered intravenously or by a nasal spray. When naloxone is used intravenously, it can be administered as a bolus, if the respiratory depression is caused by heroin or other fast-acting opiates, or in continuous infusion, if overdose is caused by a long-acting opioid such as methadone [112, 113]. It has been reported too that when naloxone is administered endotracheally, it is able to interrupt a heroin overdose, and this feature becomes especially important when the intravenous route of administration is unavailable [114]. More recently, a naloxone nasal spray has been devised to quickly administer naloxone in a needle-free system, which avoids needle-stick injuries and the risk of contracting a blood-borne pathogenic disease such as hepatitis or human immunodeficiency [115, 116]. Interestingly, when naloxone was administered nasally, it proved to be as effective as when the intravenous route was followed in a sample of 17 opiate-dependent patients, ensuring a wide margin of safety for patients and medical staff, especially in emergency situations [117]. Harm reduction programmes, over time, have aimed to reduce the frequency of fatal overdoses among heroin addicts by implementing the distribution of naloxone kits to patients and their family members. A brief overdose education has proved to be sufficient to support naloxone distribution to opioid users. During a standardized 5–10 min education programme, patients were trained to recognize an overdose and to respond to it by administering naloxone. As a result, patients were able to identify and correctly respond to a mean of 13.7 out of 16 overdose scenarios foreseen by the study [118]. Other harm reduction programmes have stressed the need to provide overdose education and naloxone rescue kits to those family members of opioid users who are motivated to receive training. This was, incidentally, true of the support groups for family members in Massachusetts [119]—a state that later extended the application of this policy to the more recent nasal naloxone spray formulation [120].

In the light of these observations, it can be stated that opioid antagonism, although the treatment of choice for opiate overdose, is not a good tool for achieving abstinence and recovery. NTX as a therapy possesses only limited efficacy on heroin-dependent patients presenting a low level of severity of both addictive and psychiatric symptoms, a high level of social adjustment, and a strong motivation to be treated. Conversely, opioid blockade can be ineffective and even harmful in heroin addicts who suffer from their addictive disease in a severe form and present a comorbid psychiatric disorder.

1.4.2.1 When Are We Not Allowed to Use Opioid Antagonists in Dual Disorder Patients?

A past or current history of opiate addiction stands, in our opinion, as an absolute contraindication to the use of opioid antagonists, regardless of the kind of comorbid psychiatric disorder that may be involved. In patients tolerant to opiates, opioid antagonists would induce a withdrawal symptomatology, while in abstinent patients they would exacerbate the post-withdrawal syndrome, so facilitating relapses.

All affective states that are distinguished by the prevalence of depressive symptoms should be considered a contraindication to the use of opioid antagonists, as they might exacerbate anhedonia and delay the recovery process.

We discourage the use of opioid antagonists for any first psychotic episode with prominent positive manifestations, as opioid antagonism has proved to be ineffective on that kind of symptomatology.

Full-blown anxiety disorders should be considered a contraindication to the use of opioid antagonists, as they might exacerbate anxiety and precipitate a panic attack.

The obsessive-compulsive disorder (OCD) should be considered a contraindication to the use of opioid antagonists, as they might exacerbate thoughtfulness, especially in predominantly obsessive patients.

Opioid antagonists should not be included in the pharmacotherapy of anorexia nervosa, as they have proved to be ineffective and might be harmful to anorexic symptomatology.

It is our conviction that opioid antagonist-based detoxification and maintenance programmes should be implemented only in cases where opioid agonists are unsuitable, bearing in mind that only those patients whose condition is less severe and who are motivated to receive treatment are candidates for giving a good response.

1.5   Future Perspectives

In the future, it will be advisable to modify the mental health and addiction treatment programmes, organizing them in such a way as to really meet the needs of DD patients with. For the success of the programmes, the following aspects must be kept in mind.

1.5.1   Recruitment

Recruitment is understood to be the phase in which patient participation in treatment is encouraged. In general, it includes "'attraction' measures, such as the provision of resources to support patients' quality of life and medical assistance or the removal of any obstacles to the treatment and adaptation of the programme to individual needs (e.g. opening of the outpatient clinic in particular time slots). Patient recruitment can also be facilitated through additional measures, which may seem to be related only indirectly to the patients' pathology, such as the organization of a childcare service, when the patient follows the activities of the programme, consulting for the work and free time. Recruitment is a long-term process that aims to keep patients in the programme and help them manage the problems that arise. Establishing a personalized relationship with patients, maintaining it for a long period of time, and focusing on individual needs are the three fundamental aspects of recruitment. In DD cases, it is appropriate to adapt recruitment techniques to the nature, severity, and degree of functional impairment resulting from the dual pathology. The insertion in treatment of a patient with panic attack disorder and episodic alcohol misuse requires a different approach than that provided for a schizophrenic, homeless, and with polysubstance use. In severe cases, such as a psychotic disorder, or violent behaviour, it is possible to resort to coercive recruitment methods, such as mandatory medical treatment.

1.5.2   Retention in Treatment Rate

Keeping the patient in treatment for as long as necessary is an essential point of every programme. In fact, for many patients, participation in treatment takes place in different places: even in integrated programmes, participation in various subprogrammes is often necessary, depending on the stage of illness. For this reason, it would be appropriate to include a CM programme for DD patients during the treatment, to limit these inconveniences to a minimum.

1.5.3　Treatment Globalization

Being able to treat all DD patients depends on the availability of specific programmes for psychiatric pathology and substance use, aimed at better recruitment of patients, to provide differentiated services based on the degree of severity and functional impairment, as well as patient motivation and compliance, to guarantee the availability of the treatment in all its various phases. It would be advisable to ensure, to all patients, the possibility of access to programmes aimed at reducing substance use, and to those for which the 'drug-free' condition constitutes a prerequisite for entry, and for those where a long-term drug treatment programme is expected.

1.5.4　Stages of Treatment

Commonly, with the term 'acute phase', in the medical sense, those phenomena with sudden onset are indicated, which require a prompt response. Intervening in the acute phase of a DD patient means confronting medical, psychiatric, and toxicological emergencies that may include intercurrent illnesses, states of intoxication, withdrawal symptoms, suicidal behaviours, and episodes of violence, impulse dyscontrol, and psychotic disorders. Stabilizing a patient in the acute phase often means detoxifying him in the hospital or outpatient clinic or starting a methadone or buprenorphine treatment. The presence of a severe psychotic episode, violent or with impulsiveness, requires emergency hospitalization in a psychiatric ward, while the treatment of patients with less severe pictures can be started also in day-hospital. After the acute phase, there may be a sub-acute phase. For example, it is common for insomnia and anxiety to occur in recently detoxified patients, even for several days or weeks. On the other hand, in patients with DD, these symptoms can be interpreted both as a sub-acute expression of withdrawal and as a sign of relapse of a concomitant mood disorder. Even though the sub-acute phase is not considered as crisis, ignoring these symptoms, not evaluating, or treating them can favour their aggravation and decompensation and, therefore, lead to the exacerbation of the SUD. When the symptoms of intoxication or withdrawal have disappeared, it is advisable to carry out a new diagnostic evaluation and plan the rehabilitation intervention, paying attention to the problems related to the patient's quality of life. Long-term stabilization treatments are generally outpatient or residential. In the most serious cases, in the presence of a DD, the role of the CM is essential. An alternative procedure guides the patient through a four-part group therapy. At the beginning, a CM intervenes in a personalized manner to introduce the patient to the goals and the philosophy of treatment, to assist him during the crisis moments, in the search for accommodation and work. The second step involves the so-called 'persuasion groups', which can help patients who deny the existence of a SUD and poorly motivated ones. However, it is a good idea not to deal hard with the patient, especially in the early stages of treatment. After this stage, the patient is placed in the so-called 'active treatment groups' characterized by the presence, within them, of patients who have achieved the goal of reducing/suspending substance use and have reached an acceptable stabilization of the DD. In these groups, through 'peer' comparison techniques, it is possible to develop a psychoeducational-behavioural approach. Finally, when the patient has achieved the objectives described above, he/she can be placed in a group in which the subjects develop all the resources available in order to maintain the condition of substance non-use and prevent relapses.

Mood Disorders in Dual Disorder Heroin Use Disorder Patients

2

2.1 Clinical Aspects

2.1.1 Epidemiology

Depression as a syndrome is certainly a common psychiatric issue among HUD patients (see Table 2.1 for details).

According to several studies, one out of three HUD patients can be diagnosed as depressed [121–126], and lifetime evaluations have revealed prevalence rates varying between 60% and 90% [127–131]. Personality disorders are very commonly associated [132–138], but depressive syndromes mostly belong to the area of mood disorders [129, 130, 134, 137, 139–150].

An index episode of moderate depression characterized one patient out of three, among those entering methadone treatments [121, 125, 151], and similar rates are quoted by surveys among large groups of subjects treated in drug-free settings. One good example is that depression was assessed in as many as 30% of patients who followed drug-free rehabilitation programmes in therapeutic communities in a totally drug-free regimen [152]. Correlations between depression rates and the natural history of HUD are reported in Table 2.2.

Depression or dysthymia often reaches a level of 50%, and 60% has been recorded when lifetime prevalence is considered [129, 134]. Major depressive episode follows detoxification treatments with a frequency of 25% [153], whereas as many as 62% of methadone-maintained subjects develop one major depressive episode during, or shortly after, methadone tapering.

According to Rounsaville [137, 154–157], index and lifetime prevalence rates for major depression among HUD patients vary between 17% and 23%, and between 48% and 70%, respectively. Subjects who spontaneously enter methadone treatment are more likely to display major depression (34% vs. 14% among untreated subjects). Depression is found in over 50% of street addicts [130].

© The Author(s), under exclusive license to Springer Nature
Switzerland AG 2023
I. Maremmani et al., *Dual Disorder Heroin Addicts*,
https://doi.org/10.1007/978-3-031-30093-6_2

Table 2.1 Mood disorder/heroin use disorder epidemiology

Diagnosis	%	Studies
Major depression		
Index episode	33	Wieland & Sola, 1970; Lehman & De Angelis, 1972; Robins, 1974; Weissman et al., 1976; Rounsaville et al., 1979; Dorus & Senay, 1980; Steer & Kotzer, 1980; Senay, 1981
	42	Brienza et al., 2000
Lifetime	60–90	Hendriks, 1971; Khantzian & Treece, 1979; McLellan et al., 1980; Jainchill et al., 1986; von Limbeek et al., 1992
Atypical depression	12.4	Rich et al., 1989
Non-bipolar depression	13.4	Maremmani et al., 2000, 2000a, 2000b
Manic episode	<0.1	Rounsaville et al., 1982a
Manic episode after methadone maintenance	0.015	Gold et al., 1982
Hypomanic episode		
Index episode	0.9	Rounsaville et al., 1982a
Lifetime	7.0	Rounsaville et al., 1982a
Cyclothymia	5.5	Mirin et al., 1988; Mirin & Weiss, 1991
Bipolar 1–2	5.5	Rounsaville et al., 1982a; Mirin et al., 1988; Mirin & Weiss, 1991
Bipolar 1	55.6	Maremmani et al., 2000, 2000a, 2000b
Bipolar 2	51.8	Maremmani et al., 1994

Table 2.2 Major depression and natural history of heroin use disorder

Diagnosis	%	Studies
Before treatment	14	See studies about methadone maintenance
In the street	54	Brienza et al., 2000
At treatment entry	34	See above
During treatment		
Drug-free	46	Dorus & Senay, 1980
	30	Clerici et al., 1987
Methadone maintenance, index episode	12.6	Chatham et al., 1995
	17–23	Rounsaville et al., 1980, 1981, 1982, 1982a, 1983, 1983a, 1985, 1986, 1987; Rounsaville, 1985; Rounsaville & Kleber, 1986; Humeniuk et al., 2000
Methadone maintenance, lifetime	48–70	See above
During detoxification	62	Dackis & Gold, 1983
After detoxification	25	Dackis & Gold, 1983

As regards mood elation, full-blown manic episodes are quite unlikely (0.9% of the Yale Study population) [157]. On the other hand, hypomanic features occur with a frequency reaching 7% and as many as 5.5% of these addicts can be assessed as suffering from bipolar 1 or 2 disorders [137]. Interestingly, 3 patients among the 200 examined developed manic episodes after methadone discontinuation [158].

Similar results are provided by another study, which reported rates of 12.4% for major depression, whether typical or atypical, and 5.4% for bipolar disorders, including cyclothymic disorder [159, 160].

In the 1990s original data from a PISA-V.P. Dole Research Group study suggested that the rate of bipolar 2 disorder was far higher, at least among non-psychiatric patients. Interestingly, only 20% of patients who had initially been classified as suffering from major depression, single episode, without psychiatric antecedents, maintained the same diagnosis through time. On the other hand, 7.5% had been through major depression, single episode, and were in remission at the time of the study and 2.5% were assessable as recurrent major depression. The remaining 37.5% of major depressive episodes were part of pictures either of bipolar 1 (2.5%) or bipolar 2 (35%) disorders, based on a history of mood elation episodes, whether spontaneous or iatrogenic. Both cyclothymic and dysthymic disorders proved to be infrequent; psychotic episodes, whether mood-congruent or incongruent, were uncommon, too. Melancholic depression was rarely found. By contrast, 87.5% displayed significant hyperthymic (62.5%) or dysthymic (25%) temperamental features, so documenting the prevalence of the bipolar spectrum [161].

In a different study performed by the same team, 45 consecutive HUD patients were assessed for the presence and quality of concurrent psychiatric disorders, which were divided into four major clusters: affective, anxious, psychotic, and showing polydrug use. The affective clusters comprised bipolar 1 disorder, depressive phase (55.5%), dysthymic disorder (13.3%); the anxious cluster (4.4% of the total) included panic disorder with or without agoraphobia, and obsessive-compulsive disorder; psychotic syndromes (11.1%) and impulse control disorders were classified together in the psychotic cluster; polydrug use comprised cases of anxiolytic drug (4.4%) and/or alcohol dependence (11.1%), and received as much attention as DD, accepting the interpretation that polydrug use is the result of an underlying panic or social phobic disorder [54, 162].

Our research group has long supported the hypothesis that mood disorders are more frequent in SUD than in schizophrenic spectrum disorders. This has been shown for opioid and cannabinoid users [162]. Lately, in research projects with our Canadian partners, from a sample of 497 subjects drawn from an At Home/Chez Soi study, 146 and 94 homeless individuals were identified as having bipolar disorder and schizophrenic spectrum, respectively. In the previous 12 months, a greater proportion of bipolar disorder homeless reported greater use of cocaine, amphetamines, opioids, hallucinogens, cannabinoids, and tranquilizers than schizophrenic spectrum. Cocaine and opioids were significantly associated with bipolar disorder homeless, illustrating the relationship between substance use and bipolar disorder in a vulnerable urban population of homeless people affected by adverse psychosocial factors and severe psychiatric conditions [163]. In the same study, homeless individuals were selected for lifetime unipolar depression and lifetime bipolar depression, and patterns of substances used in the previous 12 months were identified with the Mini-International Neuropsychiatric Interview. No significant differences were observed between unipolar depression and bipolar disorder homeless demographics. Bipolar disorder homeless patients displayed a higher percentage of central nervous system (CNS) stimulants and opioids as compared with the unipolar depression homeless individuals. CNS stimulant was the only predictor within the bipolar disorder homeless group [164]. In conclusion, bipolarity seems to be closely correlated with substance use; this correlation has also been verified in a homeless population.

At this point no further data are required to definitively assess the actual prevalence of bipolar disorders compared with unipolar ones among HUD patients. The low occurrence of full-blown mood elation appears to be inconsistent with the well-known euphoric effects of opioids. On neurochemical grounds, an increase of endorphins has been documented during manic states; similarly, on clinical grounds, data have been reported that allow antimanic properties to be attributed to the opioid antagonist naloxone [165]. The same agent is consistently ineffective in depressed patients. In psychodynamic terms, it may be noted that the denial of sorrowful aspects of reality, the emphasis on factual and emotional contingency, and an attitude of omnipotence, all of which are outcomes of heroin use, resemble the psychological features of manic states, though definite manic themes or full-blown manic behaviours may be missing.

2.1.2 Substance Use and Bipolarity. The Bipolar Spectrum Concept

By now there is a new momentum in the field of addictions from pathophysiological and therapeutic perspectives [166]. Bipolarity is basically excluded from such perspectives in the addiction literature. Yet bipolar spectrum disorders, substance non-medical use, and addiction often co-occur in the community [167] and constitute reciprocal risk factors that, we would argue, can be viewed in a unitary perspective. They also co-occur in clinical populations [84]. We express the conviction that such a unitary perspective could provide a better clinical understanding and management of patients with co-occurring bipolar spectrum and addictive disorders, bringing significant benefits to the fields of mood disorders, addiction, and DD [168].

Bipolar spectrum disorders are a group of chronically recurring disorders of varying and fluctuating intensity, all of them characterized by intermittent or prolonged affective instability, states of inhibition, and excitement of various mental functions such as mood, cognition, and psychomotricity [169]. Swinging between depression and elation is typical, and episodes can even occur in which opposite symptoms of excitement and inhibition are combined (irritable or anxious mixed states). Mood swings vary in severity, duration, and sequence. Excitement, irritability, and/or euphoria following life events and, at a much later stage, ushered in by substances, have recently been conceptualized as signs of bipolar disposition, thus superseding the dichotomy between spontaneous and induced euphoria [170]. In other words, the notion of 'substance-induced mood disorder' in the DSM-IV Manual [171] disregards the subthreshold mood changes associated with antecedent cyclothymic and hyperthymic temperaments [84, 172, 173]. Likewise, the notion of an 'independent' mood disorder in drug and/or alcohol addiction in the manual tends to disregard the relevance of antecedent bipolarity at a temperament level in DD patients.

In the last few decades, the unipolar–bipolar dichotomy [174] of manic-depressive illness has been widespread, and it has proven to be of heuristic value for clinical and therapeutic research. This nosographic approach, however, left many affective conditions undefined, in the interface zone between unipolar and bipolar disorders. In particular, bipolar 2 forms have been described on the basis of the presence of severe depressive episodes requiring hospitalization, alternating with hypomanic periods that do not require hospitalization [175]. Although hospitalization might be considered an artificial criterion for a correct definition of the diagnostic threshold for mania, this conceptualization meant taking an important step forward towards recognition of the large universe of bipolar patients whose excited periods remained at the sub-manic level. More recently, Akiskal [176] and Akiskal and Mallya [177] proposed a broader conceptualization of the 'soft' bipolar spectrum that modifies the foregoing definitions of bipolar 2 by incorporating depressions with hypomanic episodes, whether protracted or brief in duration, whether showing cyclothymic or hyperthymic traits, while including those with familial bipolarity (Fig. 2.1).

Another important question for clinical practice is posed by hypomania, which initially manifests in response to pharmacological treatment with antidepressants, alcohol, or stimulants. Although an extensive literature strongly supports the inclusion of such patients under the heading of bipolar disorders [178], DSM-5 and ICD-10 [179] have denied bipolar status to these patients. This is an unfortunate decision, considering that depressive episodes followed by pharmacological hypomania seem to represent a subtype of the bipolar 2 pattern that some authors describe as bipolar disorder, type 3 [84]. In prospective observations, nearly all adult patients who have antidepressant-associated hypomanic episodes progress months or years later to bipolar states with spontaneous hypomania or mania [180]; this also appears

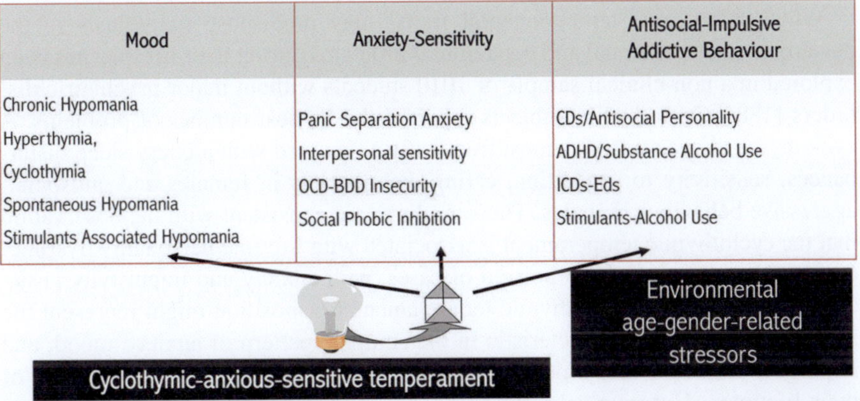

Fig. 2.1 Bipolar spectrum according to Akiskal and Mallya

to be true of adolescent depressives [181]. Moreover, patients developing mood switches with antidepressants, especially at the beginning of treatment, often present with a family history of bipolar disorders and a high susceptibility to rapid cycling [182]. Interestingly, antidepressant-associated hypomania is not limited to major depressions. It can occur in dysthymic patients [183] and personality disorders [184], as well as social phobic, obsessive-compulsive, and other anxiety states [185]. In brief, the depressive phase of bipolar patients can, in a significant minority of patients, be replaced by subthreshold depressive trait personality, socially anxious or obsessive inhibitions.

The issue of comorbidity between bipolar disorder and anxiety, impulse control, eating, substance use, and personality disorders is very complex and prone to different pathogenetic interpretations. It is likely that the affective dysregulation of bipolar disorder extends beyond elation and depression to include, among others, such negative affective arousal states as anxiety, panic, irritability, impulsivity, and mood liability. This syndromic complexity, if occurring jointly with early age at onset during adolescence, high frequency of recurrence of episodes, and a high incidence of separations and/or divorces, school or job difficulties, isolated antisocial types of conduct, and substance non-medical use, tends to produce an unstable, unpredictable, and stormy life [185, 186].

Many patients within the bipolar spectrum, especially when recurrence is high and the inter-episodic period is not free of affective manifestations, may meet the recognized criteria for personality disorders. This is particularly true of cyclothymic bipolar 2 patients, who are often diagnosed as having borderline personality disorder because of their extreme mood instability [172]. Cyclothymic mood instability and impulsivity might be related; each of these is, in fact, marked out by environmentally induced periods of uninhibited or facilitated thinking and behaviour, poor insight or ego-syntonicity, and marked changes in mood state between dysphoric and pleasurable affects. Because mood lability is a common characteristic of both sets of disorders [186, 187], DSM-IV criteria for cyclothymia and borderline disorder seem to describe a related psychopathological picture from different points of view, as in the case of social phobia and avoidant personality disorder.

Whether 'extreme temperamental traits' may predispose individuals to the development of emotional and behavioural problems during their lifespan has been explored in a non-clinical sample of 1010 students without major psychiatric disorders [188]. Cyclothymic subjects reported the highest number of problems. A cyclothymic disposition was most frequently associated with anxiety-sleep disturbances, sensitivity to separation, eating disturbances in females and antisocial-aggressive behaviour in males. These findings are consistent with the observation that the cyclothymic temperament is associated with lifetime personality dysfunction [172] and, in a high proportion of cases, with anxiety and impulsivity [189–191]. We submit that cyclothymic temperamental disposition might represent the mediating underlying characteristic in the complex pattern of anxiety, mood, and impulsive disorders that bipolar spectrum patients display throughout much of their lifetimes. Unfortunately, the current formal diagnostic rules (ICD-10 and

DSM-IV) are almost exclusively based on state symptomatology and do not take into consideration temperamental dispositions or their associated psycho(patho) logical traits.

The core elements of addictive psychopathology take the form of craving and loss of control over instinctual drives, which are quite common in general psychiatry. Craving, for instance, is recognizable as a powerful urge to attain an objective, such as a drug, or some non-chemical form of stimulation, such as food or sex [192]. Adopting a psychopathology-based perspective, craving-related urges, and substance-bound behaviours closely resemble the (hypo)manic excitement of bipolar patients; the substance itself is a dominant theme and aim, and it is pursued with an overwhelming appetitive drive. Thus, beyond the similarities between their clinical picture, (hypo)mania and addiction share a common ground of excitement and impulsive hyperactivity.

There has been a progressive increase in the evidence that lifetime heroin use is not uncommon among bipolar patients [159, 193–198]. The frequency of heroin use is, in fact, often as high as 20% during depressive episodes and may reach 25% during manic episodes [199]. Yet some studies report lifetime heroin use in patients with a history of mania to be far lower, no more than 5% [200].

The association between mood disorders and substance use has been observed for over 2000 years. Plato pointed to alcohol as being one of the causes of mania [201]. Sorano, around 100 B.C., stated that the excessive drinking of alcohol often induces manic states [202]. Around 90 B.C., Aretheus noted that mania, which he describes as a transient delusional condition, may be produced by the excessive consumption of wine or opium [203]. Early in the twentieth century, Kraepelin asserted that alcohol non-medical use, which can be observed in as many as 25% of patients suffering from manic-depressive psychosis, is the outcome of a state of psychomotor excitement [204].

The use of cannabinoids may elicit psychotic syndromes with excitement and hypomanic features, which tend to achieve resolution more rapidly than they do in spontaneous psychotic states [205]. Cases of hypomania have been described as being due to the disulfiram–marijuana combination [206], and manic syndromes have been documented in which marijuana non-medical use followed the consumption of prescribed fluoxetine [207].

Among cannabis-abusing chronic psychotics, bipolar disorders are much commoner than schizophrenia. On clinical grounds, cannabis-abusing bipolar psychotics show higher levels of aggressiveness and a lower degree of emotional flattening [162]. A strong relationship has been reported between cocaine non-medical use, attention deficit disorder with hyperactivity, and bipolar disorders [208, 209]. Hypomanic features are often observed in cocaine users [210]. Cocaine is the second most commonly used substance among bipolar patients (30%), after alcohol (80%); it is followed by sedatives-hypnotics (21%) and opioids (13%) [211]. Mood disorders are a risk factor for substance non-medical use, especially in forms of bipolar disorders that are distinguished by their early onset and the recurrence of mixed-manic episodes or states.

A further sign of bipolarity, according to our research group, is the presence of familiarity for affective disorders in patients with mood disorders. It is therefore important to also evaluate the familiarity of affective disorders in HUD patients.

Up to 19% of cocaine users and 7.5% of opioid ones have a first-level family history of mood disorders [212]. First-level relatives of cocaine users are at greater risk of both unipolar and bipolar disorders, compared with the relatives of non-users [212, 213]. Siblings of HUD patients whose parents have suffered from depression are characterized by a high rate of mood and/or anxiety disorders. Siblings of depressed HUD patients are more likely than siblings of non-depressed addicts to develop antisocial personality disorder and display impaired social and intellectual functioning.

In the PISA-V.P. Dole Research Group sample of HUD patients, a first- or second-level family history of psychiatric illness was found in as many as 70%. Of that 70%, 30% did not suffer from any axis I psychiatric disorder but displayed an affective temperament (hyperthymic or depressive). The remaining 40%, besides having a family history of psychiatric illness, were themselves affected by a major psychiatric disorder [161].

Studies on monocorial twins have mostly focused on alcohol-related problems: twins score the same as regards the prevalence of alcohol-related issues, concurrent non-medical use/dependence of other substances, and forerunning present antisocial conduct (often in childhood or adolescence). In monozygotic twins, a family history seems to carry weight for the co-occurrence of major depression and alcoholism, but not for other kinds of non-medical use. Some authors point out, however, that the possible discrepancy between the environmental backgrounds of the monozygotic and dizygotic twins examined limits the reliability of results [214–216].

An evaluation of depressive features in addicted patients should always consider the relationship that links depressive symptomatology with addictive states. Dysphoria, for instance, may be a salient item either in opioid intoxication or withdrawal [217, 218]. Research has investigated the possible impact of addiction on spontaneous depressive states, in an attempt to distinguish substance-induced features (such as apathetic mood or exhaustion) or withdrawal-related items (such as sleep or appetite disorders), from others, which are closer to the core of an independent depressive disorder (such as chronic dysphoria or hopelessness) [219]. The three nuclear features of depression as an illness are anhedonia, psychomotor excitement or inhibition, and suicidal thoughts. Anhedonia, according to Rounsaville, clinically resembles hypophoria, which Martin singled out as a prominent mood feature in HUD patients [220]. Hypophoria seems to be crucial, first in initiating substance non-medical use, and, again, as part of the secondary withdrawal syndrome, which can persist for years or become important after years of abstinence, by acting as a significant risk factor for relapses into addiction. Separately, a minority of depressed addicts display suicidal thoughts, so suggesting that suicidal thoughts develop independently of drug addiction and other widely manifested depressive features among HUD patients. The prevalence of depressive features in HUD patients cannot be explained merely as being due to intoxication or withdrawal conditions [149]. The average severity of the symptoms displayed is comparable with that of non-addicted depressed patients who would like to commit, or who attempt, suicide [145]. In conclusion, the relationship between heroin addiction and depression appears to be quite a complex issue.

Several authors recommend observing patients over a drug-free period, before assessing any psychiatric comorbidity or resorting to specific therapeutic instruments. Mood and anxiety symptoms can, in fact, often be explained in terms of states of intoxication or withdrawal. In AUD patients, for example, the drug-free observation of abstaining alcoholic beverages is recommended for as long as 4 weeks before judging any comorbid condition to be present, and, therefore, starting the patient on some psychotropic treatment [221]. A hypothesis of dysthymia requires a 6-month-long observation period for correct evaluation. As a rule, when a family history of psychiatric disorders is found in subjects with a doubtful diagnosis, psychotropic treatment provided in line with current clinical judgement is appropriate [222–225].

2.1.3 Hypothesis that Depressive Symptomatology May Be Independent of the Presence of Dual Disorder

In one of our studies [83] we aimed to provide new information about (1) the mental status of HUD patients who apply for treatment of their HUD and (2) the degree of association of their baseline mental status with age, gender, substance non-medical use history, duration of dependence, and any other addictive, autonomous psychiatric disorder(s) not falling into the category of SUD (actual 'DD'). The study included 1090 HUD patients, who had requested treatment during the years 1983–2005 at the PISA-V.P. Dole Research Group of Santa Chiara University Hospital in Pisa, Italy. All patients received a diagnosis of opioid dependence with physical dependence according to the diagnostic criteria proposed in in various DSMs.

Of the participants, 45.8% reported depressed mood and 40.1% spoke of their preoccupation with somatic functions or experience of spontaneous anxiety. Sleep disorders were reported by 34.3%, and (hypo)manic or mixed excitement was displayed in a prominent way by 24.0% of the patients at the time of evaluation; 21.1% felt or showed aggressive behaviours and/or had been violent recently; 8.9% had engaged in self-injurious acts. Appetite had increased or decreased in 15.9% of the subjects. Memory disturbance occurred in 12.8% subjects. The least featured symptoms were delusions (7.0%), altered states of consciousness (6.4%), and hallucinations (4.7%).

Principal component factor analysis of the mental status items of Drug Addiction History Questionnaire (DAH-Q) yielded a three-factor solution. The first factor reflected a 'depressive-anxious' dimension (illness awareness, anxiety state, depressed mood, sleep and eating disturbances), which accounted for 31.1% of the variance. The second factor, accounting for 11.9% of the variance, reflected a psychomotor excitement dimension (hypomanic/manic or mixed state, aggressiveness and violence, suicidality). The third factor, which reflected a 'psychotic state' dimension, included memory deficits, altered consciousness, delusions, and hallucinations, so accounting for 10.3% of the total variance. Based on the highest z-scores obtained for each factor (dominant factor), we clustered all the subjects into three groups. The dominant 'depressive-anxious' group comprised 506 subjects (46.4%), the dominant 'psychomotor excitement' group 421 (38.6%), and the dominant 'psychotic state' group 163 (15.0%). Comparison of these groups revealed significant differences (Fig. 2.2).

Depressive-anxious HUD patients had milder somatic impairment, used fewer (other) substances, and underwent fewer types of treatment attempts. Their average educational level was lower, their economic conditions were better, heroin use was daily or less than daily for most, rather than 'more times a day' as in other groups. The addictive mode (i.e. the kind of lifestyle most common in those while using heroin) was typically a 'stable' one, that is, maintaining productivity and not engaging in street crime despite major individual and relational impairment. Nevertheless, a majority in this group had undergone a series of relapses and repeatedly failed to maintain abstinence (because they were in the 'revolving door stage'). The prevalence of concurrent use of alcohol, unprescribed BDZs, cocaine, and cannabis was lower. Social adjustment was impaired to a greater extent in dominant 'psychomotor excitement' patients. Lastly, dominant 'depressive-anxious' patients were less likely to be rated as having a 'DD'. In other words, it can be stated that the global weight of addiction-related impairment was lower in predominantly 'depressive-anxious' patients than in predominantly 'psychomotor excitement' or 'psychotic state' peers. Baseline conditions in which psychomotor excitement and psychosis predominated were those most likely to correspond to the otherwise assessed presence of an addictive and autonomous psychiatric disorder (DD). In summary, we

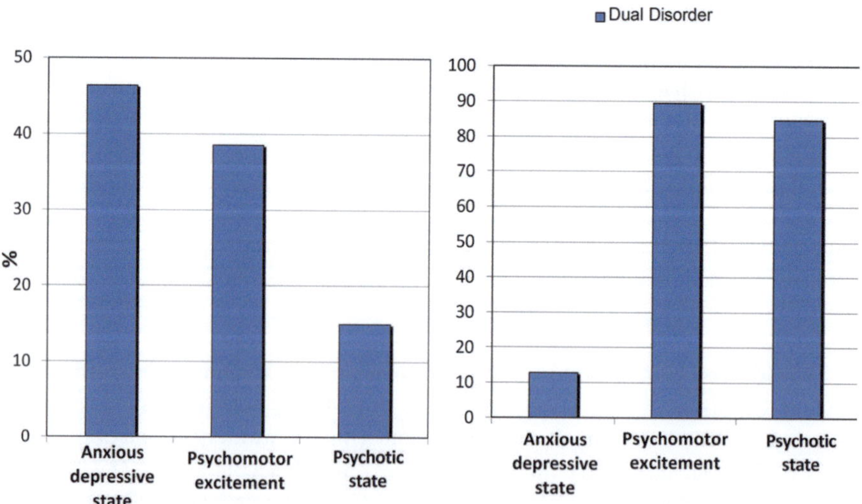

Fig. 2.2 Independence of depressive symptoms from the presence of a dual disorder: Psychopathological syndromes at treatment entry (left side) and correlation with the presence of a dual disorder (right side)

found that depressive features were the most frequent psychiatric symptoms among HUD patients looking for treatment, and part of the most frequently represented clinical state (depressive-anxious). It should, in any case, be pointed out that the depressive features of HUD patients were associated with anxiety rather than with suicidality, while a dominant depressive-anxious state was linked to a lower severity of drug addiction history. Conversely, psychomotor excitement and psychosis predicted the presence of polydrug use and an actual DD. It is therefore very important for clinicians to be able to identify major as well as minor psychomotor excitement and psychotic symptoms in HUD patients presenting for treatment, because it is likely that these patients are affected by another independent mental disorder (DD) that deserves specific clinical attention and treatment. By contrast, the presence of depressive features in the clinical presentation of HUD patients appears to be an unreliable indicator of general psychiatric severity. It could, in fact, be classified as a common comorbid condition of the average addict, often developing at lower levels of addiction severity, along with the early course of the addictive disease. In conclusion, our data indicated something opposite to the general trend of identifying DD from baseline depression patients and ascribing psychomotor excitement or psychosis to intoxication from psychoactive substances. Depressive-anxious symptoms are more likely to be parallel to addiction as a non-specific form of psychic disturbance, whereas psychomotor excitement and psychotic ones are likely to be part of a DD.

We then replicated this result in a sample of Slovenian HUD patients [226]. In a sample of 591 Slovenian HUD patients, psychomotor excitement was the most frequent psychiatric symptom; it was linked with a lower severity of drug addiction history. By contrast, the presence of depressive features in the clinical presentation appeared to be a reliable indicator of general addiction severity. Psychomotor excitement and psychosis, but not depression, predicted the presence of an actual DD, providing further support for the view that it is important for clinicians to be able to identify major as well as minor psychomotor excitement and psychotic symptoms in HUD patients presenting for treatment.

2.1.4   Primary or Secondary Nature of Comorbid Mood Disorder in Relation to HUD

The higher incidence of mood disorders among HUD patients does not seem to be attributable to heroin non-medical use. In fact, the recurrence of depressive episodes is common throughout the history of addicted patients, even when those episodes forerun the onset of substance use. During methadone treatment, depression is still common, though less so than in untreated addicts [227]. A group of addicts examined using the Beck Depression Inventory displayed depressive features in 60% of cases when starting methadone treatment, but only half that proportion (30%) while on methadone. Among methadone-maintained subjects, depression mostly occurs within the first 2 months; from then on, the occurrence rate falls progressively, so suggesting that most cases of depression develop in reaction to a severe addictive condition, rather than being opioid-induced. The presence of depression in HUD patients seems, however, to have a negative prognostic implication. Patients who are depressed when entering treatment are those that will display enduring psychostimulant non-medical use while in treatment, even at a 6-month term [228]. The likelihood of the onset of major depression occurring after methadone discontinuation has been estimated as being as high as 4% [158]. It must be remembered that, before psychotropics were developed, laudanum used to be resorted to for the treatment of depression, with results that were especially satisfactory in cases of agitated depression [229]. Electroconvulsive therapy produces a release of endorphins, both in animal and human samples [230]. A higher methadone dosage is required to achieve stabilization in addicted patients with comorbid mental diseases (mostly corresponding to mood disorders) [56].

It can be awkward to discriminate between drug-induced symptoms and primary psychopathology, because a considerable overlap is found, even on pathophysiological grounds, between substance non-medical use and mood disorders [231]. Cholinergic and aminergic systems influence mood, feelings, and psychomotor activity, so that mood disorders themselves may be supposed to stem from an abnormal interaction between these systems, as well as a state of cholinergic-muscarinic hypersensitivity [231]. Presumably, drugs prescribed for the treatment of mood disorders can counteract that abnormality. Accepting this point of view, drug non-medical use may be read as an attempt at self-medication directed at autonomous psychiatric disorders.

Several factors make it difficult to distinguish heroin-induced mood disorders from autonomous equivalent pictures. These are the extensive symptomatological overlap between mood disorders and SUDs, the awkwardness involved in obtaining clear and exhaustive information about past psychopathology and past patterns of substance non-medical use, and the differences between treatment settings and populations from which data are gathered (drug-free outpatient services, methadone clinics or treatment centres, therapeutic communities, and emergency units) [152, 231, 232].

In one of our studies (Fig. 2.3) [233] we explored, in DD/HUD patients, the temporal relationship based upon the age at onset of various diseases. When the onset of HUD was at least 1 year prior to the associated mental disorder, the patient was described as 'primarily affected by HUD', while when the onset of mental disorder was at least 1 year prior to the associated HUD, the patient was described as 'primarily affected by mental disorder'. If there was less than 1 year between diagnoses of either condition, then the patient was not assigned to either category. On this basis, this study has examined the correlations between mood disorders and the chronology of illness in DD/HUD patients. A total of 506 consecutive outpatients were enrolled in the study. Mean age ± SD was 29.61 ± 5.9 years (ranging from 17 to 45 years). Most patients were males ($n = 376$; 74.3%), had never married ($n = 369$; 72.9%), and reported an educational experience lasting less than 9 years ($n = 330$; 65.2%). As many as 217 (42.9%) were unemployed at the time of clinical assessment. One hundred and nine (21.50%) reported poor economic status; 76 (15.0%) were living alone. According to the age of onset of HUD and of

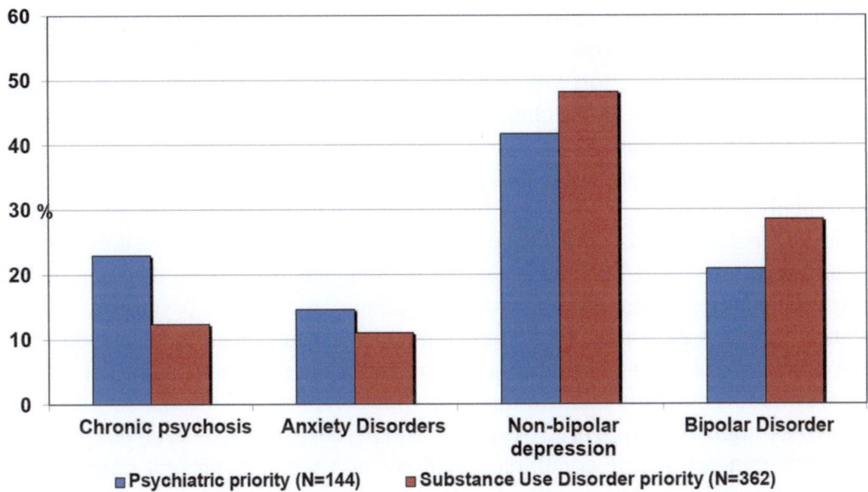

Fig. 2.3 Dual disorders and temporal priority

mental illness 362 (71.5%) were HUD priority patients and 144 (28.5%) mentally ill priority patients.

In our study, approximately 72% of our consecutive DD/HUD participants developed a mental disorder after heroin addiction. This finding differs from the results reported in the available literature on this topic, which express a consensus that mental disorders generally precede drug non-medical use [234–237]. One difference is that our study was restricted to those with a primary diagnosis of HUD, the high incidence of polydrug use, we may assume that the clinical progression observed was not dependent on heroin non-medical use alone. Our data suggest, rather, that patients with mood disorders were initially affected with drug addiction and that the most important predictors of progression from heroin use to psychiatric comorbidity were a diagnosis of mood disorders, repeated treatment failures, and physical complications, which is consistent with the previous literature [238, 239]. In contrast, psychosis was more likely to be a prevalent diagnosis in mentally ill priority patients—a conclusion that supports Khantzian's self-medication theory [143]. Our primarily psychotic patients might find heroin a substance that can, initially, ease psychotic symptoms and fragmentation anxiety [240, 241]. Conversely, in our sample we observed progression from substance non-medical use to mood disorders. In this connection, we cannot rule out the possibility that emotional dysregulation may be a predisposing factor to drug addiction [79, 186]. It may be speculated that in these subjects the presence of a premorbid state (cyclothymia, anxiety, impulse dyscontrol) alongside polydrug use could destabilize their psychopathological condition, so predisposing the onset of a diagnosable mood disorder [36].

In summary, it is reasonable to think of a self-therapeutic use of heroin at the start of 'toxicomanic career' in the lives of psychotic patients, with a worsening during the long-term use of heroin. Regarding heroin-addicted patients with concomitant mood disorders, we cannot definitively rule out the possibility that these patients use heroin in a self-therapeutic manner, but the possible but unprovable initial beneficial effect exerted by the substance on emotional instability would soon be followed by a mood-destabilizing action, which would then accelerate the course of the illness and ultimately lead to a worse clinical presentation, both on the addictive and on the psychopathological plane.

The chronology of illness in DD patients has important clinical implications. A commonly held view supposes that most patients with a dual disorder present primarily with a mental disorder that becomes more complex over time as drug dependence deepens [234]. This suggests that treating the psychiatric disorder might prevent the onset of drug dependence. Furthermore, treating the psychiatric condition as a priority, even in the presence of concomitant drug dependence, may resolve the addiction when the psychiatric condition has been effectively controlled.

Our data, only partly confirm this view, however. Most of our patients demonstrated a progression from drug dependence to psychiatric disorder, so that treating the comorbid psychiatric condition would not be enough to prevent drug dependence. Moreover, our data suggest that the theory set out above can be applied to the treatment of patients affected by psychosis; but it would be hard to consider extending it to patients affected by mood disorders. We suggest, therefore, that in all cases where DD is present, drug dependence should be treated first [49]. Further studies are now required to enable researchers to check whether these data can be confirmed and verify if this approach is also valid for dependence on substances other than heroin.

2.1.5 Impact of Comorbid Mood Disorders on the Natural History of HUD

Depressed addicts report a higher rate of recent alcohol and opioid use than their non-depressed peers. Consistent with this, psychosocial and legal problems arising from substance use are more severe among depressed addicts. Several studies have found that depression is often associated with recent stressful life events, familial disharmony, financial troubles, as well as working and legal problems [219]. The combination of depression and maladjustment is likely to drive addicts towards requests for treatment, whereas troubles related to substance non-medical use alone are not likely to promote treatment-seeking behaviours [219]. As a rule, it is only when legal and psychosocial troubles are brought about those addicts become motivated strongly enough to ask for medical intervention. Addicted patients entering treatment—an event that usually marks a critical phase in addictive history—have higher levels of depression than peers already in MMT [242, 243]. DeLeon defined this depressive syndrome of the addict as 'circumstance-related depression' [244, 245]. It is interesting to note that no correlation has been found so far between levels of cannabis consumption and the severity of the depressive symptoms displayed.

Dysphoria can be a crucial issue in leading addicts to ask for treatment. As regards therapy, data are available that indicate the possible effectiveness of antidepressant pharmacotherapy and psychotherapy in depressed addicts.

According to data gathered by the PISA-V.P. Dole Research Group, no difference emerges between addicts with or without comorbid mood disorders as regards somatic issues, typology of lifetime used substances, number of past treatments, or clinical aspects of the addictive disease (e.g. patterns of drug use, periodic abstinence, and addictive dynamics). Addicts with mood disorders do, however, display poorer psychosocial functioning, but it should be recalled that depression itself, even without concurrent substance non-medical use, is associated with psychosocial deterioration and the impairment of free time. As far as family adaptation is concerned, it is addicts who have no comorbid mood disorders who appear to do best. In fact, depression seems to favour family relationships, or, rather, to improve them with respect to the standards of addicted patients. In other words, the disruptive potency of addiction is attested by the corrective effect of comorbid depression, which adds to the damage.

Addicts with mood disorders report a less satisfactory sexual life, consistent with the nature of the disease, and a greater number of legal problems. Addicts with an index episode of depression tend to receive greater therapeutic care (with several therapeutic approaches combined), at least at the beginning [242, 243]. As for the chronology of addiction, it took less time for HUD patients with mood disorders to develop their addiction: in fact, although these subjects are, on average, quite old when first using the substance, they start regular substance use earlier. In addition, HUD patients with comorbid mood disorders prove to have been addicted for a shorter time when they first ask for treatment [246].

2.1.5.1 Most Discriminant Characteristics of Bipolar 1 DD/BIP1-HUD Patients at First Opioid Agonist Treatment

In one of our studies [247] we compared the clinical characteristics and natural history of heroin addiction between bipolar 1 and NDD/HUD patients at their first agonist opioid treatment. Our supposition was that DD/BIP1-HUD patients, compared with their non-dual disorder peers, showed a more severe psychopathological condition and a shorter, less severe drug addiction history at treatment entry. If borne out, this interpretation would support a 'self-medication' approach to heroin use, not only in our psychotic patients, but also in DD/BIP1-HUD ones. In that case, bipolar 1 patients would start using heroin to limit mood instability, after which the addictive process could frustrate the subjectively beneficial effect of heroin. From this perspective, it is likely that patients may have sought in methadone and/or buprenorphine treatment as an alternative compensation for their discomfort.

We selected patients who requested their first agonist opioid treatment. The sample consisted of 46 HUD patients who, after psychiatric screening, had received an additional diagnosis of bipolar 1 disorder. Most of these patients were males. As control group we selected 214 patients who underwent psychiatric screening and showed the absence of any psychiatric disorder. The two groups were homogenous in their age and gender structures.

With respect to demographic data, no differences were observed regarding marital status, occupation, income, and living situation. DD/BIP1-HUD and NDD/HUD patients significantly differed over education. About 50.0% of DD/BIP1-HUD patients and 73.7% of controls showed a relatively short duration ($\leq$8 years) of education.

No differences were observed as regards somatic comorbidity, social adjustment, and combined treatments. Compared with controls, DD/BIP1-HUD patients showed a higher percentage of subjects with altered mental status, as well as legal problems and polydrug use. No differences were found regarding age at first contact with heroin, dependence length, age at onset of the continuous use of heroin, and age at first agonist opioid treatment. DD/BIP1-HUD patients presented shorter dependence duration, either considering time from initial heroin use, or from the onset of the continuous use of heroin. DD/BIP1-HUD patients showed significantly greater frequency in their use of alcohol, CNS depressants, CNS stimulants, hallucinogens, cannabinoids, and inhalants. The concomitant use of other opioids, such as painkillers and illegal methadone, was a topic where no significant differences emerged. DD/BIP1-HUD patients more frequently showed an unstable modality of heroin use and typically presented psychopathological antecedents. By contrast, controls showed the following characteristics: stable modalities of use; they typically did not present any psychosocial or psychopathological antecedents.

Based on the logistic regression analysis, the odds of being a DD/BIP1-HUD patient were significantly higher in the case of patients who reported the presence of polydrug use and legal problems with an unstable modality of use. A longer lapse of time from the onset of HUD to its treatment turned out to be a good predictor of belonging to the control group.

With respect to substance-use modalities, DD/BIP1-HUD, at a higher frequency than that of their non-dual disorder peers, present an unstable modality of heroin use and psychopathological antecedents. It is notable that an unstable modality of heroin use has proved to be typical of those HUD patients who present aggressive behaviours [85]. Aggressiveness has, in fact, been found to be associated with a bipolar 1 diagnosis [248]. We submit that the unstable modality of heroin use might be due to mood instability, which, in the long term, is, of course, exacerbated by the chronic use of a short half-life opioid agent such as heroin. It remains unclear whether bipolar patients experience a certain mood-balancing action, at least in the early phases of heroin use. Despite this, the fact that the stage of the addictive illness has proved unable to differentiate bipolar HUD patients from controls casts further shadows over the self-therapeutic hypothesis as a way of accounting for heroin addiction in bipolar patients. If bipolar HUD patients used heroin in a self-therapeutic manner, we would expect that to occur at an early stage of the addictive disease, as observed among DD/PSY-HUD patients. The self-reported presence of polydrug use and legal problems accompanying an unstable modality of heroin use implies the greatest likelihood of belonging to the bipolar group of HUD patients. A greater time interval from the onset of HUD to its initial treatment predicts a patient's belonging to the control group.

We cannot definitively rule out the possibility that bipolar HUD patients use heroin in a self-therapeutic manner, but any unprovable initial beneficial effect exerted by the substance on emotional instability would soon be followed by a mood-destabilizing action. That would accelerate the course of the illness, and ultimately lead to a worse clinical presentation, both on the addictive and the psychopathological plane.

2.1.5.2 Differentiating Between the Course of Illness in Bipolar 1 and Chronic DD/PSY-HUD Patients at Their First Agonist Opioid Treatment

Bipolar disorders and chronic psychosis are a frequent form of comorbid DD in heroin-addicted patients. One possible explanation for this comorbidity is provided by the 'self-medication hypothesis', according to which substance non-medical use may function as an attempt to alleviate emotional suffering brought about by the psychiatric illness. Assuming that street-heroin use can be interpreted as an attempt to supply self-care for psychotic symptoms and mood instability, the non-therapeutic use could be revealed by the presence of a more severe heroin-addiction history (in terms of its course and gravity) in DD patients, especially at their first AOT request. A naturalistic comparative cohort study was designed with the aim of comparing the clinical characteristics of 283 heroin-addicted patients presenting for their first AOT, after dividing the group according to the absence ($n = 214$) or presence ($n = 69$) of DD (with the group of 69 comprising 23 chronic psychotic and 46 bipolar 1 patients; Table 2.3) [249].

Table 2.3 Drug addiction history questionnaire variables in heroin-dependent patients at AOT entry (only significant differences are reported)

	NDD	PSY	BIP1		
	$N = 214$	$N = 23$	$N = 46$	$F/\chi2$	p
2a. Altered mental areas ($M \pm SD$)	1.27 ± 1.1a	6.21 ± 2.1b	5.95 ± 1.4b	361.91	0.000
7. Legal problems, presence (N, %)	30 (14.3)b	2 (8.7)a	13 (28.3)c	6.47	0.039
8. Polydrug use, presence (N, %)	45 (21.2)a	10 (43.5)ab	26 (56.5)b	25.57	0.000
8a. Comorbid used substances, n ($M \pm SD$)	1.18 ± 1.5a	2.34 ± 1.8b	2.89 ± 1.8b	24.33	0.000
10. Combined treatment, presence (N, %)	169 (79.0)a	13 (56.5)b	34 (73.9)ab	5.97	0.051
Addiction latency (age at first use–age at onset) ($M \pm SD$)	6.92 ± 6.1b	2.88 ± 3.3a	5.78 ± 5.6ab	4.05	0.018
79. Dependence length (years) ($M \pm SD$)	4.29 ± 1.4b	3.00 ± 3.1a	2.36 ± 1.3a	3.17	0.000
58. Modality of use (unstable) (N, %)	29 (15.8)a	7 (36.8)ab	23 (56.1)b	31.28	0.000
59. Periodic self-detoxification (N, %)	157 (87.7)a	11 (64.7)b	28 (75.7)ab	8.49	0.014
60. Stages of heroin dependence (stage 3) (N, %)	121 (67.6)a	3 (17.6)b	23 (56.1)a	17.18	0.000
61. Without stressors before use (N, %)	127 (74.3)a	5 (27.8)b	18 (46.2)b	23.69	0.000

Each letter denotes a subset of categories whose column proportions do not differ significantly from each other at the 0.05 level

We found differences between DD patients after dividing the whole group into psychotic (DD/PSY-HUD) patients, bipolar 1 (DD/BIP1-HUD) ones, and NDD patients. At AOT entry, altered mental status areas were, of course, significantly fewer in NDD patients than in DD patients; polydrug use was more frequent in DD/BIP1-HUD patients than in NDD ones. DD/PSY-HUD patients had an intermediate position. Dependence length was longer in NDD patients. The addiction latency (time elapsing between first use and continuous use) was shorter in DD/PSY-HUD patients than in NDD ones (with DD/BIP1-HUD patients in an intermediate position). An unstable modality of heroin use was found more frequently in DD/BIP1-HUD patients than in NDD ones (with DD/PSY-HUD patients in an intermediate position). Periodic self-detoxification was found more frequently in NDD patients than in DD/PSY-HUD ones (with DD/BIP1-HUD patients in an intermediate position). At AOT entry, fewer DD/PSY-HUD patients and DD/BIP1-HUD ones were in stage 3 of the illness. DD/PSY-HUD and DD/BIP1-HUD patients were also distinguished by the absence of psychosocial stressors before their first use of heroin.

Comparing DD with NDD patients, the duration of HUD (in years) and the absence of polydrug use were the most discriminant characteristics of NDD patients. In contrast, DD patients were distinguished by an unstable modality of heroin use, together with a higher number of comorbid used substances and the presence of legal problems.

Comparing DD/PSY-HUD with DD/BIP1-HUD patients, the fact of reaching stage 3 of the illness is, overall, a strong predictor of a patient who belongs to the DD/BIP1-HUD patient group, as well as the presence of polydrug use. On the other hand, a lengthy duration of dependence is the most discriminant characteristic of DD/PSY-HUD patients (Table 2.4).

Compared with NDD patients, our DD/PSY-HUD patients, at first treatment entry, were characterized by areas of more strongly altered mental status, a shorter length of dependence, and a very short addiction latency (i.e. the time that elapses between the first use of heroin and its continuous use). By themselves they were

Table 2.4 Most important characteristics of NDD- and DD-HUD (bipolar 1 and chronic psychotic) patients

	STEP	Exp(B)	95% CI for Exp(B)	p
Most important predictors of the group of DD patients				
Duration of dependence (years)	1	0.50	0.37–0.67	0.000
Modality of use, unstable	2	3.12	1.35–7.23	0.008
Polydrug use, presence	3	2.94	1.30–6.60	0.009
Legal problems	4	2.67	0.99–7.18	0.051
Most discriminating characteristics of bipolar 1 heroin-dependent patients at first AOT				
Chronic psychotic HUD patients		1.00		
Stage of illness (stage 3)	1	556.72	2.72–113,625.81	0.020
Duration of dependence	2	0.46	0.24–0.98	0.021

incapable of stopping their heroin use, not even periodically. They were in stage 2 (the intermediate or 'dose-increasing' phase) of illness and reported more stressors before their first use of heroin. Their shorter duration of heroin addiction, not reaching stage 3 of the disease (known as the 'revolving door phase') and less polydrug use differentiated them from DD/BIP1-HUD patients. To sum up the main differences, heroin addiction was more severe in DD/BIP1-DD patients and less severe in chronic psychotic patients than in heroin-addicted patients without any form of DD.

One of the possible implications of these data is that DD/PSY-HUD patients are requesting AOT as a way of searching for the antipsychotic properties of agonist opioid medications. Their heroin addiction history is not, in fact, as compromised as that found in NDD patients. Despite this, the use of street heroin has always been continuous, and the shorter duration of their dependence is the only factor that prevents them from reaching stage 3 of the illness. NDD/HUD patients do request treatment at this stage.

In conclusion, the differences found between chronic psychotic and bipolar 1 heroin-addicted patients in the course and severity of their addictive disease, considering the limited severity of the addictive disease in chronic psychotic patients at their first AOT entry, do not justify the exclusion of a therapeutic use of heroin, at least at the beginning of such a patient's toxicomanic career, so limiting the progression of the addictive disease. This pattern of development seems to be excluded for bipolar 1 heroin-addicted patients, who come to their first AOT with a more severely addictive disease.

2.1.5.3 Clinical Presentations of Substance Use in Bipolar HUD Patients at Time of Treatment Entry

In one of our studies [85], patients included in the PISA-DATASET (dataset from previous studies on AOT carried out in Italy and used in previously published articles) were selected on the basis of the following characteristics:

- Diagnosis of bipolar 1 or 2 disorders according to DSM-IV TR and various DSM criteria
- Diagnosis of opioid dependence with physical dependence according to DSM-IV TR and various DSM criteria
- Being at their lifetime first hospitalization
- Not receiving medication for the treatment of bipolar disorders
- Using at least two substances (heroin included) at study entry

Patients using opioid agonist medications or illegally obtained methadone were excluded to limit the confusing effects of this medication on clinical psychiatric presentation.

This study included 150 consecutive bipolar HUD patients. The mean age of these patients was 29 ± 6 years old (range 17–50). Of these 150, 91 (60.7%) were male; 85 (56.7%) were single, 104 (69.3%) had experienced less than 9 years of education, and 70 (46.7%) were unemployed. As to drug addiction history, 127 (84.7%) patients reported physical complications. One hundred (66.7%) were unemployed, 92 (61.3%) were part of a family, 53 (35.3%) had an ongoing romantic relationship, 81 (54.0%) enjoyed social leisure, and 72 (48.0%) encountered legal difficulties. Eighty-six (57.3%) were polydrug users (three or more substances). Within the whole sample group, 120 (80.0%) had experienced past treatment failures.

In order to obtain groups of patients differing in their clinical presentation at hospitalization, study participants were divided into four groups based on their episode polarity. As many as 103 patients (68.6%) showed a major depressive episode; 22 (14.7%) a hypomanic episode; 5 (3.3%), a full manic episode; and 20 (13.3%) a mixed episode, according to DSM-IV TR or various other DSM criteria.

We compared the demographic and clinical characteristics of our patients according to their current episode polarity. No statistically significant differences among the four groups were observed as regards age, gender, educational level, marital status, job, or financial needs. Nor were any statistically significant differences observed either among most of those who had a drug addiction history or who displayed questionnaire factors (somatic comorbidity, altered mental status, work, family, romantic involvement, social leisure and legal problems, the status of being a polydrug user, associated treatments).

Obviously, no statistically significant differences were observed regarding the non-medical use of heroin.

Patients experiencing a depressive episode at clinical presentations showed a more frequent use of unprescribed anxiolytic hypnotics. During a hypomanic episode, patients more frequently used cocaine-amphetamines, while, during a manic episode, patients more frequently used cannabis and cocaine-amphetamines. The associated use of alcohol, cocaine-amphetamines, and cannabinoids was more frequently encountered during a mixed episode (Fig. 2.4).

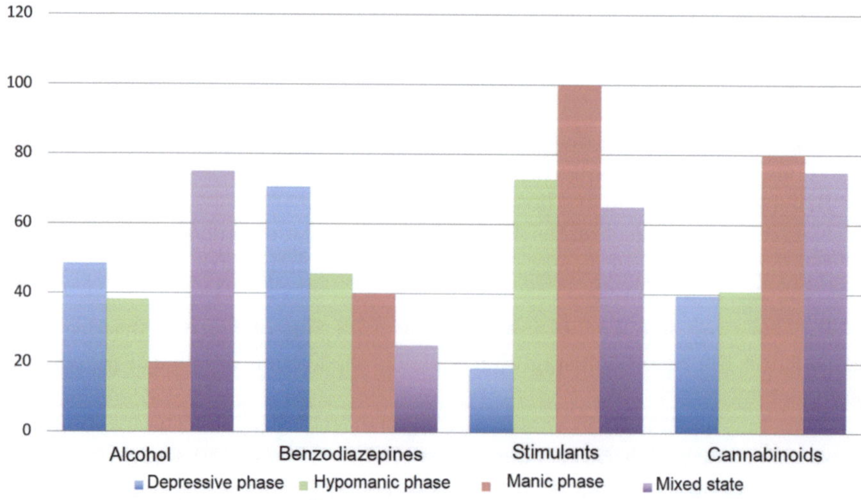

Fig. 2.4 Secondary used substances in DD/BIP1-HUD patients according to the phase at hospitalization

In the case of depressed patients, the use of CNS depressants is consistent with their toxicological status. It should be noted that BDZ use in HUD patients may be correlated with a condition of opioid dependence improperly compensated by street heroin [75]. From a psychopathological standpoint, depressants may aggravate the slowing of cognitive and physical functions caused by depression, but it remains true that these medications are effective in treating insomnia and anxiety, which are often symptoms of depression. Also, patients may not be seeking an actual 'lift' of their depression but be searching for a state of 'oblivion' in which the pain of depression is cancelled. In depression, what is seen is not a higher use of stimulant substances, but the use of CNS depressants that may sometimes relieve some aspects of depression (or may not do so)—a situation that fails to provide support to Khantzian's hypothesis.

More clearly, Khantzian's hypothesis does not seem to be supported by the other three kinds of clinical presentations. Patients during a hypomanic, manic, or mixed episode, despite experiencing a state of excitement, tend to continue their non-medical use of psychostimulants, further reinforcing and elevating their mental state. This is consistent with a proposed bipolar-stimulant spectrum where sub-threshold bipolar traits are aggravated by stimulant non-medical use [79].

If we focus on HUD patients, the concomitant use of cocaine is reported to be a serious phenomenon that will determine negative consequences on social adjustment and outcome. When heroin and heroin-cocaine users have been compared, a direct relationship has been found between cocaine non-medical use and the frequency of psychiatric disorders, together with a correlation with the severity of self-rated psychopathology [250]. We do not know if this lack of awareness of psychopathological symptoms is due to the use of cocaine or to the underlying excitement that sustains cocaine use. Moreover, if cocaine use ensures the self-enhancement of one's level of hypomania, cyclothymia, or hyperthymia, the craving for hypomania is likely to be particularly strong in HUD patients, whose level of excitement is lowered by heroin use [70]. In addition, cocaine has been reported to induce a higher frequency of mixed states when used by bipolar patients [251]. This evidence suggests that some bipolar patients, after deciding to use cocaine instead of being excited, may have shifted from a manic or hypomanic to a mixed episode.

During a manic episode, our bipolar patients show a high level of consumption of stimulants and cannabinoids. In the literature, the non-medical use of cannabinoids in bipolar patients has been found to induce manic symptoms [252], so it is possible that, in our manic patients, as with cocaine use, they may use cannabinoids to optimize their level of excitement. To date, cannabis use is also considered to be one of the most important risk factors for schizophrenia, thanks to its ability to precipitate or exacerbate psychotic symptoms [253–258]. In line with this assumption, in our sample, cannabis is mainly used in manic and mixed states that, unlike depressive and hypomanic episodes, are often characterized by the presence of psychotic symptoms. Whatever the causes of the use of cannabis, Khantzian's hypothesis is not supported in its application to cannabis use. For many subjects, ending cannabis use is difficult to achieve, not only because of prior habits of use, but also because of the attendant psychotic symptoms, including poor insight and judgement, lack of impulse control, and cognitive impairment. Most of these subjects are unable to understand that cannabis use is connected with the onset of symptoms [26].

One widely debated issue is whether Khantzian's hypothesis is a suitable instrument for interpreting alcohol dependence. In examining patients with a mixed episode, we found that, besides their non-medical use of cocaine-amphetamines and cannabinoids, and in contrast with the other three clinical presentation groups, they often resort to alcohol use. Patients experience their mixed mood as something undesirable and unpleasant, but they continue to consume substances that tend to preserve their mixed, dysphoric state. Craving for substances and dependence creates a loop, a senseless vicious circle in which patients obtain neither satisfaction (mood elation) nor physical benefit (relief). In line with this observation, a past or current alcohol use disorder has proved to raise the likelihood of a switch from depressive to manic, mixed, or hypomanic states in patients with bipolar disorder [259]. Nervousness in alcoholic patients has been hypothesized to be the only negative mood state to predict increases in alcohol consumption later in the day. Further examination of this within-person relationship has demonstrated that men were more likely to consume alcohol when nervous than were women, but this association is unrelated to family history of alcoholism, problem drinking patterns, or traits of anxiety and depression. Consistent with the self-medication hypothesis, alcohol consumption has been associated with lower levels of nervousness, but this effect varies in a way dependent on several demographic and clinical variables [260]. Almost one quarter of individuals with mood disorders use alcohol or drugs to relieve symptoms, with the highest prevalence of self-medication in bipolar 1 disorder. After checking the effects of SUDs, self-medication has been associated with higher rates of comorbid anxiety and personality disorders than those found in individuals who do not self-medicate [261]. On the basis of these data, we believe that, in the case of alcohol, Khantzian's hypothesis accounts for anxiety disorders more satisfactorily than mood disorders, although it must be added that it actually explains controlled rather than addictive use. In fact, enduring use, despite the worsening, or the inadequate balance, of symptoms, is inconsistent with a current self-medicating explanation, although that explanation may have been appropriate in a previous stage of controlled use. It should also be remembered that patients were assessed for mood during current drug use, thus ruling out the ambiguity between spontaneous mood swings and substance-induced intoxication. In fact, our patients had been displaying affective dysregulation for some time before being diagnosed and had been engaged in substance use, which was bound to worsen the affective core of their clinical pictures (i.e. stimulants during excitement and depressants during depression). The hypothesis of symptomatological overlap between temporary substance-related intoxication and mood states is superseded in this way.

After reviewing our data, we speculate that, setting aside depressive and mixed episodes, the non-medical use of substances in hypomanic and manic episodes of bipolar disorder is more probably due to patients' desire to maintain their current affective state rather than to resolve depressed mood.

These considerations also provide a possible explanation for the fact that bipolar patients tend not to comply with therapy during hypomanic, manic, and mixed states [262–264]. In the literature, patients' lack of compliance with prescribed therapy has been principally associated with their lack of insight into their mental illness [265–267]. We go beyond that in suggesting that, during hypomanic and manic phases, bipolar patients do not comply with prescribed therapies and tend to exacerbate their mental status by means of substances, not only because they are unaware of their mental illness, but also because they somehow live the current episode as a pleasurable and rewarding experience (in cases of addiction to mania).

The obvious limitations of this study are as follows: this is a retrospective analysis carried out on a small cohort of patients, rather than a study specifically designed to elucidate this issue. Assessments of the same subject in various clinical presentations of the natural history of this illness would have provided a better level of information. In addition, we must consider the difficulty in determining whether the substance use modifies the mood, or the mood state determines the substance used. It is possible that stimulants are seen in those with mania or hypomania because the stimulant produced the mood state. They could have been depressed without it. Lastly, we have no information about the temperament of our subjects. So, we cannot exclude the presence of a depressive temperament that is able to moderate the nature of patients' substance non-medical use; that would set up the need to modify our hypothesis. One of our earlier findings, however, was that heroin users mainly have a cyclothymic temperament [78].

In summary, our data do not support Khantzian's hypothesis, if we exclude the use of CNS depressants during a depressive phase to alleviate anxiety. Also in this case, it can be said that CNS depressants are able to alleviate insomnia and anxiety, but, more generally, may aggravate the slowing of cognitive and physical functions caused by depression. Khantzian's hypothesis, more evidently, does not seem to be able to account for the use of psychostimulants and cannabis during a hypomanic, manic, or mixed state. In fact, the use of these substances leads to the further destabilization of mood. On alcohol use we have to say that alcohol use, in our subjects, is concomitant with a mixed state. Conversely, we would have expected the use of alcohol during hypomanic and manic states to limit the euphoric condition. Lastly, apart from the expected result of a prominent use of CNS stimulants during a depressive phase of bipolar patients, in line with Khantzian's hypothesis, this study showed that they were used more prominently during hypomanic or manic phases. This apparently supports an alternative hypothesis—that mood elation is a pleasurable and rewarding experience that, in bipolar patients, can be started or prolonged using CNS stimulant drugs.

2.1.6 Addiction and Suicidality

In addiction treatment the first objective is prompt intervention when a patient displays homicidal behaviours and/or suicidal thoughts, and/or is pharmacologically unstable. The first two situations require immediate hospitalization in a psychiatric department. The third can sometimes be managed in non-psychiatric hospital departments. Alcohol-related mood alterations and depressed mood are strong predictors of suicidal acts. Only after these conditions have been checked can any treatment for addiction be started.

The epidemiology of suicide in drug addiction is reported in Table 2.5.

Of addicts, 90% with a history of suicidal acts also have a history of depression [268]. According to the San Diego Suicide Study (SDS Study) [269], HUD patients are at greater risk of suicide when they have concurrent mood disorders, 29% of

Table 2.5 Heroin use disorder and suicidality

Diagnosis	%	Studies
Substance use and dependence in general population	11–18	Robins, 1974
Substance use and dependence in suicidal people		
Before 1970s	5	Dorpat & Woodhall, 1960; Barraclough et al., 1974
During 1980s	58	San Diego Suicide Study, 1989; Pages et al., 1997
<30 years	67	San Diego Suicide Study, 1989
>30 years	46	San Diego Suicide Study, 1989
>40 years	14	San Diego Suicide Study, 1989
Suicide in general population	0.3E−4	Miles, 1977; Humeniuk et al., 2000
	0.82E−4	
Suicide in hard-core street SUD patients	3E−4	Galanter & Castaneda, 1985
	8.2E−4	
Suicidal thoughts in heroin use disorder patients	31–75	Deykin & Buka, 1994; Rossow & Lauritzen, 2001
Suicidal attempts in heroin use disorder patients	7–25	Ward & Schuckit, 1980; Stimmel et al., 1983; Galanter & Castaneda, 1985; Krausz et al., 1996
	28–61	Deykin & Buka, 1994
Heroin use disorder patients who attempted suicide		
History of depression	87	Murphy et al., 1988
Atypical depression	29	San Diego Suicide Study, 1989
Short duration depressive symptoms	100	Hasin et al., 1988
Heroin use disorder patients who committed suicide		
Polysubstance users	92	
With psychosocial difficulties	12.6	San Diego Suicide Study, 1989; Kosten, 1988; Bukstein et al., 1993; Chatham et al., 1995; Mezzich et al., 1997; Mino et al., 1999; Hill et al., 2000
Heroin mono-users	8	Flower et al., 1986

which correspond to atypical depression. Transient depressive features are quite frequent too in patients diagnosed as 'pure addicts' (on average they display 4.1 depressive symptoms): addicts' suicidal behaviours may therefore be equivalent to full-blown depressive states, with rapid onset and intense symptomatology, but lasting for too short a time (under 15 days) to meet the diagnosis of major depressive episode [270]. In any case, addiction itself carries a high risk of suicide.

The relationship between alcoholism and suicide has been known for a long time, but recognition of the link between suicide and opioid addiction is quite recent [271, 272]. Studies performed before the 1970s reported a suicide rate as low as 5%, probably due either to a defective surveying methodology or the low degree of severity of the incipient phenomenon. The SDS study, surveying 283 consecutive cases of suicide in San Diego County between 1981 and 1983, reported a 58% prevalence rate of alcohol or substance-related problems [269, 273–275], which is far higher than that of the general population (11–18%) [123].

The suicide rate among addicts (between 8.2 and 30 per 100,000) was 11 times higher than in the general population [276–278]. The lifetime prevalence rate for suicide attempts varies from 7% to 25% among addicts [276, 279, 280]. Addicts usually first commit or attempt suicide below the age of 40—a younger age than that for AUD patients or the general population [281]; 50% of addicts first commit or attempt suicide at an age below 28 [282]. Again, the SDS study reported that 67% of young people (below 30 years of age) who committed suicide were HUD patients, whereas suicidal addicts were only 46% of older-than-30 suicide committers and 14% of older-than-40 ones.

Early psychosocial difficulties, as witnessed by living in institutions, fostering families, a diagnosis of attention deficit disorder with hyperactivity, a positive family history for suicide, alcohol dependence, and depression, all seem to be risk factors for suicidal acts among HUD patients, especially for those displaying prominent disruptive behaviours [279, 283, 284]. Polydrug use, especially of sedative-hypnotics and alcohol, is also a risk factor for suicide among HUD patients, due to either narcotic potentiation or aggressive dyscontrol [279, 283, 285]. Suicidal HUD patients recorded a recent use of 3.6 different substances on average; 84% had been using alcohol, heroin, and psychotropics together, while only 8% had been pure drinkers, and 8% had been be pure opioid addicts [285]. Suicidal thoughts may be present in non-depressed addicts too, especially when addiction is combined with a lack of family support, severe psychosocial maladjustment, and polydrug use [286]. As regards polydrug use, it should be pointed out that the non-medical use of cannabis or hallucinogenic drug carries a lower risk of suicide than combined alcohol, heroin, cocaine, and tobacco non-medical use [287, 288]. Features of suicidal HUD patients vary according to gender: female suicidal addicts tend to use prescribed medications, display borderline features, have a history of past suicide attempts, and declare suicidal intentions. In DD suicidal addicts, the axis I comorbid disorder usually foreruns addiction [289].

As regards which kind of mood disorder is at greatest risk of suicide, it can be noted that bipolar 1 patients, unless a record of mixed episodes is prominent, display a tendency to be at high risk of polydrug use but are unlikely to commit suicide.

By contrast, depressed and dysphoric patients, whether non-bipolar or bipolar 2 or bipolar 1 with mixed features, are suicide-prone [288].

On therapeutic grounds, an effective antidepressant treatment lowers the likelihood of suicide among depressed HUD patients [290]. According to the observations of the PISA-V.P. Dole Research Group, NTX-treated patients seem to be at higher risk of suicide, whereas methadone treatment appears to offer some protection against it [291].

While most of the studies on suicidal risk factors have investigated the correlation between these factors and the likelihood of completed suicide [292–296], others have focused on suicidal ideation and suicide attempts [297–300]. The latter do not necessarily predict death by suicide, yet their strong correlation with completed suicide [292, 294, 301, 302] makes their investigation a priority in the clinical assessment of suicidal risk. In one of our studies then we aimed to provide new information [303] on:

The prevalence of suicidal ideation in HUD patients who present for treatment for opioid addiction.

The degree of association of these thoughts with psychopathology, socio-demographic characteristics, and drug addiction history.

The study included 616 subjects, who had requested treatment during the years 1995–2003. All of them received a diagnosis of opioid dependence with physical dependence (according to DSM-IV criteria) and gave their informed consent for study participation.

The average age of the patients was 29 ± 6 years (range 16–51). Most of them were male (77.5%), single (69.3%), with less than 9 years of education (77.6%), and unemployed (50.6%).

Suicidal thoughts, during the past week, were reported by 199 (29.1%) patients. According to the 4-level severity range of the Symptom Checklist-90 (SCL90) items (not at all—a little bit—moderately—quite a bit—extremely), 17 (2.8%) showed the maximum degree of thoughts of ending one's life (serious suicidal intentions). When present, suicidal thoughts were light or moderate in about one-fifth of the sample. Depression and hostility were the only psychopathological dimensions that turned out to be correlated with suicidal thoughts. Regarding socio-demographic characteristics, unemployment, receiving public welfare benefits, coming from blue collar or unemployed families, and living alone were significantly associated with suicidal ideation. Other variables such as age (less than 25 vs. 25 or more years), gender (males vs. females), marital status (single vs. others), education (less than 8 years vs. 8 or more), income (poor vs. sufficient) did not prove to be significantly correlated with suicide ideation. As regards psychiatric comorbidity, mood disorders, whether depressive or bipolar spectrum, were significantly correlated with suicidal ideation. Statistically significant differences were not observed for somatic comorbidity in terms of major illnesses (absence vs. presence), HIV positiveness (negative vs. positive), AIDS—acquired immune deficiency syndrome (absence vs. presence).

Some aspects of social adjustment, such as family problems, problems in affective relationships, and leisure activities yielded significant association with the presence of thoughts of ending one's life. Others, like work problems (minor/no problems vs. major problems) and legal problems (absence vs. presence), did not turn out to be correlated with suicidal ideation. Regarding the concurrent use of other substances, no statistically significant association with alcohol, stimulants, hallucinogens, or cannabinoids was found, whereas a significant association was found between the presence of thoughts of death and the use of central nervous system depressants and, especially, with the presence of polydrug use.

Regarding substance non-medical use history, suicidal ideation did not correlate with patterns of heroin use (presence of periodic self-detoxification vs. uninterrupted use), frequency of intake (daily vs. sporadic), age of first substance use (under 17 years vs. 17 or more years), or age at first treatment. On the other hand, the association between length of addiction and thoughts of ending one's life turned out to be statistically significant.

At multivariate analysis level, the odds of having thoughts of ending one's life were higher for subjects receiving welfare benefits (OR 1.69), those affected with bipolar spectrum disorder (OR 1.42), for the unemployed (OR 1.37), those with early HUD onset (OR 1.36), those living alone (OR 1.33), those with problems in organizing social contacts and free time (OR 1.28).

The high rate of comorbid depression/bipolar spectrum disorders as well as the strong relationship between these and current suicidal ideation in our heroin addicts has important clinical implications. Suicidal ideation, suicide attempt, and completed suicide are three different, but overlapping categories: suicidal ideation strongly predicts both attempted and completed suicide, and suicide attempt is the most powerful predictor for future suicide, particularly in the presence of mood disorders [292, 294, 296, 299, 301, 302, 304, 305]. On the other hand, however, the vast majority of suicide attempters come from a population of persons who have permanent suicidal thoughts, while suicide attempt without any previous suicidal ideation is extremely rare [299]. Major mood disorders and SUDs are the two most common axis I diagnoses among suicide victims and attempters, and the frequently observed comorbidity between mood and substance-use disorders further increases the risk (and lethality) of suicidal behaviour [295–299, 306]. Since major mood disorders and substance-use disorders are independent and interactive risk factors for suicidal ideation and suicide attempts in persons with unipolar depression [307] and with bipolar disorder [288], our study further indicates that patients with heroin addiction are at a particularly high risk of suicide. Early detection and rigorous treatment of comorbid and/or underlying mood (particularly bipolar spectrum) disorders seems to be an important part of suicide prevention in this population.

2.1.7   Heroin Addiction and Its Consequences on Mood

Opioids usually produce mood disorders during intoxication, while chronic opioid use induces a fall in CNS noradrenergic firing. Unlike other used substances, opioids are very unlikely to cause psychotic symptoms. Substance use during manic episodes may depend on loss of inhibition, impulsiveness, impairment of judgement, or lack of caution. Patients with mixed episodes are twice as likely to use substances than normal subjects.

The switching phase can be intensely unpleasant and lead to substance use as a form of self-medication. Taking the opposite view, some authors judge that mood liability develops because of CNS neuroadaptation to chronic exposure to heroin. The leading hypothesis is that heroin-induced depression stems from functional alterations in the endorphinergic, noradrenergic, and hypophysis-adrenal gland system. Adaptation to the protracted use of heroin may continue for several months after detoxification and come to underlie what is clinically described as hypophoria [220]. Since 1942, detoxified HUD patients have been described as showing a 'protracted withdrawal syndrome', or a 'post-withdrawal syndrome', which features chronic residual and often invalidating withdrawal symptoms [80, 308–310]. The clinical picture is dominated by an organic mood syndrome, which is sensitive to methadone and represents the crucial risk factor for relapse into heroin use.

Dysphoria, in fact, is usually associated with an increase in craving and substance-seeking behaviours. Relapse into heroin use followed by a soothing of dysphoria works to refuel the vicious circle of addiction, even when other features of early or protracted withdrawal are absent. Mood disorders also develop during opioid detoxification. Depression seems to occur more frequently among addicts who have gone through methadone tapering (60%) than among those entering methadone treatment after heroin discontinuation (25%) [153]. This can easily be explained by considering that addicts with mood disorders tend to join methadone treatment programmes, as this is the only treatment that has proved effective in restoring the heroin-related opioid imbalance and controlling the associated psychopathology. So, it is quite likely that mood alterations, which led subjects to undergo methadone treatments, will re-emerge after therapeutic stabilization has been achieved.

2.1.7.1 Exploring the Depressive Syndrome of DD/BIP1-HUD Patients (Dual Depression)

In the previous 10 years, some studies by our research group tried to describe the psychopathology specific to SUD [311] by clearing up the issue of how this information could be utilized for treatment choice [43] or monitoring outcome [41].

We identified five main domains: (1) the 'Worthlessness/Being trapped (W/BT)' dimension that assembles depressive, obsessive-compulsive, and psychotic symptoms; (2) 'Somatic Symptoms (SS)', which is characterized by several somatic and anxious features, and resembles opioid withdrawal; (3) 'Sensitivity/Psychoticism (S/P)', which features psychoticism and sensitivity; (4) 'Panic Anxiety (PA)', which can be described as a fear of travelling by train or bus (agoraphobia), going around alone, sensations of dizziness or fear of feeling sick, and the experience of critical anxiety; (5) 'Violence/Suicidality (V/S)', comprising aggressiveness against others and/or self-directed aggressiveness with anger, rage, and breaking things up [40].

As mentioned above, the SCL90 factor W/BT brings together depressive, obsessive-compulsive, and psychotic symptoms. Treatment-seeking addicts who display depressed mood usually report feelings of uselessness and the feeling of being trapped in a corner. These patients feel abandoned, sad, with no goal or interest; they are excessively preoccupied with difficulties, and report feelings of guilt, while experiencing a low sexual drive, too. Obsessive-compulsive symptoms include difficulties in making decisions, completing a task, and concentrating, along with worries about one's ineptitude, an 'empty mind' sensation, and an incapacity to dominate one's thoughts. Other symptoms, such as the need to check out actions several times or act slowly to avoid making mistakes, are not featured. Compulsions and memory impairment do not appear in any factor. Thought disorders consist of feeling alone even when with other people, the thought that one's mind is not working properly, while never feeling close to others. Lastly, these subjects report a feeling of inferiority, are easily hurt (interpersonal sensitivity), do not like being alone (phobic anxiety), and often feel nervous and upset ('free' anxiety). On the whole, this factor is essentially made up of depressive, obsessive, and psychotic features, dominated by feelings of uselessness and of being trapped in a corner (Table 2.6) [40].

The W/BT syndrome does not seem to be influenced by the continued use of heroin versus detoxification treatment or by the lifetime presence of psychiatric

Table 2.6 Symptomatologic characteristics of dual depression

	Load	Type
79. Feelings of worthlessness	0.69	DEP
22. Feelings of being trapped or caught	0.68	DEP
29. Feeling lonely	0.66	DEP
30. Feeling blue	0.66	DEP
54. Feeling hopeless about the future	0.64	DEP
32. Feeling no interest in things	0.63	DEP
77. Feeling lonely even when you are with people	0.60	PSY
41. Feeling inferior to others	0.57	INT
46. Difficulty in making decisions	0.54	OC
28. Feeling blocked in getting things done	0.53	OC
89. Feelings of guilt	0.53	
55. Trouble in concentrating	0.52	OC
71. Feeling everything is an effort	0.52	DEP
90. The idea that something is wrong with your mind	0.52	PSY
88. Never feeling close to another person	0.50	PSY
10. Worried about sloppiness or carelessness	0.48	OC
31. Worrying too much about things	0.47	DEP
34. Your feelings being easily hurt	0.45	ANX
05. Loss of sexual interest or pleasure	0.44	DEP
51. Your mind going blank	0.44	OC
26. Blaming yourself for things	0.43	DEP
57. Feeling tense or keyed up	0.43	ANX
03. Unwanted thoughts, words, or ideas that won't go away	0.41	OC
75. Feeling nervous when you are left alone	0.40	PHOB
Eingenvalue	26.8	
Variance	29.9	

DEP depressive symptomatology, *PSY* psychoticism, *INT* interpersonal sensitivity, *OC* obsessive-compulsive symptomatology, *ANX* anxiety, *Phob* phobic anxiety problems—not even by the kind of substance used [37–39, 312]. It is, however, influenced by age (being more marked in older opioid addicts), the setting of the treatment, and the flow of time [313, 314]. Its presence in opioid addiction can be better understood by considering the close link between mood disorders and addiction, in terms of neurobiological background, psychological and psychopathological risk factors, and the epidemiology of the two conditions [79, 315–329]. The involvement of some brain systems, such as the reward, motivational, stress, and inhibitory control systems in the physiopathology of addiction, may justify the presence of symptoms such as worthlessness, feeling lonely, blue, and hopeless about the future. We know that an amotivational status is consistent with the chronic changes observed in the mesolimbic dopaminergic system, including a steep fall in the dopaminergic tone and the activation of the CREB/dynorphine pathway [213, 316, 330–336], as well as in the neuroendocrine stress system, which is implicated both in affective regulation and addictive behaviour [337–341]. Our failure to find any association of this dimension with depression or bipolar spectrum disorders [342], together with the lack of any significant correlation with some aspects of craving-related behaviour [343], is consistent with the presence of an inhibitory component in the reward deficiency syndrome [316]. The positive association of this dimension with access to AOT rather than to therapeutic community (TC) treatment calls into question the severity of addiction-related disruption to various areas of life (e.g., the family, work, legal matters), with inevitable consequences on psychological well-being and the urgent need for recuperation, most easily obtained by AOT. Moreover, consistent with a manageable condition, this dimension seems to be influenced by the flow of time after detoxification, which, again, may link this dimension with the condition of active substance use [344].

In one of our studies, we compared 972 HUD patients with 504 major depression (MD) patients based on our five SCL-90 dimensions, with the purpose of estimating the magnitude of the differences, in terms of psychopathological symptoms. We observed that prominent psychopathological domains were more frequent in HUD patients, in particular, W/BT, SS, and S/P. The V/S dimension was more frequent in MD patients, while the PA dimension fails to differentiate between the two groups. The prominent psychopathological groups were the most important factor in significantly differentiating between the two groups, when drawing comparisons based on age, male gender, and the severity of psychopathological symptoms. Our results suggested that the five psychopathological dimensions found seemed to confirm the trait, instead of the state, nature of our proposed psychopathology of heroin addiction. In any case, the psychopathological symptoms of HUD and MD patients seem to differ quantitatively and qualitatively [42].

In another study we clustered the W/BT symptoms characterizing depressed HUD patients (W/BT-HUD) when compared with non-depressed ones and with NDD depressed ones (NDD-MD) [345].

Compared with non-depressed HUD patients, W/BT-HUD ones were distinguished by the presence of the following depressive syndrome. They were females, feeling blue, worried about sloppiness or carelessness, feeling lonely, feeling everything is an effort, and never feeling close to another person. Conversely, non-depressed HUD patients were characterized by worrying too much about things. Compared with NDD-MD patients, W/BT-HUD ones were distinguished by the presence of the following depressive symptomatology. They were worried about sloppiness or carelessness, with their feelings being easily hurt, feeling lonely even when they are with people, with feelings of guilt, with their mind going blank, having difficulty in concentrating, unwanted thoughts, words, or ideas that won't go away. Lastly, these people have the problem of feeling blocked in getting things done. By contrast, NDD-MD patients were marked out by the following stereotype. They spent much of their time feeling lonely, up against feelings of worthlessness, feeling tense or keyed up, having to worry too much about things, with loss of sexual interest or pleasure, blaming themselves for things, and upset by feeling being trapped or caught.

In Fig. 2.5 are reported several depressive symptoms belonging both to the NDD/MD syndrome and to the W/BT-HUD syndrome. The W/BT psychopathological dimension also includes the item 'feelings of guilt' which is not normally included in any of the standard dimensions in the SCL90 questionnaire, considering standard factor analysis. The symptom 'feelings of guilt' does not correlate with the depressive symptoms listed in the W/BT dimension. This item appears to be a specific symptom included in the depressive syndrome of W/BT-HUD patients rather than a depressive MD symptom. MD and W/BT-HUD patients share as many as 10 items, considering the whole dimension of symptoms: 'feelings of worthlessness', 'feeling of being trapped or caught', 'feeling lonely', 'feeling blue', 'feeling hopeless about the future', 'feeling no interest in things', 'feeling everything is an effort', 'worrying too much about things', 'loss of sexual interest or pleasure', and 'blaming yourself for things'. On the other hand, three depressive symptoms listed in SCL90 are specific to the depressive MD syndrome and fail to show any correlation with the W/BT-HUD

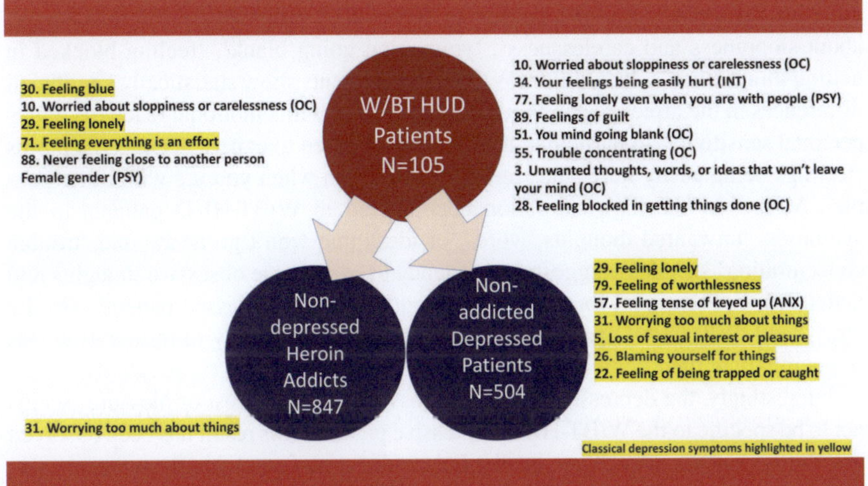

Fig. 2.5 Differences among W/BT-HUD, non-depressed/HUD, and NDD-MD patients

syndrome: 'feeling low in energy or slowed down', 'thoughts of ending your life', 'crying easily'. Finding none of these three symptoms during the clinical evaluation of HUD patients should not rule out a diagnosis of depressive syndrome in HUD subjects.

'Worrying too much about things' is a depressive symptom, but its presence is more frequent in non-depressed HUD patients. On the other hand, W/BT-HUD patients show psychopathological symptoms that are not only related to a merely depressive clinical picture, but also linked to various affective dimensions, such as emotional reactivity/interpersonal sensitivity ('never feeling close to another person') and affective resonance with the consequences of their clinical condition ('worried about sloppiness and carelessness'), suggesting that these two subdimensions may be important features of the depressive syndrome in W/BT-HUD patients. What is more, in these patients the presence of a cognitive dimension related to the affective resonance features is also confirmed by the high saturation found in the symptoms 'feeling blue' and 'feeling lonely'.

Unsurprisingly, W/BT-HUD patients shared their depressive syndrome with NDD/MD ones, but, according to our results, some symptoms turned out to be more frequent and more severe in W/BT-HUD patients, and some others in MD ones. In particular, 'feelings being easily hurt', 'feeling lonely even when you are with other people', 'feelings of guilt', 'the mind going blank', 'trouble concentrating', 'unwanted thoughts', 'words, or ideas that won't leave your mind', 'feeling blocked in getting things done' identified W/BT-HUD patients. Conversely, 'feeling lonely', 'feelings of worthlessness', 'feeling tense or keyed up', 'worrying too much about things', 'loss of sexual interest or pleasure', 'blaming yourself for things', 'feelings of being trapped or caught' were more representative of MD patients.

Based on our results, there are other clinical considerations that now need to be discussed. Compared with MD patients, W/BT-HUD patients show statistically significant differences in the psychopathological items related to the cognitive subdimension of depressive pictures. W/BT-HUD subjects tend to show a high degree of affective resonance with the consequences of their clinical condition ('worried about sloppiness and carelessness', 'your mind going blank', 'feeling blocked in getting things done'). In addition, W/BT-HUD patients show statistically significant differences in the affective subdimension associated with emotional reactivity/interpersonal sensitivity; in particular, they tend more often to experience the symptoms 'feelings being easily hurt' and 'feeling lonely even when you are with other people'. Moreover, the high saturation encountered in W/BT-HUD patients in the symptoms 'unwanted thoughts, words, or ideas that won't go away' and 'trouble concentrating' seems to suggest the tendency to experience obsessive thoughts and deficiency in attentional focus more frequently than in depressed patients. On the other hand, W/BT-HUD patients tend to experience deficiency in infuturation less frequently than their depressed peers.

Interestingly, the depressive symptom 'loss of sexual interest or pleasure' seems not to be specific to the W/BT-HUD depressive picture. This result has been observed in previous studies. More specifically, Baharudin et al. found that there was no significant correlation between depression and erectile dysfunction among men in MMTP suggesting that the causal relationship between depression and erectile dysfunction is probably bidirectional [346]. It has also been assumed that depression may be a consequence of erectile dysfunction or that, vice versa, depression may cause erectile dysfunction [347, 348]. Past studies showing data on depression and erectile dysfunction are inconsistent. Spring et al. found that patients in MMT with a lower Derogatis Sexual Functioning Inventory score had a higher level of depression on the Hamilton Rating Scale. They concluded that the sexual dysfunction recorded may have been due to psychiatric problems rather than to treatment with opioids [349]. Our findings are consistent with those earlier findings, besides suggesting that sexual problems are more specific to MD patients than to W/BT-HUD ones.

With reference to the severity of depressive psychopathology, the results of our study reveal some coherence with the data regarding the frequency of the symptoms found. W/BT-HUD patients show not only that they experience symptoms related to the cognitive subdimension of depression more often than the MD patients and the HUD ones, but also that they tend to display those symptoms in a more severe way ('worried about sloppiness and carelessness'). In other words, 'worrying about sloppiness or carelessness' (both in its frequency and severity) was the most important symptom in differentiating W/BT-HUD patients from their non-depressed peers, but also from depressed patients without a history of substance use. The symptom 'worrying about sloppiness or carelessness' tends to be most specific to a clinical variant of depression that seems to affect heroin addicts.

It is worth adding that, when W/BT-HUD patients are compared with NDD/MD ones, our study has shown that some depressive symptoms tend both to be more frequent and more severe. W/BT-HUD patients show not only more frequent, but also more severe symptoms related to the emotional reactivity/interpersonal sensitivity subdimension of depression ('feelings being easily hurt', 'feeling lonely even when you are with other people').

Lastly, the symptom 'difficulty in making decisions' seems to belong to a 'deficiency in decision-making' subdimension that W/BT-HUD patients appear to experience in a more severe way than MD and HUD non-depressed ones.

To sum up, our findings show that W/BT-HUD patients feel less trapped, more emotionally responsive, more cognitively impaired, and less sexually disinterested than depressed, drug-free patients. Moreover, the clinical impact of the two depressive subdimensions 'emotional reactivity/interpersonal sensitivity' and 'cognitive/ affective resonance' tend to be more severe in W/BT-HUD patients than in depressed, drug-free ones. The depressive syndrome of W/BT-HUD patients can differentiate W/BT-HUD patients from drug-free depressed ones, so confirming its specificity to HUD. These findings seem to be consistent with the concept that W/BT-HUD patients experience a clinically different variant of MD (dual depression).

2.1.7.2 Dual Depression and Its Relationship with the Reward Deficiency Syndrome and the Post-Withdrawal Syndrome

Looking more deeply now into the depressive psychopathology that is most likely to be found and is most severe in W/BT-HUD patients, we may assume that, from a clinical viewpoint, some clinical features appear to overlap with the symptoms of the 'Reward Deficiency Syndrome'.

The Reward Deficiency Syndrome (RDS) is a brain disorder distinguished by a clinically significant deficiency of dopamine (DA) in the brain's reward circuit—more specifically, the midbrain and prefrontal cortex. It is primarily acquired genetically, but may otherwise result from prolonged stress [350], and is caused by a decreased DA sensitivity in the areas of the brain that are involved in the mediation of encoding for attention, reward expectancy, disconfirmation of reward expectancy, and incentive motivation [351]. It has been suggested that individuals with a hypodopaminergic state are at risk of seeking reward from RDS behaviours to satisfy their lack of natural rewards [352].

Core symptoms of the RDS are the loss of emotional reactivity, drives, and aims, and the inability to experience or anticipate any pleasure [316]. In other words, what is clinically relevant in people with RDS is a sort of hedonic dysregulation—or anhedonia. Anhedonia is a condition that leads to the loss of the ability to experience pleasure in response to natural reinforcers like food, sex, and exercise, and social activities [351]. It has been shown that anhedonia, when accompanied by hyporesponsive reward circuits [353], is an important characteristic of many neuropsychiatric syndromes, such as SUDs [354].

On the other hand, the clinical features shown by W/BT-HUD patients appear to resemble the Post-Withdrawal Syndrome (PWS) described by Martin as an enduring pathological state in abstinent detoxified opiate addicts [220, 355, 356], and clinically described, more recently, as a late-onset condition in HUD distinguished by protracted abstinence from heroin use. PWS features some psychopathological symptoms such as feelings of hypophoria (lack of drive, motivation, and reactivity with respect to what that individual regards as being satisfactory), dysphoria, extreme sensitivity to pain, inability to complete even simple tasks, and inability to experience pleasure through recreational or natural stimuli (i.e. precisely what is meant by the term 'anhedonia') [220, 357].

Hypophoria and anhedonia are two distinctive clinical features of the PWS. Within the framework of the 'three-stage model' of toxicomanic history, it has been demonstrated that the hedonistic-euphoric dimension, which was prominent at the beginning, tends to be gradually replaced by a counterpolar state, which is, precisely, distinguished by anhedonia and hypophoria. From a withdrawal-related point of view, through each detoxification cycle the patient passes from the acute withdrawal state (counterpolar to intoxication) to a later and more enduring drug-free state featuring symptoms of hypophoria, which looms as an acquired state of discomfort related to the absence of drug-related stimulation [358–360].

In other words, at the end of the natural history of addiction, most drug addicts experience a condition of predominantly depressive affective valency, characterized by hypophoria, otherwise known as 'secondary or late withdrawal syndrome' or PWS (alternatively, 'hypophoric syndrome'). This situation persists for a long time and is attributable to a reward deficit which remains at super-criminal levels over time. Moreover, this syndrome closely resembles the subthreshold symptoms of dysthymia and the residual symptoms of chronic bipolar disorder [361] and also recalls the symptoms of the RDS described as a sequela of alcohol and stimulant chronic use [359, 362, 363], considering that a 'late-onset depressive psychopathological model' may be valuable not only for HUD but also for the natural history of SUD in general, regardless of the related drugs.

2.1.7.3 Addiction Anhedonia: Towards a Depressive Syndrome Specific to Substance Use Disorder Patients (Dual Depression)

There is an entire diagnostic category in the DSM that is dedicated to substance-induced mental disorders [171]. According to this model, the finding of a depressive syndrome in drug addict patients would not only be independent of the presence or absence of a coexisting drug addiction picture; it would be present with clinical characteristics indistinguishable from those of major depression. According to what has been mentioned supra it is clear that this is not actually correct. W/BT-HUD patients, for example, do not seem to share some of the core symptoms expressed by depressed non-drug addicts, such as loss of libido and coarctation of infuturation. In addition, this variant of the depressive syndrome often manifests itself over time, not infrequently following the suspension of the use of opiates (whether illicit or as a medication) [220, 355].

This form of depressive syndrome is distinguished by a variety of neurobiological, clinical, and prognostic features unlike those of major depression. W/BT-HUD patients experiencing a prominent depressive syndrome feel less trapped, more emotionally responsive, more cognitively impaired, and less sexually disinterested than depressed, drug-free patients. These symptoms are more severe and more frequent in W/BT-HUD patients than in depressed, drug-free ones. What is more, the anhedonia they experience seems to differ in its features from that experienced by depressed, drug-free patients. In fact, it develops in parallel with the whole unfolding of the addiction disease [358, 359] and seems to display greater severity too, judging by the greater number of treatment failures than those the same patients had previously experienced [153]. Possible confirmation of greater severity comes from the fact that it does not always recede in response to treatment with antidepressant drugs, though on this topic the available data are ambiguous and largely depend on the category of antidepressant class prescribed—with imipramine showing the most satisfactory success rate [228, 364, 365]. These findings reinforce the idea that the depressive syndrome present in addicts—anhedonia, in particular—would be more the consequence of the addiction process on mood than an episodic symptom linked to an affective phase. We may propose the idea that this variant of 'anhedonia' related to the depressive syndrome of W/BT-HUD patients is an 'addictive anhedonia'. That would be consistent with the D2 down-regulation model used by Gold et al. to describe the RDS symptoms [351] and with the evidence that D2R availability in the putamen is inversely correlated with years of opiate use [366].

It is also known that specific neurobiological long-term modifications in the reward and motivational system occur in patients with SUD. Among them, the finding of the activation of the transcription factor CREB is of remarkable interest due to the consequently intensified expression of dynorphine, which is a high-efficacy k-opioid receptor endogenous agonist. In recent years, it has been demonstrated that the activation of k-opioid receptor mediates anxiety- or depressant-like, anhedonic or dysphoric effects after either stress or chronic drug exposure [330, 367, 368].

What is more, the neuroendocrine stress system is likewise involved in the regulation of mood in SUD patients [341, 369].

The importance of recognizing this clinical condition in HUD patients lies in the fact that it is considered a good indicator of relapse, that it is sensitive to opiate agonists, and that it is aggravated by administering opiate antagonists [137, 370–372]. Moreover, this depressive syndrome shows a weaker prognosis than the depressive syndrome of non-drug users [364].

To sum up, the depressive syndrome of W/BT-HUD patients seems to be a specific variant of the depressive syndrome that occurs because of the addiction process. As a result, it can neither be attributed to the presence of a dual disorder, nor assessed as an independent depressive-anxious picture.

2.1.7.4 Therapeutic Implications

As mentioned earlier, opioids have been demonstrated to have properties typical of antidepressant medications, so suggesting that opioid use may start as a form of self-medication for depressive symptoms, according to Khantzian's theory [143, 373, 374]. This fact supports the endorphinergic hypothesis for dysthymic disorders. According to the PISA-V.P. Dole Research Group, over-standard long-acting opioid dosages (i.e. methadone up to 120 mg/day) are useful in treating most of the cases of depression in HUD patients.

The use of antidepressant medications should be resorted to only as a partial clinical response to depressive symptomatology in patients receiving a MMTP. In these patients the risk of relapse is high [149, 375].

Tricyclic antidepressants (TCA) (i.e. imipramine and clomipramine), which are dopaminergic agents (i.e. bupropion), which, like trazodone, are helpful medical resources during methadone tapering, at the end of a successful programme, or, in the first 6 months following the successful accomplishment of a programme. In the latter situation, those medications play a therapeutic role as anti-hypophoric agents, limiting mild withdrawal symptoms (including protracted withdrawal states, or enduring insomnia) in drug-free subjects in MMT. Clinical trials on the effectiveness of tricyclic antidepressants have given ambiguous results. Despite this, according to the PISA-V.P. Dole Research Group, TCA medication dosage of around 150 mg/day may be useful in treating those clinical conditions.

As regards serotonergic system reuptake inhibitors (SSRIs), their effectiveness and safety have been documented by the PISA-V.P. Dole Research Group on subjects displaying recurrent depression by maintaining on average methadone dose of 100 mg/day. SSRI bioavailability rises in methadone-maintained patients. Both fluoxetine and fluvoxamine may increase methadone blood levels significantly (by up to 200%, in the case of fluvoxamine). Therefore, methadone doses should be used carefully, especially when SSRIs are added in the induction phase [376, 377]. Stimulating properties of MAOIs ((monoamine oxidase inhibitors), which have been documented even in depressed non-SUD patients, make them unfit for use with HUD patients, because of their proneness to misuse.

Interestingly, in one of our recent clinical studies it has been shown that high-dosage trazodone (300 mg/die) might find a clinical use in the post-detoxification phase. We found that trazodone is probably able to improve depressive-anxious symptomatology (and cocaine craving) in cocaine use disorder patients who had previously voluntarily stopped cocaine use. Before being treated, these patients showed hypophoric symptoms and were at high risk of early relapse, but 6-month treatment with trazodone showed its capacity to avoid early relapse into cocaine use in these patients [365].

2.1.8 Possible Trajectories of Addictions: The Role of Bipolar Spectrum

Drug addiction is a chronic disease affected by a combination of genetic, environmental, and drug-induced factors [378, 379]. Researchers involved in addiction medicine have been used to facing single-drug use disorders (e.g. 'mere' heroin or cocaine addiction), even though, in a longitudinal perspective, patterns of substance use that include 'drug switching' and mixed addictions are commonplace [380, 381]. Current real-world practice induces us to deal with polydrug use disorders and trajectories of addictions that show considerable heterogeneity [381–384].

Focusing on genetics, cocaine, and heroin addictions, for instance, often implies studying a situation made heterogeneous by differences in chemical classes, primary targets, routes of administration, metabolic pathways, and psychopharmacological effects, but the varied situations under review may share some biological mechanisms [385, 386]. There may be distinct genetic risk factors that apply to heroin and/or cocaine addiction, but the presence both of shared and distinct genetic liability for precisely these two addictions has been suggested [387, 388].

Shifting to a clinical perspective, trajectories of drug use progression and outcome vary, depending on the primary drug of non-medical use. Our current and previous studies pointed out a cluster of AUD patients characterized by a former history of HUD (FHUD) who, if not adequately treated for their HUD, tend to transit into a severe form of AUD [76].

In previous studies we indicated a specific relationship between bipolar disorder and HUD or AUD [70, 71] even at the level of temperaments [77, 78]. In the case of our HUD patients, we suggested the need for a more complex model linking cocaine and bipolarity. Subthreshold bipolarity, including irritable and cyclothymic temperaments, seems to activate a predisposition to heroin addiction, but craving for the suppressed hypomania, could, in its turn, lead to cocaine non-medical use, which eventually unmasks a frank bipolar disorder—in some cases leading to mixed state, severe mania, as well as psychosis beyond mania. Returning now to our AUD patients, we hypothesized that cocaine use was an attempt to maintain a baseline level of mood elation like a hyperthymic temperament or hypomanic state. Alcohol use, especially in youngsters, may be an instrument to cope with chronic dysphoria corresponding to an affective temperament. The attempt to induce and maintain hypomania by cocaine use would, on this hypothesis, lead to full-blown bipolar disorders. In this context, alcohol use may favour involvement in cocaine use by cyclothymics owing to its sedative effect but would eventually become a further pro-dysphoric factor.

This topic required us to further examine those who were FHUD-AUD, by additionally focusing on concomitant cocaine use disorders (CUD). We compared prevalence, and clinical characteristics (diagnosis, addiction, and treatment history), between FHUD-AUD patients—those with and those without CUD.

In one [74] of our studies, we designed a comparative cohort study to compare the demographic, diagnostic, and clinical characteristics, together with the addiction and treatment history, of consecutively ascertained FHUD-AUD patients with and without comorbid CUD. Since 2004, the Centre for the Assessment and Treatment of Alcohol-Related Pathology, La Sapienza University, at the Umberto I University Hospital in Rome, has been using a clinical protocol that comprises a detoxification unit, which may be followed by a long-term outpatient psychopharmacological approach to prevent relapses. We considered all consecutive AUD patients, according to DSM-IV TR criteria, who had been referred for treatment to the outpatient clinic, during the years 2004–2007. Previous studies had been performed with this sample [71, 76, 389]. All patients were evaluated after the resolution of acute withdrawal to avoid, in the diagnostic process, possible interferences arising from the acute phase of their illness.

The sample consisted of 60 FHUD-AUD out of 448 consecutive AUD patients. Sample mean age was 26 ± 5 (range 16–37 years). The majority were male ($N = 50$, 83.3%), single ($N = 37$, 64.9%), with educational level < 8 years ($N = 31$, 651.7%), employed ($N = 31$, 51.7%) living with their families ($N = 39$, 65.0%). For clinical and history details see [76].

In all, 45 (out of a total of 60 FHUD-AUD patients taking part in the study) were found to combine the FHUD feature with concomitant CUD. Of these, 37 (82.2%) were male. Mean age was 43 ± 6 years. A total of 15 former heroin use-alcohol use disorder patients had never used cocaine (i.e. were FHUD-AUD only). Of these, 13 (86.7%) were male. Mean age was 43 ± 5 years. Thus, the prevalence of FHUD-AUD with concomitant CUD in these patients was 45/60 (75%), when reviewed cumulatively in 2007.

Distinguishing FHUD-AUD patients between those with and those without CUD, no differences emerged as to age, gender, civil status, unemployment rates, level of education, or living situation. Problematic social adjustment and physical complications did not allow differentiation between the two groups. Patients with FHUD-AUD concomitant with CUD showed a more severe concomitant BDZ and cannabinoid use disorder. No differences emerged regarding any concomitant hallucinogen use disorder. No differences emerged either for presence of a psychiatric diagnosis ($p = 0.262$), while FHUD-AUD with CUD show a greater presence of the bipolar spectrum. As to AUD history, no differences were found between the two groups regarding age at first use of alcohol, duration of drinking habit, age at AUD onset, or duration in years of alcoholism. FHUD-AUD/CUD patients reached a higher maximum level of daily alcohol consumption ($p = 0.040$), while no differences were found between the two groups in the daily amount of alcohol intake at the onset of their dependence history ($p = 0.109$). The two groups of patients did not show statistically significant differences in the items: age at onset of HUD, dependence length, or prevalence of 'stage 3' HUD. The development of addiction may be considered to consist of three stages: (1) acute (immediate) drug effects (honeymoon stage); (2) transition from recreational use to patterns of use consistent with addiction (increasing dose stage); and (3) end-stage addiction, which is distinguished by an overwhelming desire to obtain the drug, a diminished ability to control drug-seeking, and reduced pleasure from biological rewards (revolving door stage) [213].

No differences were observed either regarding past AOT (with methadone) or numbers of years spent in treatment. Neither the prevalence of blocking dosages achieved, nor methadone maximum dosage permitted differentiation between the two groups. According to Dole and Nyswander theory, the methadone blocking dosage is the dosage that blocks, in a patient, the action of heroin in his/her brain and so makes it possible to live as a normal citizen in the community. This dosage is generally above 60 mg/day; in our experience it is, more specifically, at least 80 mg/day in the case of methadone or 16 mg/day in the case of buprenorphine [66, 88, 390]. We consider that standard treatment has been performed when the Dole and Nyswander methodology is followed.

Regarding the most important predictors of FHUD-AUD with CUD patients, concomitant cannabinoid use disorder and the presence of bipolar spectrum are correlated with formerly having had a heroin-alcohol use disorder and now running concomitantly with cocaine use disorder.

In this study, the presence of a bipolar disorder, considered in its full-blown clinical expression, cannot differentiate between our poly-addicted subjects—i.e. by distinguishing between those with and those without CUD. The intriguing consideration that emerges from these data is that only subjects affected by bipolar spectrum transit to comorbid CUD. Bipolar spectrum and addiction often co-occur and constitute reciprocal risk factors. In particular, patients whose disorders fall under the bipolar spectrum—and its hyperthymic and cyclothymic temperamental substrates—are at increased risk for substance use, possibly moving towards full-blown addiction through exposure to intrinsically dependence-producing substances [49, 70, 79, 360, 391]. For that reason, bipolar spectrum and SUD are best considered under a unitary perspective.

Our previous study [76] highlighted a specific cluster of former heroin-alcohol use disorder patients, who were not AUD during heroin use, but who seem to have been inadequately treated for their HUD following a non-standard procedure, and have subsequently developed a more severe form of AUD. In this case the trajectory from HUD to AUD seems to be due to an unbalanced opioid endogenous system that spontaneously or iatrogenically (due to a non-standard AOT) trends towards substituting opioid use with cross-tolerant drugs (e.g., alcohol or BDZ) [392]. The next step towards cocaine use disorder suggests that this cluster of patients appears to be more complicated and less immediately open to understanding. Current findings suggest that only patients with bipolar spectrum disorder show concomitant CUD. In line with this, following our proposed pathophysiological model, the

Fig. 2.6 Addiction possible trajectories. The bipolar spectrum role

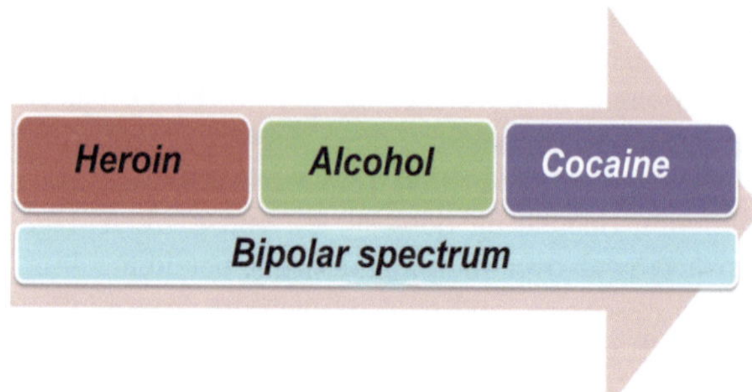

presence of subthreshold bipolarity could initially have created a predisposition to heroin addiction, but it could then have led to cocaine non-medical use due to the onset of craving for the suppressed hypomania [70, 391].

Contrary to our previous finding in which non-standard AOT methodology or the preference for drug-free regimens are examples of interventions that may directly favour, or fail to counter, a switching evolution of HUD towards alcoholism [392], variables related to AOT are unable to differentiate between the two types of FHUD-AUD patients—those with and those without concomitant CUD. These results forced us to look at addiction from a different perspective. Current 'official' nosology (e.g., DSM) is largely limited to physical manifestations of addiction that can be objectively observed and are well suited to maintaining an 'atheoretical' perspective, by considering the psychiatric symptoms of addiction as being mere 'comorbidities' [36]. Beyond DD, several papers contributed by the PISA-V.P. Dole Research Group have pointed out that addiction may show a specific and proper psychopathology [38–40, 393] underlying the complexity that surrounds a brain disease, addiction, that clinicians tend to fail to perceive in its entirety. This brings fascination to the suggestion that bipolarity could be strictly related to trajectories moving between mixed addictions. As shown in Fig. 2.6, the proposed model of progression gets entangled with subthreshold bipolarity and SUDs in an almost inextricable way.

Clinicians should pay more attention to mood disorder in subjects affected by SUD. Other than the full-blown expressions of psychiatric illness that are frequently related to SUD, the recognition and treatment of bipolar spectrum could be useful in preventing the transition through addictions.

2.2   Treatment of Mood Disorders in DD/BIP1-HUD Patients

The reduction of opioid use may itself induce the onset of psychiatric disorders (mania, depression, psychosis) that put the subject at risk of a relapse into heroin use. When mood disorders are unrelated to substance non-medical use, psychiatrists should be careful about using agents associated with non-medical use liability and consider possible interactions with other psychotropics (e.g. BDZs). MAOIs should be avoided, so as to prevent interactions with cocaine, heroin, or other psychotropic drugs [394–396]. Rapidly acting BDZs (diazepam, alprazolam) should be avoided, as they have a high addictive potential. Slowly acting BDZs (oxazepam, clorazepate), which ensure a lower non-medical use liability, are safer to use, at least in selected patients and under medical supervision. Any other psychotropic should be evaluated by urinalysis. In methadone-maintained patients who are dependent on heroin and BDZ, clonazepam, a long-lasting, potent, and slow-acting BDZ, which is therefore free of addictive properties, can be resorted to as a replacement for other compounds [75, 397–401].

One frequent complication of opioid addiction is dependence on alcohol, cocaine, or other substances. Of methadone-maintained patients, 60% were using cocaine when they entered treatment. Cocaine non-medical use is found in as many as 40% of HUD patients, alcohol non-medical use is problematic in 15–30% of cases, and BDZ non-medical use is quite common [402–405]. No comparable data on NTX-maintained patients are available. Even so, it does seem that polydrug use is common among patients who enter NTX treatment without fitting it, but who refuse or are denied better-fitting options due to environmental pressure or cultural bias [406].

Special care is required when treating addicts suffering from additional psychiatric disorders, as intervention on heroin addiction alone, even when successful, cannot be expected to resolve the non-medical use of other substances. Such patients require closer monitoring (daily alcohol test, twice-a-week urinalyses), more frequent counselling sessions, direct access to self-help groups (e.g. Alcoholics Anonymous), and specific pharmacotherapy (e.g. disulfiram) [407].

Two studies have shown that high-dose methadone treatment, when combined with frequent medical controls, is likely to favour a decrease in cocaine use. As a rule, patients addicted either to heroin or other substances, CNS depressants in particular, should be stabilized on methadone and gradually detoxified from other substances. Attempts to treat all different kinds of non-medical use at once are bound to fail. The recommendation is that non-medical use issues should be faced one by one [407].

2.2.1 Antidepressants

Despite the frequency of depressive disorders among HUD patients, few reports are available in the literature on the use of tricyclic antidepressants in these patients. When doxepin was administered at doses ranging between 25 and 150 mg once a day in the evening, an improvement in the data on anxiety, depressive features, and anxiety-related insomnia [408] was documented. Amitriptyline partly controls withdrawal symptoms in abstaining volunteers [408]. In a double-blind, placebo-controlled study of doxepin in depressed addicts, a significant improvement was documented along the Zung and Beck Hamilton rating scales. Although a lot of probands dropped out, retained subjects showed a decrease in craving [409]. Later studies performed on methadone-treated subjects failed to show any greater improvement for imipramine-treated subjects (doses ranging between 150 and 225 mg/day) vs. placebo, but a general decrease in depressive symptoms was documented [228]. The conclusion could be drawn that methadone treatment accounts for the improvement of depressive symptoms, no further advantage being provided by imipramine. In cases of severe depression, the parenteral administration of clomipramine (25–50 mg) ensures fast and significant improvement, showing impressive results after just 1 week of treatment [227]. The natural course of depressive symptoms after methadone initiation is marked by a gradual decrease in severity that continues through the first 8 months [121, 137, 149, 410, 411]. Tricyclic agents should therefore be resorted to only when depression shows no significant improvement in response to methadone treatment and when, consequently, the estimated risk of relapse stays high [121, 137, 149, 410, 411]. Caution is also needed in the light of several cases of tricyclic non-medical use that have been documented in the literature [412, 413]. According to the PISA-V. P. Dole Research Group, a dose of 150 mg/day is effective in treating most of the cases of depression in HUD patients. Stimulant tricyclics, bupropion, vortioxetine, and trazodone contramid can be used alongside methadone tapering, at the end of a successful programme, or to favour abstinence in drug-free subjects in the first 6 months after the successful accomplishment of a programme, due to their property of controlling mild withdrawal symptoms (enduring insomnia or protracted withdrawal states) [365].

On the whole, clinical trials on the effectiveness of tricyclic antidepressants have provided ambiguous results. This may be partly attributed to the difficulty of retaining abstaining addicted patients in any unspecific treatment. To sum up, it may be said that trials on doxepin have agreed in showing its efficacy in methadone-maintained patients, at doses ranging between 25 and 100 mg. Otherwise no significant efficacy has been ascertained for either imipramine or desimipramine. However, desimipramine blood levels are higher than expected in methadone-maintained subjects.

As regards serotonergic system reuptake inhibitors (SSRIs), their effectiveness and safety have been documented by the PISA-V.P. Dole Research Group on subjects displaying intermittent depression while maintained at average methadone doses of 100 mg/day. It must be remembered, though, that SSRI bioavailability rises in methadone-maintained patients. In fact, both fluoxetine and fluvoxamine may cause methadone blood levels to increase significantly (by up to 200%, in the case of fluvoxamine) [376]. Sertraline increases methadone blood levels during the first 2 weeks of administration [414]. Methadone doses should therefore be pondered carefully, especially if SSRIs are added on during the induction phase. Interestingly, fluvoxamine has proved useful in improving the bioavailability of methadone over a 24-h period, in high dose-treated patients, who report withdrawal symptoms before each new administration (probably due to a fast metabolism). Patients who show an unsatisfactory response to 100–150 mg/day methadone can definitely benefit from the addition of fluvoxamine [377, 415].

Stimulating properties of MAOIs, which have been documented in depressed non-addicts too, make them unfit for use with HUD patients, due to their non-medical use proneness. Moreover, the likelihood of cheese-effect accidents is supposedly too high in patients such as addicts, who are known to have hardly any control over their consumption of chemicals, food, or alcohol. In prognostic terms, the presence of affective symptoms predicts poorer control over non-medical use conducts, heavier psychosocial impairment, and a greater suicidal risk.

2.2.2 Mood-Stabilizing Drugs

Bipolar syndromes are probably the most frequent psychiatric disorders among HUD patients. As mentioned above, 39 out of 40 consecutive HUD patients entering methadone treatment were diagnosed as suffering from bipolar 1 or bipolar 2 disorder, or displayed hyperthymic temperament, or else had a family history of bipolarity [161]. The use of mood stabilizers is appropriate in patients with bipolar disorders or borderline personality disorder, which are both categories that often involve substance non-medical use. However, neither lithium nor carbamazepine has been clearly shown to be suitable for HUD patients with bipolar disorders [414]. Moreover, it should be recalled that the normalization of basal mood does not ensure control over true addiction, once the revolving door phase has been entered. Mood stabilization may be crucial for the control of substance use in the honeymoon phase, or in subjects who can stay persistently abstinent after the accomplishment of detoxification. Bipolar users have a poorer outcome than non-using peers. Their response to lithium is predictably poor, whereas better results can be expected if anticonvulsants, especially valproate, are used. However, lithium may reasonably be attempted in bipolar cocaine addicts [416–418].

Lithium–methadone interaction have been suggested on an experimental basis, but has not yet been clinically confirmed [419, 420]. Phenytoin, carbamazepine, and phenobarbital strongly decrease the bioavailability of methadone, so causing opioid withdrawal [414]. Valproic acid and the latest anticonvulsants do not seem to have this effect.

2.2.3 Opioidergic Agents

2.2.3.1 Agonists

Antidepressant properties have been reported for opioids, so suggesting that opioid use may develop as a form of self-medication for depressive symptoms, on one hand, and to support the endorphinergic hypothesis of dysthymic disorders, on the other. The administration of opioids to depressed patients has showed some efficacy, though failures have been reported too. In two trials, beta-endorphins were successful in treating depression in a few non-addicted depressed patients (there were two responders in one trial and three—out of six—in another) [374, 421]. The efficacy of beta-endorphins was confirmed vs. placebo, whereas no greater efficacy over placebo was documented for morphine or methadone, on non-addicted depressed patients [422]. In opioid addicts, higher methadone doses (over 100 mg/day) are needed to stabilize patients with prominent features of depression and aggressiveness at programme entrance [50]. In a 2-year follow-up, MMT seemed successful in achieving major mood stabilization in bipolar 1 patients [54]. Though contrasting data do exist [423], some neurobiological observations are consistent with that orientation. Opioid receptors and endorphins are highly concentrated in hypothalamic and limbic areas, as both are involved in the physiology of affective states; and opioid systems have been shown to interact with catecholaminergic systems, which are themselves involved in the pathophysiology of depressive disorders. This is in agreement with Extein's hypothesis that 'a decrease in endorphinergic activity may be the pathophysiological basis of depression' [424].

Table 2.7 shows pharmacological interactions and dosages in HUD patients with mood disorder psychiatric comorbidity as recorded in the experience of our research group.

2.2.3.2 Opioid Antagonists in Mood Disorders

The effects of opioid antagonism on mood are far from having been elucidated; investigations have been carried out both on healthy subjects and psychiatric samples [425].

The antimanic properties of morphine have been used in the past to control agitation. More recently, new-onset mania, psychosis, and irritability have been observed in heroin addicts, following heroin detoxification and NTX maintenance [426, 427]. In particular, a retrospective study has examined the clinical features of mania triggered by opioid withdrawal, in a sample of 45 patients admitted to a psychiatric hospital during a 3-year period. Twenty-eight patients were at their first manic episode and 17 had a previous history of bipolar disorder. Most cases had a long history of opiate dependence [428]. The emergence of mania following opioid withdrawal supports the mood-stabilizing effects of opioid agonists rather than the antimanic properties of an opioid blockade.

It has been hypothesized that NTX might induce dysphoric states by blocking the stress-response and well-being effects associated with opioid peptides. A double-blind, placebo-controlled study has assessed the effect of NTX on 36 non-addicted, healthy individuals, who underwent an 8-week trial with frequent mood assessments. No significant differences on mood scales were noted for either subject group, but one subject was discontinued from the study because of a severe dysphoric reaction. Authors concluded that subpopulations of patients under physiological or psychological stress might react to NTX by displaying dysphoric symptoms [429]. Another double-blind, placebo-controlled study examined the effect of NTX on the mood and cognitive functioning of overweight male subjects who were involved in an 8-week trial. Unexpectedly, the chronic administration of a high dose of NTX (300 mg/day) did not significantly affect mood or cognition among overweight adult men [430].

Switching now from healthy subjects to psychiatric samples, NTX has been mainly studied in the field of addictive disorders. A review of the pharmacological properties of NTX in alcohol, opiate, and nicotine studies failed to reveal dysphoria as a serious side-effect produced by NTX treatment, but suggested combining such treatment with antidepressant drugs [431]. If we focus on the case of opiate addiction, the evidence is not unanimous and, to some extent, is in conflict with what has been observed for other substances. In a 6-week, placebo-controlled crossover

Table 2.7 Principal drug interactions and methadone dosages in the experience of the PISA-VP Dole Research Group in MD/HUD patients

| | Dosage (mg/day) | |
	Mode	Range
Bipolar patients		
Methadone (stabilization dose)	120	50–320
Carbamazepine	510	400–800
Valproic acid	480	318–1000
During depressive phase		
Fluoxetine	20	10–40
Fluvoxamine	120	50–200
Paroxetine	28	20–40
Sertraline	100	25–200
Citalopram	20	5–60
Escitalopram	10	5–30
During manic phase		
Haloperidol	7	3–9
Clozapine	50	25–100
Risperidone	4.5	1.5–6
Olanzapine	10	5–20
Quetiapine	200	100–300
Aripiprazole	15	5–20
Asenapine	20	5–20
Lurasidone	40	15–80
Non-bipolar depression and dysthymic HUD patients		
Methadone (stabilization dose)	120	60–200
Imipramine	80	50–150
Clomipramine	100	50–150
Trimipramine	75	25–150
Fluoxetine	30	20–40
Fluvoxamine	150	100–200
Paroxetine	30	20–40
Sertraline	100	50–200
Citalopram	20	10–60
Escitalopram	10	5–30
Vortioxetine	10	10–20

Caution during the induction phase for the methadone plasmatic concentration increase, both with tricyclic and with serotonergic drugs. Reassess the dosage if the patient is already on treatment. Consider the QTc prolongation action of anti-D2 drugs. Beware of tachycardia and serotonin syndrome, characterized by mental confusion, diaphoresis, myoclonus, hyperreflexia, hypertension, cognitive deficits. Carbamazepine reduces plasma concentrations of methadone

design study, NTX was used to prevent relapse among former opioid addicts who had been free of opioids for 9 to 44 months. The reaction ranged from dropping out with abstinence-like symptoms to a dysphoric reaction during NTX administration [432].

With regard to kappa-opioid receptor ligands, their potential use in the treatment of affective disorders is a still more controversial issue. The kappa-opioid receptor system has been hypothesized to contribute to the pro-dysphoric and aversive consequences of stress, suggesting the anti-dysphoric and mood stabilizer effects of k-opioid receptor antagonists. Other authors disagree with this theory and suggest that k-opioid receptor antagonists might be useful in treating depression rather than dysphoria. For instance, Emrich et al. indicated the possible antidepressant effects of buprenorphine [433]. Only the mood-stabilizing properties of k-opioid partial agonists are generally accepted [434].

In summary, opioid antagonists have not been shown to possess antimanic properties on either current or former opiate addicts. The well-known antidepressant properties of opiates [435], and the common finding of depressive states after rapid opiate detoxification, might lead us to assume some antimanic action for opioid-antagonist agents [436]; even so, the absence of data on non-addicted bipolar subjects prevents us from predicting their specific effects on pure manic patients.

Although opioids are known to produce euphoric states, and spontaneous states of elation are associated with high CNS levels of endorphins, a low incidence of manic states has been reported among HUD patients. Naloxone, an opioid antagonist which has no apparent effect on depressed patients, has proved to have antimanic properties [165]. It has been hypothesized that NTX has a negative influence on basal mood, on the basis of observations on addicted or non-addicted patients. One bulimic patient treated with NTX developed panic attacks [437]. Of 80 NTX-maintained patients who were also receiving psychosocial treatment, 13 experienced an overdose accident during the first year of treatment. Four overdoses were lethal, including one case of suicide. Of nine non-lethal overdose cases, four were classified as attempted suicide [291].

In one of our study we aimed to investigate the predictors of failure in a NTX maintenance treatment programme [44]. Treatment failure was defined by treatment discontinuation along relapsing behaviour. One hundred and forty-nine subjects diagnosed as HUD patients along DSM-IV criteria and selected as opioid non-tolerant by a baseline naloxone test were recruited along a 54-month period. Mean age was 26 ± 5 (range 16–37 years) and approximately half of the patients were younger than 25 years. The majority were male, never married, with low educational level, employed mostly as workers, coming from families living on direct income from either blue- or white-collar work, living in urban environment with their families. A small minority can be rated as poor.

Before the treatment, a naloxone test was performed in order to ascertain the level of opioid tolerance, in order to avoid the long-acting opioid antagonist NTX being administered to tolerant individuals. After a 1-week induction phase, NTX was administered with the supervision of a family member, 100 mg on Mondays and Wednesdays, 150 mg on Fridays. The clinical status was updated along monthly evaluations. Treatment outcome was rated as positive if substance non-medical use had stopped. Non-abusing patients might be either judged to need ongoing treatment or be allowed to go off NTX. Otherwise, the outcome was negative when treatment was discontinued arbitrarily, when relapse followed treatment discontinuation, or when ongoing treatment failed to prevent substance use.

Negative outcome is predicted by the presence of job major problems and/or by the unemployed job situation at study entry. Subjects tend to stay longer in treatment, who have no work problems and a helpful relationship with their families. Some of the considered areas of psychopathological impairment (insight, consciousness, memory, anxiety, mood, feeding, aggressiveness, thought, perception) seem to affect NTX treatment suitability: depressed or dysphoric mood is predictive of treatment discontinuation together with aggressive or self-injuring behaviours, and delusional thought [44]. By contrast, bipolar patients with a low craving for opioids are those who seem to benefit from NTX maintenance, as witnessed by the satisfactory retention rate among this subgroup compared with uncomplicated addicts or non-bipolar addicts. The use of fluoxetine as add-on to NTX maintenance has been shown to improve patients' outcome, so suggesting that NTX has an anti-reward property, which is specifically reversible through fluoxetine's antidepressant effects [359, 370].

2.2.4   The Long-Term Outcomes of DD/BIP1-HUD Patients After Admission to Enhanced MMTP

In one of our studies we compared the long-term outcomes of treatment-resistant NDD/HUD patients with DD/BIP1-HUD ones [52]. We decided to evaluate whether comorbid psychopathology was able to influence methadone treatment outcomes in patients who had previously failed in first-line, low-threshold treatment facilities, when those patients were included in a high-threshold, maintenance-oriented, high-dose methadone programme.

The hypothesis of the study was that bipolar 1 psychiatric comorbidity would not affect treatment outcomes if patients with comorbid disorders received higher, individualized doses of methadone and that a favourable outcome would be related to long-term ongoing treatment (retention).

To test this hypothesis, a group of treatment-resistant HUD patients, with bipolar 1 or without psychiatric comorbidity, were followed in a naturalistic approach for a minimum of 0.5 and a maximum of 8 years in the context of the maintenance high-threshold, high-dose Pisa Methadone Maintenance Treatment Programme (PISA-MMTP), using retention in treatment and rates of heroin use as the main end-point parameters. All 104 consecutive patients were admitted to the programme over an 8-year time period (from January 1995 to May 2003) and followed for up to 8 years. The length of the prospective observation was 3 years on average (min. 0.5, max. 8); follow-up evaluation was carried out monthly, from the beginning of treatment.

In Italy, low-threshold facilities for drug addicts are available in each territorial district. In those settings, when opioid agonists are employed, dosage and duration of treatment are usually limited, regardless of clinical indication [86, 438], which suggests the value of increased dosage or treatment duration [439–442].

Patients are allowed to negotiate the lowering of dosages regardless of urinalyses and to have their medication tapered earlier than advisable on the basis of the scientific literature.

All the patients participating in the study were recruited from the PISA-MMTP, which belongs to the Pisa University Department of Psychiatry. Since 1993, the PISA-MMTP has been using a clinical protocol that has the characteristics of a high-threshold treatment facility for opioid addiction focusing on pharmacological maintenance. After patients at the PISA-MMTP have been safely inducted into treatment with methadone, their doses are gradually increased until the point is reached where there is no more than one urine drug screen which is positive for illicit opioids, cocaine, or BDZs in the previous 60-day period. Once this requirement is fulfilled, the patient is defined as having been 'stabilized', and the dose at which this goal has been accomplished is referred to as the 'stabilization dose'. No upper limit for dosage exists. Nevertheless, one time limitation is present in this setting: patients who cannot achieve stabilization within 1 year are terminated, to be transferred to local treatment units. The dosage is increased to reflect the results of urinalyses, and evidence of improvement on social grounds is not enough by itself to justify dose stability as long as the urinalyses stay positive for opioids. Patients are not allowed to raise or lower the dose by themselves. Take-home doses, without limitations, and at most for a 7-day period, are allowed once patients have shown complete compliance with the rules of the programme. Urine samples for toxicology analyses are collected randomly almost once a month, to allow evaluation of the metabolites of illicit drugs and BDZs.

In our programme patients are required to be actively involved in treatment by attending the clinic whenever that is scheduled, participating in the development of their treatment plan, working towards treatment goals, meeting with medical and case management staff, and attending groups when needed.

Patients with psychiatric comorbidity are also treated with psychoactive drugs (mood stabilizers, antipsychotics, or antidepressants) and supportive psychotherapy, as needed. All physicians working in the PISA-MMTP are psychiatrists who have been trained for at least 2 years in the treatment of addictive disorders.

To be referred to the PISA-MMTP, patients should have:

A diagnosis of heroin dependence according to DSM-IV criteria. We selected those with bipolar 1 psychiatric comorbidity (DD/BIP1-HUD patients) and those without concomitant DSM-IV axis I psychiatric disorders (NDD/HUD patients). Axis II diagnoses were excluded from the study, since a wide range of personality disorders are usually displayed by substances users, which makes it very difficult to define axis II diagnostic subgroups.

Resistance to previous first-line, low-threshold methadone treatment programmes attended at local addiction treatment units. Criteria for treatment resistance included at least two unsuccessful treatments in the 2-year period before being referred to our programme. Patients had been treated with the standard protocols for heroin dependence (MMT with dosages up to 100 mg/day) and were discharged because of persisting positivity for opioid metabolites at urinalyses.

Their baseline characteristics were average age 30 ± 6 (min 18, max 46); mostly male (74.0%), single (83.2%), and currently unemployed (45.1%), with a low educational level (68.3%).

The toxicological urinalyses were expressed using two indices: %CU (per cent clean urines) and CU/TS (per total specimens' clean urines). %CU represents the percentage ratio between urinalyses proving negative for the presence of morphine and the total number of urinalyses carried out for each patient during the treatment period. TS-CU is the percentage ratio between the number of urinalyses testing negative for the presence of morphine and the number of urine analyses that the protocol has envisaged throughout the process. In this case the reference number was 386 (the theoretical maximum number of urine samples per patient, considering an 8-year period). %CU tends to give a preference to patients who remain 'opioid free', but who terminate the study in advance, for reasons not correlated with the study (for example, imprisonment). TS-CU too considers how long the patient remains in the protocol but gives less precedence to these patients. These two indices represent the two extremes, and the results tend to balance out.

Regarding the demographic, clinical and addiction history data of the sample at the beginning of treatment, DD/BIP1-HUD patients turned out to be different from NDD/HUD patients in their educational level. The two groups did not differ significantly in the other demographic variables investigated (age, gender, marital status, work). Moreover, DD/BIP1-HUD patients seemed to indicate a lower frequency for 'daily or more' heroin intake and to have had a lower duration of addiction, besides having a lower age at first treatment. Patients belonging to the two groups did not differ significantly on work, family problems, romantic concerns, legal problems or illness severity, and general social adjustment. No significant differences were observed, even in age at first use of heroin, in age at onset of dependence or presence of polydrug use. Using Cox regression life table statistics, the following variables were not related to retention rate: 'daily or more' heroin intake and age at first treatment. A better retention rate was found for highly educated patients and those with a longer duration of dependence. DD/BIP1-HUD patients had been hospitalized for their illness at least once (1.72 ± 0.8, range 1–6) during the 2-year period preceding admission to our programme and had been treated with a variety of psychoactive drugs (typical and atypical antipsychotics, antidepressants, mood stabilizers, and BDZs).

Regarding the outcome of patients, as related to bipolar 1 psychiatric comorbidity, at the end of the observational period, 19.0% of NDD/HUD patients and 19.5% of DD/BIP1-HUD patients completed their rehabilitation programme and left the treatment or were referred to another programme as a 'stabilized patient'. About 50.8% of NDD/HUD patients and 36.6% of DD/BIP1-HUD patients had failed to achieve stabilization within a year, or relapsed into heroin use during the programme, so they were terminated and referred to their local treatment services. None of the patients were dismissed for violence; none gave up the treatment for side-effects; none were imprisoned and only one was re-hospitalized. About 30.2% of NDD/HUD patients and 43.9% of DD/BIP1-HUD patients were 'stabilized' and were still in treatment at the end of the period of observation. These differences were not statistically significant.

The severity of illness and the global assessment of functioning showed different significant trends in our patients. DD/BIP1-HUD patients reported, at the end-point evaluation, lower severity of illness than NDD/HUD patients. Time effect and group-time effect were significant. Interestingly, the severity of illness was equal in the two groups, at baseline. These differences were not related to the outcome.

At the end-point evaluation DD/BIP1-HUD patients reported a better social adjustment than NDD/HUD patients. Time effect and group-time effect were both significant. At baseline, social adjustment was better in NDD/HUD patients. These differences were not related to the outcome.

Neither NDD/HUD nor DD/BIP1-HUD patients relapsed into addictive behaviour after 4 years of treatment. The cumulative proportion of NDD/HUD patients surviving at the end of the observational period was 0.44. The proportion for DD/BIP1-HUD patients was 0.58. The higher survival rate for DD/BIP1-HUD patients was due to the greater number of subjects who stayed in treatment rather than to a difference in the number of patients who left the programme with a positive outcome (detoxified after a period of MMT or referred, once stabilized, to other programmes), as the latter parameter was not modified by the presence or absence of dual disorder. Females and males showed similar retention rate. DD/BIP1-HUD and NDD/HUD males showed no different retention rate. DD/BIP1-HUD females showed higher retention rate than NDD/HUD ones. This difference was statistically significant.

On average, DD/BIP1-HUD patients needed a higher methadone dosage in the stabilization phase (135.85 ± 65.7 mg/day) compared with NDD/HUD patients (119.46 ± 67.3 mg/day). This difference was not statistically significant (Fig. 2.7).

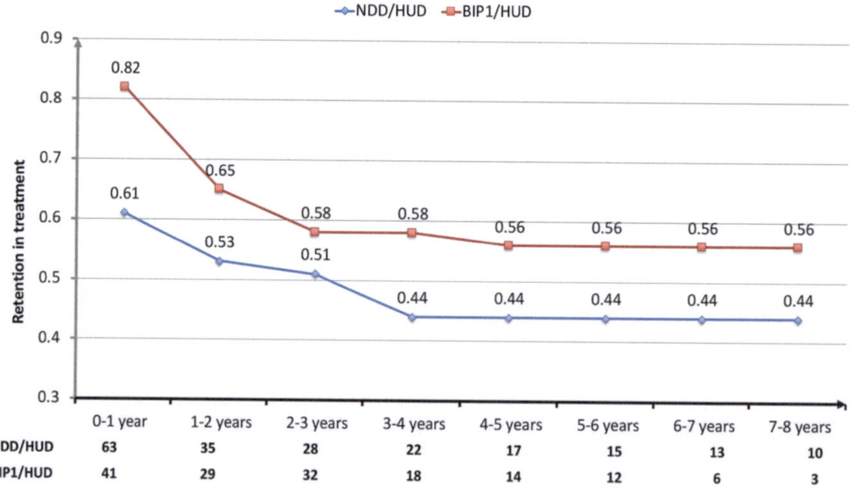

Fig. 2.7 Retention in treatment of DD/HUD with bipolar 1 (DD/BIP1-HUD) and without dual disorder (NDD/HUD)

Differences were, of course, observed according to the outcome and according to the group-outcome effect. Comorbid group was treated systematically with valproate maintenance as the first-line regimen, dosages ranging between 300 and 900 mg/daily b.i.d. Lithium and carbamazepine are usually avoided because lithium treatment requires patients to be compliant with stable dosing and regular follow-up, and because carbamazepine is difficult to employ, since it enhances metabolism of opioids [443]. In any case priority was given to methadone dosage adaptation [49]. Psychotropic medications were not systematically used for the non-comorbid group.

On average, 77.31% of samples tested negative for morphine. No patient provided positive samples for the entire duration of treatment. No patient provided exclusively negative samples. In patients who left the programme with a positive outcome the %CU index was 90.75 ± 3.9; in patients with a negative outcome, it was 62.26 ± 8.6; in patients still in treatment, it was 89.16 ± 5.0. These differences were statistically significant in all comparisons. No differences were observed between DD/BIP1-HUD and NDD/HUD patients. The group–outcome interaction was not significant, either.

The CU/TS index revealed differences between different outcomes: positive, negative, still in treatment. No differences were observed between DD/BIP1-HUD and NDD/HUD patients. Similarly, the group–outcome interaction was not significant. In summary, no differences were found regarding urinalyses for morphine between DD/BIP1-HUD and NDD/HUD patients during the observational period.

In summary, we examined treatment retention and outcomes for DD/BIP1-HUD and NDD/HUD treatment-resistant, methadone-maintained patients. We observed that:

DD/BIP1-HUD and NDD/HUD patients differed at baseline in terms of their educational level, duration of their heroin addiction, level of heroin use, and age at first addiction treatment, but these differences did not appear to be related to the better retention or better outcome of the DD/BIP1-HUD patients.

DD/BIP1-HUD patients were retained in treatment for longer especially if women.

DD/BIP1-HUD patients showed no differences in rates of opioid-negative urine specimens.

DD/BIP1-HUD patients tended to require higher doses of methadone than NDD/HUD patients.

The main conclusions to be drawn from our results are:

In the presence of problematic non-compliant patients with a bipolar 1 diagnosis, a flexible dosing regimen that permits the administration of higher doses may lead to higher retention rates. The relevance of the present data becomes clearer when we consider that between a third and a half of all opioid addicts suffer from additional mental disorders [157, 444, 445].

DD/BIP1-HUD treated with higher dosages may have outcomes that are as satisfactory as those of uncomplicated HUD patients, as long as they are maintained on their medication in the long term.

2.2.5 Proposals

We propose the following strategies when treating DD patients with affective disorders:

- Antidepressant pharmacotherapy alone cannot extinguish addictive behaviour in HUD patients.
- Long-acting opioids have antidepressant properties.
- Over-standard dosages of methadone (over 120 mg/day) are needed.
- Antidepressant medications (especially SSRIs) increase blood levels of methadone.
- SSRIs must be used in rapid metabolizer patients on methadone.
- Caution is needed during the MMT induction phase.
- SSRIs are not useful during the detoxification of patients with HUD.
- Craving increases during manic phases. Switching antidepressants must be avoided. Anti-craving antidepressants (fluoxetine or sertraline) in depressed HUD patients must be preferred.
- Avoid the inhibitors of the monoamine oxidase, because of their interaction with cocaine (disulfiram effect).
- BDZ for treating comorbid anxiety must be avoided (long-acting opioids have anxiolytic properties).
- The co-use of clomipramine and methadone can reduce the latency of the antide-pressant effect.
- Tricyclic stimulant antidepressants, bupropion, vortioxetine, and trazodone, can be used after opioid detoxification for at least 6 months as anti-hypophoric agents.
- In HUD patients it is possible to find tricyclic use (especially amitriptyline) and tricyclic withdrawal syndrome.
- Mood stabilizers are useful in DD/BIP-HUD patients, but mood-stabilizing therapy alone does not extinguish addictive behaviour in HUD patients.
- Caution with carbamazepine is needed. Methadone dosage must be increased if carbamazepine is necessary. This increase is not necessary with valproic acid. Lithium can be used only in compliant cocaine user HUD patients.

Anxiety Disorder in Heroin Use Disorder Patients

3

3.1 Clinical Aspects

Most addicted patients display symptoms of anxiety at some time during their addictive history [206, 245, 446–451]. In AUD patients, as much as 50–70% of that symptomatology can be described as generalized anxiety, panic disorder and phobic syndromes. The occurrence of anxiety features is even more common among specific groups of cases featuring withdrawal or intoxication syndromes, where that frequency rises to 80%. A genetic link between anxiety and addictive disorders has been postulated; some authors have interpreted that link as depending on a self-medicating dynamic. Although it is hard to tell whether anxiety is of a primary type or springs from a substance non-medical use/addiction course, it can be agreed that comorbid anxiety disorders in AUD patients or drug addicts deserve specific clinical attention and therapeutic intervention.

Any of the *DSM-5* anxiety disorders can become manifest during a phase of intoxication or withdrawal, whatever the substance used. The most common pictures are those typical of phobias, panic disorders and generalized anxiety. *DSM-IV* indicates syndromes such as substance-induced anxiety disorders and states that prominent symptoms comprise free anxiety, panic attacks, obsessions and compulsions. The onset of symptoms can come less than 1 month after an episode of intoxication or withdrawal and may endure for months, so causing significant psychosocial and working impairment, as well as difficulties in managing private life. Comorbid anxiety disorders sometimes represent a true dual disorder, but their features are not distinguishable from drug-induced ones. Despite this, *DSM-IV* provides useful criteria for drawing a distinction: the likelihood of an anxiety disorder being primary rises when anxiety symptoms forerun the onset of substance non-medical use; when symptoms endure far beyond an episode of intoxication or withdrawal; or when they exceed what might be expected from the severity of the toxic state. Lastly, a history of anxiety disorders unrelated to any condition of use/dependence makes a diagnosis of primary anxiety disorder more likely.

© The Author(s), under exclusive license to Springer Nature Switzerland AG 2023

I. Maremmani et al., *Dual Disorder Heroin Addicts*, https://doi.org/10.1007/978-3-031-30093-6_3

3.1.1   Epidemiology

According to the 1994 National Comorbidity Survey [452], 24.9% of the general population is affected by some anxiety disorder, whereas alcohol dependence only occurs in 13.7%. AUD patients or drug addicts with a comorbid panic-agoraphobic disorder or social phobia display severe anxiety, and the degree of severity of their anxiety symptoms appears to strengthen their drive towards alcohol consumption. In this context, higher anxiety levels are predictive of heavier drinking or drug-taking. The rate of anxiety disorders among addicted patients does not exceed that expected for the same disorders in the general population. Moreover, the rate of comorbidity for alcohol or drug dependence among people affected by anxiety disorders is not particularly significant when compared with that for the general population. Consistent with this, the risk of alcohol use/dependence developing among social phobia patients is high only in a subgroup showing features of bipolarity, type II.

Anxiety symptoms are the rule during stimulant intoxication or CNS depressor withdrawal due to an increased release of catecholamines. Administering sodium lactate is effective in eliciting panic attacks not only in patients suffering from panic disorder but also in AUD patients. Moreover, lactate serum levels increase during alcohol intoxication in AUD individuals. Anxiety symptoms forerun the onset of alcohol use in as many as 40–60% of AUD patients with comorbid anxiety disorders. On the other hand, it is far more common to recognize the use of alcohol as the background for many anxiety disorders. It is still controversial whether, once detoxification has been achieved, anxiety symptoms can be expected to shoot up or, conversely, dwindle. Certainly, anxiety disorders that have a favourable outcome are expected to take quite a long time to achieve resolution.

In monocorial twins born of AUD patients, anxiety is marked only among subjects who drink heavily, so suggesting there may be a link between the degree of exposure to alcohol and the likelihood of developing clinically relevant anxiety. It has not so far been demonstrated, however, that a high risk of drug addiction or alcohol dependence correlates with a correspondingly high risk of anxiety disorders. The risk of alcohol dependence in subjects with panic disorder, phobias or generalized anxiety does not differ from that of the general population. Lastly, one possibility not to be ignored is that the development of anxiety disorders in AUD individuals is itself the sign of a genetically determined proneness to anxiety that is independent of alcohol use.

HUD patients very commonly report anxiety-like symptoms, and several studies have reported features of anxiety and neuroticism as being strongly represented among them, but only a minority of patients can actually be diagnosed as affected by any anxiety disorder outside the context of opioid withdrawal. At least one anxiety disorder affects up to 12% of patients, with a lifetime prevalence of only 6% [137, 156]. Average rates for phobias are very low, though the range is between 1% [148] and 9.5% [453].

Clinical pictures that resemble episodes of panic disorders are not infrequent during MMT or methadone tapering, with a recorded frequency of between 1% and 2% [158, 159, 206]. In such cases, scholar phobia and separation anxiety are commonly reported as early precursors of current full-blown anxiety. These data indicate that the spontaneous panic disorder of HUD patients might actually be the result of an opioid dysfunction, with a consequent lack of endorphinergic inhibition on the ascendant noradrenergic firing [158].

As regards OCD, the only data available are those in the Yale study by Rounsaville and colleagues, who report an index and lifetime rate of 10% and 20%, respectively [454]. OCD-affected patients tend to concentrate their negative expectations on an object that becomes their feared object, and they structure their daily life around an avoidant attitude. Similarly, though not symmetrical, drug addicts structure their lives around the compulsive pursuit of a single object, the drug, and concentrate the whole body of meanings and expectations of their own existence on it. In this way, the drug may be viewed as an invulnerable defender against underlying phobic preoccupations. Wurmser put forward the suggestion that 'in most addicts, a phobic core can be identified, which can be typically described as the phobia (and desire at the same time) of being trapped, captured, enchained within boundaries, institutions, jail, either physical restriction or affective ties'. The drug would then gain the value of a counterphobic shield: it is compulsively craved for as strongly as the phobic object is avoided [455].

3.1.2 Panic Disorder and Opioid Use

Critical anxiety over somatic symptoms has been highlighted in pharmacovigilance studies about buprenorphine and tramadol but is probably attributable to an acute imbalance of opioid tolerance in subjects with a medium-high level of opioid addiction [456, 457]. Panic attacks, without the presence of withdrawal syndrome, are documented in non-addicted subjects after the intake of opioid antagonist agents [437, 458] and opioids with k-agonist activity [459] or Vicodin (a codeine-based painkiller). A naloxone test on patients with panic attacks, instead, gave negative results [460], suggesting the heterogeneity between interference with the μ-agonist system, linked to instinctive-like phenomena, and psychopathological phenomena such as psychosis and critical anxiety that are predominantly related to other receptor involvement. The prevalence of the independent panic disorder in opioid addicts or users has been found around 2% [461].

The increase over time in the prevalence of panic attacks from 1% to 6–13% in MMT patients seems to be at least partly attributable to the increase in cocaine use [462]. In a group of 9279 subjects receiving prescriptions for opioid-containing preparations, 282 subjects, all of them reporting regular opioid use, presented an association between psychiatric disorders such as depression, dysthymia, generalized anxiety disorder, panic disorder and alcohol and other substance non-medical use [463]. This fact affects subjects without highly interfering pain, for whom the intensity of pain is the most likely reason for the regular use of opioids. In opioid-tolerant subjects, we must differentiate critical anxiety from acute opioid withdrawal or from intoxication by other substances. In both cases, the person experiences subjectively urgent and alarming symptoms and reacts in an agitated and ready-to-rescue manner. Usually, the scare related to the experience of panic refers to a general feeling of imminent death or imminent risk of an explosive and uncontrollable illness. Otherwise, opioid withdrawal syndrome is recognized by the brain as a substance in which the patient is looking for specific remedies (an opioid or a substitute drug). However, it is possible that panic attacks begin in the patient's post-addiction era and that, due to a form of cognitive conditioning, the brain manifests the somatic and behavioural reactions typical of a withdrawal syndrome even behind stimuli of a different nature that complicate the feasibility of making a correct diagnosis. Moreover, the subjective variability of opioid withdrawal highlighted during rapid detoxification procedures may also refer to the panic mechanism, which fictitiously increases the withdrawal severity due to its overlap with a 'central' alarm state [436, 464, 465]. The response to opioids does not help, since both opioid withdrawal and panic attacks generally benefit from acute opioid intake.

Crampiform pain, diarrhoea (and not pseudo-diarrhoea—defined as increased stool frequency, with a normal daily stool weight of less than 300 g), congestion of the nasal mucous membranes with rhinorrhoea and chills are indicative of opioid abstinence. A phenomenon of doubtful interpretation will also clearly be of anxiety, rather than part of withdrawal matrix, if it resolves spontaneously, leaving a post-critical state of asthenia and drowsiness. Opioid withdrawal syndrome has a gradually increasing course over the hours, and while it may fluctuate in the intensity of symptoms, it keeps the subject alert and tense.

In subjects treated with opioid effective and stable doses, above the levels of tolerance acquired during addiction processes, the onset of panic disorder is unlikely; some cases of the previous disorder are apparently in remission during the maintenance phase of methadone treatment. In these cases, however, the disorder may re-emerge during medication disengagement, on the basis of a generic anxiety diathesis: subjects with a history of heroin use, however, stabilized by methadone, are more sensitive than controls to the acute increase of synaptic norepinephrine (obtained by yohimbine) [466]. To differentiate these two conditions, it is useful to gradually reduce opioid coverage: critical anxiety symptoms reported after ongoing dosage reductions of less than 25% in stabilized patients are indicative of latent anxiety disorder rather than opioid decompensation related to acquired tolerance.

3.2   Treatment of Anxiety Disorders in Drug Addicts

Apart from conditions of intoxication or withdrawal, the treatment of anxiety in addicted patients does not differ from the treatment of simple anxiety syndromes. Anti-anxiety agents are indicated for patients who continue to display anxiety even when receiving effective treatment for their addiction. Target symptoms should always be defined and monitored, and treatment should not necessarily be thought of as chronic. This is particularly true of BDZs, which are useful only to the extent to which they prompt patients' acceptance of other treatments. Agents such as alprazolam, lorazepam or diazepam should be avoided because of their strong use liability. Diazepam is one of the most popularly used psychotropics among HUD patients, not only due to its property of soothing some of the opioid withdrawal symptoms: as addicts themselves report, it is often used to maintain euphoria or to reproduce a heroin-like euphoria when taking methadone [467], if heroin itself produces few strong sensations, or else to make a subject feel 'high' [468, 469]. Clonazepam, on the other hand, has proved suitable and safer and can be used in dosages of up to 0.50 mg three times per day, when required. These findings are consistent with the data provided by animal studies, in which diazepam has proved to heighten the effects of opioids [470]. At high doses, diazepam is mostly used to buffer withdrawal symptoms or improve the course of rapid detoxifications or prolong abstinence after detoxification has been completed. During methadone treatment too, diazepam use is a common finding, more so than among AUD patients [395, 408, 467, 471–473]. The percentage of methadone-maintained subjects using BDZs is as high as 10–20%, reaching a maximum of 30%, as reported by some authors if BDZs or hypnotics have been used during the previous week [412, 471, 474]. According to the Treatment Outcome Prospective Study, between 5% and 16% of methadone-maintained subjects have been using BDZs weekly or less often. Regular diazepam use is common too, as assessed by random urinalysis: 20% of patients turned out to be high-rate diazepam users (with more than three positive urinalyses over a 6-month period) and 46% were defined as low-rate users (with at most one positive result) [475]. It is doubtful whether BDZ use should be read as an attempt to deal with anxiety or actually looms as a form of addiction. Lately, the problem of BDZ withdrawal has been regarded with increasing concern, and cases of symptomatic withdrawal have been documented for dosages even lower than those taken on average by methadone-maintained patients [476]. Benzodiazepine-abusing methadone patients may display oversleeping, ataxia, speech difficulties and even anger attacks [467]. Over time, diazepam addiction has partly replaced the already recognized phenomenon of dependence on hypnotics, which are often carelessly prescribed by GPs for insomnia. Diazepam use can sometimes produce altered, dreamlike states of consciousness, which addicts may experience as optimum conditions for engaging in illicit behaviours.

Dreadful accidents may happen in those circumstances, so the prescription of BDZs to addicts should only be allowed when strictly necessary, and addicted patients should never be given free access to them. In particular, it is harmful to encourage addicts to decrease their methadone dosage and use BDZs to compensate for the difference: not only will patients' clinical conditions not improve, but they will also be put at risk of developing a poly-addictive disease [75].

No matter what the dynamics may be that underlie BDZ use, it can certainly be expected to worsen an addict's already delicate conditions, especially if heavy, regular use is initiated. That is why clinicians agree that the anxiety of agonist-maintained addicts should be dealt with first by regulating the agonist dosage, then, if necessary, by counselling facilities, relaxing techniques or environmental

Table 3.1 Pharmacological interactions and methadone dosages in the clinical experience of V.P. Dole Research Group in DD (anxiety)/HUD patients

Medication	Dosage (mg/day)	
	Mode	Range
Panic disorder		
Methadone, stabilization dose	80	40–90
Imipramine	30	25–50
Fluvoxamine	100	50–150
Paroxetine	20	10–30
Sertraline	100	50–200
Citalopram	20	10–40
Obsessive-compulsive disorder		
Methadone, stabilization dose	100	90–110
Clomipramine	150	75–300
Fluoxetine	30	20–40
Fluvoxamine	200	150–250
Sertraline	100	50–200

Be careful during the induction phase for the increase of methadone plasma concentration, with both tricyclic and serotonergic medications. Reassess the dosage if the patient is already on treatment. Consider the QTc prolongation by citalopram. Beware of tachycardia and serotonin syndrome, characterized by mental confusion, diaphoresis, myoclonus, hyperreflexia, hypertension and cognitive deficits

intervention. The findings emerging from our research group's experience indicate that the average methadone dosage needed to stabilize HUD patients with a dual disorder of anxiety disorder is lower (80 mg/day) than the average required to stabilize other types of DD/HUD patients, or even HUD patients without DD (100 mg/day) (Table 3.1). Consistently with such observations, NTX has been shown to elicit anxiety in non-addicted as well as addicted patients [437].

The anxiety disorders of HUD patients can also be treated successfully with antidepressant drugs and buspirone [477]. Tricyclic agents and SSRIs are effective in controlling both anxiety and depressive symptoms and are suitable for long-term treatment programmes. Imipramine and nortriptyline may cause sedation and hypotension.

Use caution during the methadone induction phase. Re-evaluate methadone dosage if the patient is already in treatment.

With the use of SSRI drugs, it is good to pay attention during the induction phase of MMT or when the tolerance of the subject is still unknown. If the patient is already in treatment, the dosage will need to be reviewed.

Fluoxetine, sertraline and paroxetine may initially increase anxiety, but this effect is very rare in HUD patients, especially when treated with methadone. SSRIs are preferred to tricyclics because of their lower potential for use and their lower toxicity in the event of an overdose. Finally, the withdrawal symptoms of tricyclics and SSRIs are much milder than those of BDZs. Buspirone at dosages between 15 and 60 mg per day, and also in combination with SSRIs, has been shown to be effective for medium-moderate anxiety.

3.3   Treatment of BDZ Addiction During Methadone Treatment

The use of BDZ by patients on MMT has the effect of complicating the clinical picture and may negatively influence treatment outcomes (poorer psychosocial adjustment, higher levels of polydrug use, more risk-taking behaviours and a shorter retention in treatment) [478–483]. A history of BDZ prescription is significantly associated with drug-dependent death [484], and intermittent BDZ use was found to be significantly associated with lower rates of opioid abstinence during MMT [485].

Benzodiazepine MMT users are more likely to have injected recently, to have used cocaine and amphetamines, to have borrowed or lent used needles and syringes and to have reported polydrug use in the preceding month. Benzodiazepine MMT users also exhibit higher levels of psychopathology and social dysfunction than other MMT patients. Benzodiazepine-using MMT patients are a dysfunctional sub-group of the methadone population, and they are likely to require more clinical intervention than other patients [486].

Some authors stress the high priority that should be given to stopping BDZ use during [487] or before entering MMT. For example, the Stockholm Centre for Dependency Disorders has suggested that BDZs should hardly ever be prescribed to patients on methadone/buprenorphine. Before entering MMT/buprenorphine treatment, the patient must be negative for BDZs taken without a prescription and, if a patient on MMT/buprenorphine becomes positive for BDZs, the MMT/buprenorphine therapy should be discontinued (Johan Franck, 2013—personal communication).

Others claim that cautiously prescribing BDZs may be a beneficial strategy, due to the reduction in overall illicit use [480].

The relative safety of BDZ use by methadone- or buprenorphine-treated patients has still not been systematically examined. BDZs may significantly alter the response to opioid substitution treatment with methadone or buprenorphine. In any case, BDZ had greater peak effects on performance measures (simple reaction time, digit symbol substitution task and cancellation time) in methadone-treated than in buprenorphine-treated patients [488].

Opioid/BDZ co-dependent patients reported less severe withdrawal symptoms during treatment with buprenorphine than with methadone [489].

While opioid medications have been demonstrated to be an effective treatment for opioid dependence, its impact on the treatment outcome of other types of illicit drug use is not as clear. Therapeutic approaches to BDZ dependence in patients in MMT have met with limited success. Clonazepam detoxification and clonazepam maintenance treatment (CMT) have been experimented. Maintenance strategy with clonazepam is a useful BDZ treatment modality for BDZ-dependent MMT patients with a long-term history of use and previous attempts at detoxification [490].

In our clinical experience, patients with severe comorbid dependence, when treated with over-standard dosages of methadone and co-treated with CMT, may have outcomes that are satisfactory as long as they are maintained on their medication in the long term [400]. We considered all the patients admitted to our programme over an 8-year time period (from January 1995 to May 2003) and enrolled in previous studies [52, 56].

We selected 14 patients diagnosed as HUD patients according to the *DSM-IV-R* diagnostic criteria (304.00); they also fulfilled *DSM-IV* criteria for severe dependence on sedatives, hypnotics or anxiolytics (F13.24). All these patients entered our CMT-MMT programme and were followed up.

Regarding demographic characteristics and heroin-addiction history, mean age of our patients was 30.14 ± 3.8 (range: 26–38). Fourteen (71.4%) were males and 4 (28.6%) females. Five (35.7%) were highly educated people (with over 8 years of education) and 9 (64.3%) had a low level of education. Twelve (85.7%) were single and only 2 (14.3%) had a partner. Two (14.3%) had a white-collar job, 3 (21.4%) had a blue-collar one and 9 (64.3%) were unemployed. Low income was found in 1 (7.1%) subject, and adequate income (sufficient to satisfy a requirement or meet a need) in 13 (92.9%) subjects. Thirteen (92.9%) had an urban birth location and 11 (78.6%) were living in an urban zone. Only 2 (14.3%) subjects were living alone. All patients were recruited from Central Italy. At treatment entry, at least one of the somatic complications that were investigated (hepatic, vascular, lymphatic, gastrointestinal, sexual, dental, HIV+ and AIDS) was observed in 13 (92.9%) subjects. Mean was 2.28 ± 1.5 (0–6 ranged). At least one of the mental status areas that were investigated (insight, consciousness, memory, anxiety, depression, sleep, eating, excitement, violence, suicidality, delusions and hallucinations) was found to have undergone alteration in all subjects. Mean was 6.28 ± 1.6 (range 4–10). Only 3 (21.4%) subjects enjoyed their job; 5 (35.7%) were unsatisfied with their household relationship, 6 (42.9%) with their erotic situation and 12 (85.7) with their social-leisure activities. Eight (57.1%) reported current or past legal problems. Polysubstance use (more than three substances of use) was occasionally present in 10 (71.4%) subjects. Mean number of occasionally used substances was 3.57 ± 1.6 (range 1–6). Only 2 (14.3%) patients had never been treated. Mean number of past different kinds of treatment was 2.71 ± 1.8 (range 0–6). We investigated various different kinds of treatment: therapeutic community; psychopharmacology; psychotherapy; short-term detoxification with opioid agonists, partial agonists and antagonists; and maintenance treatment with opioid agonists, partial agonists and antagonists. As to comorbid substance use, 9 (64.3%) patients occasionally used alcohol, 10 (71.4%) CNS-stimulants, 11 (78.6%) cannabinoids, 10 (71.4%) hallucinogens and 1 (7.1%) inhalants. Heroin intake took place at least once a day in 11 (78.6%) patients. Modality of heroin use was unstable in 12 (85.7%); periodic self-detoxification occurred in 10 (71.4%); stage 3 of heroin addiction was reached by 11 (78.6%); and psychosocial stressors, before starting heroin, were present in 4 (28.6%). Mean age at first heroin use was 20.57 ± 4.8 (range 14–31), mean age at start of continuous heroin use was 22.29 ± 4.4 (15–31) and mean age at first treatment was 25.64 ± 4.4 (17–33) years. Mean dependence length (months) was 79.79 ± 70.1 (range 12–240).

At treatment entry, mean dose of used BDZ (expressed as diazepam-equivalents) was 166.78 ± 57.6 mg/day (range 100–250). Eleven (78.6%) patients were using between 100 and 200 diazepam-equivalent mg/day and 3 (21.4%) over 200 mg/day. Severity of illness was considered moderate in 3 (21.4%), marked in 7 (50.0%) and severe in 4 (28.6%) patients. Global assessment of functioning classified 4 (28.6%) subjects in cluster 3 (inability to function in almost all areas (e.g. staying in bed all day; no job, home or friends); 3 (21.4%) in cluster 4 (major impairment in several areas, such as work or school, family relations, judgement, thinking or mood); and 5 (35.7%) in cluster 5 (any serious impairment in social, occupational or school functioning; e.g. no friends, unable to keep a job); only 2 (14.2%) showed a better-than-described social adjustment.

Regarding the survival in treatment of our patients, at the start of the first year, we had 14 subjects in treatment. During the first year, there was one terminal event (0.07%), with a survival index of 0.93. At the start of the second year, we had 13 in-treatment patients. During this year, there were 4 (31%) terminal events, with a fall in the cumulative survival index to 0.64. At the start of the third year, we had nine in-treatment patients. During the third year, one patient successfully terminated the treatment by leaving the programme in an opioid-detoxified condition and without BDZ. No terminal events were observed. At the start of the fourth year, eight patients were in treatment. During the fourth year, one (13%) terminal event was observed, and the cumulative survival index fell to 0.56. At the start of the fifth year, seven patients were in treatment. During the fifth year, one patient successfully terminated the programme, in an opioid-detoxified condition and taking only a small amount of clonazepam (2 mg/day in two doses). No terminal events were observed during the sixth or seventh years of treatment, the cumulative survival index remaining at 0.56. At the end of the seventh year, six patients were still in treatment. Figure 3.1 summarizes the situation for the survival in treatment of our patients. In summary, the outcome was 'negative' in six (42.9%) subjects and 'positive' in eight (57.1%). No patient with a 'negative' outcome voluntarily abandoned the programme, whether for side effects, altered bio exams, imprisonment, hospitalization or death. All negative-outcome patients lost their status as a 'stabilized patient' and were transferred to low-threshold programmes. Using Cox regression, only the urinary outcome significantly predicted survival in treatment (χ^2 = 12.43; df = 1; $p < 0.001$; Exp(B) = 0.001, CI 95%: 0.001–0.079).

Multivariate tests showed that global clinical impression severity of illness and global assessment of functioning demonstrated significant improvements in our patients independently of their outcome.

On average, patients with severe comorbid BDZ dependence needed an over-standard methadone dosage in the stabilization phase (190.73 ± 103.4 mg/day). Patients who had a positive outcome did not receive different stabilization dosages (Student's T-test = 0.55; $p = 0.586$). The clonazepam stabilization dosage was 21.36 ± 7.2 mg/day (min 12.50, max 32.50). After eliminating the toxicological examination performed at the time of enrolment in the programme (which was required to be positive), 2947 urine samples were analysed in all. Of these, 2554 (86.6%) were opioid-clean. In positive-outcome patients, the opioid urinalyses index was 0.90 ± 0.05; in negative-outcome patients, it was 0.64 ± 0.1 (Student's T-test =5.81; p = <0.01) (Fig. 3.2).

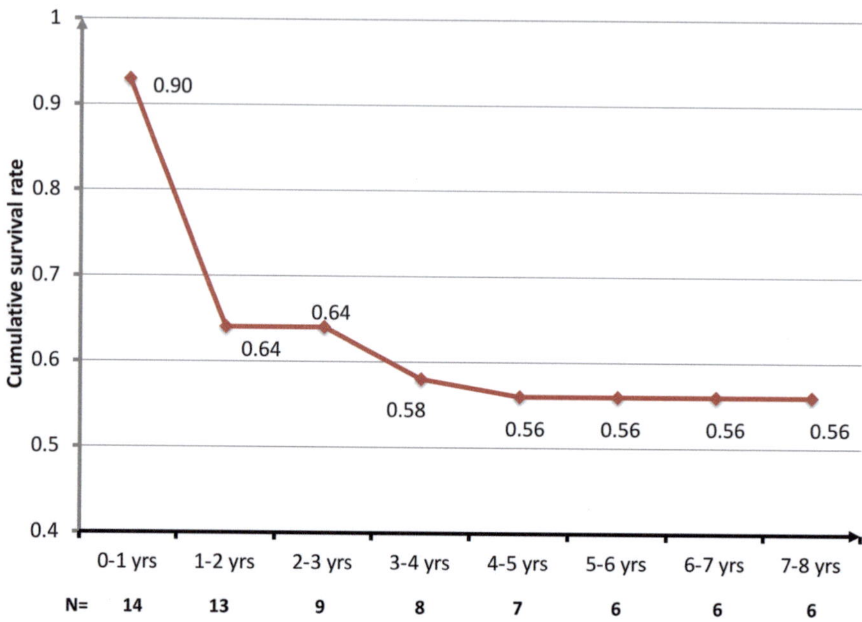

Fig. 3.1   Retention in treatment of patients with severe BDZ co-dependence

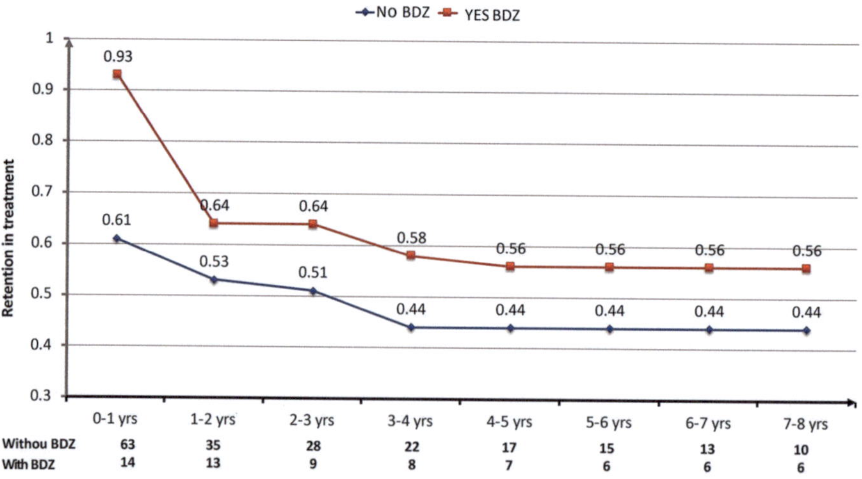

Fig. 3.2   Retention in treatment of heroin use disorder patients with and without severe BDZ
co-dependence

In our study we observed that:

- Patients were assessed at baseline, in terms of somatic and psychopathological complications, frequency of unsatisfactory social and leisure time and the presence of polydrug use.

These data agree with the observations of Drake et al. [486] on whether MMT patients with BDZ dependence can be considered to belong to a dysfunctional group. However, the characteristics found by us did not appear to be related to the patients' retention or their outcome.

- Patients with concomitant severe BDZ dependence were recorded as having been successfully retained in long-term treatment; they showed good results for opioid-negative urine specimens; they required over-standard doses of methadone.

In particular, the outcome and the percentage figures for retention in therapy of our patients did not differ from those of long-term standard MMT programmes [491–496]. The main difference between our programme and the standard Italian MMT lies in the amount of methadone administered during the stabilization phase; this ranges from 80 to 400 mg/day in our protocols and from 40 to 100 mg/day in standard protocols. A possible explanation for the need for these relatively higher doses in BDZ-dependent patients may be related to a pharmacokinetic and/or pharmacodynamic mechanism. Methadone is metabolized in the liver by the P450 cytochrome system and, more specifically, by the CYP3A4 isoform, which is involved in the metabolism of over 50% of the medical agents [497, 498]. The wide interindividual variability [499–504] recorded and the fact that CYP3A4 can be induced by several active principles [505, 506], may explain why a number of patients are under-medicated if a standard dose of methadone is used.

Unfortunately, we did not measure plasma methadone levels in our patients during the stabilization phase, so we cannot determine whether the doses used were necessary to maintain a proper therapeutic window or to control an underlying underestimated psychopathology. In our patients, the existence of a minor form of psychopathology in the other patients concealed under the main addictive symptoms cannot be excluded. There is significant overlapping between behaviours in some types of psychiatric disorders and drug-related behaviours: maladaptive behaviours, such as those commonly displayed by drug addicts, may sometimes be due to, or accentuated by, concurrent psychiatric disorders. Thus, a low degree of compliance with therapies is a common symptom of drug addiction and of several forms of psychiatric disorders [194, 507–509]. In addition, we found that the outcome of MMT patients with or without dual disorder is the same in the short [55] and long term [56].

The low score of global clinical index and the high social adjustment score values recorded for our patients and the absence of hospitalizations throughout the treatment period showed that these subjects were simultaneously compliant both with MMT requirements and with the specific BDZ therapy adopted. Cox regression suggests that the effectiveness of methadone treatment supports the results obtained with methadone–clonazepam combined treatment. Additional clonazepam for the treatment of BDZ use—medication not completely changed by the need to treat addiction—may partly explain the positive outcomes obtained in our comorbid patients, which cannot be attributed exclusively to the effects of methadone. A lack, whether of appropriately flexible methadone doses and/or of specific medications given in association with methadone treatment for these patients, could have been responsible for the conflicting results obtained by other researchers, who reported that BDZ and alcohol use were linked to worse treatment outcomes (retention in treatment) [478–483]. In addition, the psychotherapeutic support provided by our team and the high therapeutic pressure of our programme could have been responsible for good results [510]. In any case, the incisiveness of our study was limited by several factors, such as the observational nature of the protocol, the impossibility of evaluating a follow-up in the case of the patients who dropped out, the multiple interference caused by inter-individual variability (personality traits and their neurobiological correlates), the clinical setting and the temporary use of adjunctive medications. We therefore chose this kind of research because of the fact that we had little control over events and there was a contemporary focus within a real-life context. The goal of our case study was to offer new points of view and questions for further research, considering that 35% of patients who enter methadone treatment can be described as 'regular/problem users' [478].

In one other naturalistic (observational) controlled cohort study, our aim was to compare the long-term outcomes of treatment-resistant HUD patients with (HUD + BDZ) and without (HUD-BDZ) comorbid BDZ severe addiction. Sixty-three HUD-BDZ and 14 HUD + BDZ patients were monitored prospectively along with an enhanced MMTP. HUD + BDZ patients were also treated with CMT [399].

On the basis of DAH-Q-collected information, no differences were observed, at the beginning of the treatment, between HUD patients with and without comorbid BDZ severe dependence regarding gender (males, females), civil status (single, not single), education (less than 8 years, more than 8 years), occupation (student, white collar, blue collar, unemployed), welfare benefit (yes, no), income (poor, adequate) and living (alone, in family).

Table 3.2 reports significant clinical and addiction history differences between HUD patients with and without severe comorbid BDZ dependence. HUD patients with comorbid BDZ severe dependence seemed to indicate a greater number of altered mental status areas. They showed greater frequency of consciousness alterations, depressive states, sleep disturbances, excitement states and violent episodes, including suicidality, delusions and hallucination. No differences were found in insight, memory disturbances, anxious states or eating disorders. HUD patients with severe comorbid BDZ dependence seemed to indicate a greater frequency of cases of unsatisfactory social and leisure time. Their elapsed time from the onset of heroin use to initial treatment was longer, but their illness (heroin addiction) at treatment entry was less severe. Concomitant use of cannabinoids was less frequent.

Patients belonging to the two groups did not differ significantly in data for somatic complications, work, family problems, romantic concerns, legal problems,

Table 3.2 Significant differences in clinical and addiction history aspects of heroin addicts with and without comorbid benzodiazepine dependence at treatment entry

	Heroin addicts			
	Without BDZ dependence	With BDZ dependence		
	$N = 63$	$N = 14$	χ/T	p
No. mental status altered areas ($M \pm$ SD)	3.26 ± 2.0	6.28 ± 0.6	-5.97	0.000
Consciousness ($N(\%)$)	0 (0.0)	2 (14.3)	9.24	0.031
Depression ($N(\%)$)	37 (58.7)	13 (92.9)	5.85	0.015
Sleep ($N(\%)$)	29 (46.0)	11 (78.6)	4.85	0.028
Excitement ($N(\%)$)	21 (33.3)	11 (78.6)	9.65	0.002
Violence ($N(\%)$)	19 (30.2)	11 (78.6)	11.28	0.001
Suicidality ($N(\%)$)	5 (7.9)	5 (35.7)	7.82	0.005
Delusions ($N(\%)$)	3 (4.8)	4 (28.6)	7.85	0.005
Hallucinations ($N(\%)$)	0 (0.0)	3 (21.4)	14.04	0.000
Concomitant use of cannabinoids	61 (96.8)	11 (78.6)	6.28	0.012
Social and leisure, unsatisfactory ($N(\%)$)	34 (54.0)	12 (85.7)	4.80	0.036
Elapsed time from first use to first treatment (years) ($M \pm$ SD)	9.90 ± 6.7	5.07 ± 3.7	2.59	0.012
CGI-severity of illness[a] ($M \pm$ SD)	5.54 ± 0.6	5.07 ± 0.7	2.33	0.041

[a] Rated on a 7-point scale (from normal to among the most extremely ill)

polydrug use (more than three substances), past unsuccessful treatments, general social adjustment (according to *DSM-IV* GAF values), frequency of heroin intake (i.e. less than frequent, daily or more than daily), modality of use (stable, unstable), periodic self-detoxification, stage of heroin dependence (stages 1 and 2, stage 3), antecedents (without stressors, with bio-psychosocial stressors), age at first contact with heroin, age at onset of continuous heroin use, dependence length (months), age at first treatment and elapsed time from first contact to continuous use. Using Cox regression life table statistics and stepwise forward (Wald) method ($\chi^2 = 5.17$; df = 1; $p = 0.023$), a better retention rate was found for patients with satisfactory social leisure time ($p = 0.027$).

Regarding the outcome of patients, as related to severe comorbid BDZ dependence, at the end of the observational period, 12 (19.0%) patients without severe BDZ dependence and 4 (28.6%) with it completed their rehabilitation programme and left the treatment or were referred to another programme as a 'stabilized patient'. Thirty-two (50.8%) patients without severe BDZ dependence and six (42.9%) with it had failed to achieve stabilization within a year or relapsed into heroin use during the programme, so for them treatment was terminated and they were referred to their local treatment services. None of the patients were dismissed for violence; none gave up the treatment for side effects; none were imprisoned or hospitalized. Nineteen (30.2%) patients without BDZ severe dependence and four (28.6%) with it were 'stabilized' and were still in treatment at the end of the period of observation. These differences were not statistically significant ($\chi^2 = 0.65$; df = 2; $p = 0.720$).

The CGI and GAF showed different significant trends in our patients. Comorbid BDZ patients with severe dependence reported, at the end-point evaluation, lower severity of illness (1.96 ± 0.9) than patients without comorbid severe BDZ dependence (3.07 ± 0.8). Time effect (F = 1816.51; df = 1; p = 0.000), time-group effect (F = 19.23; df = 1; p = 0.000) and time-outcome effect (F = 40.42; df = 1; p = 0.000) were significant. Time-group differences were not related to the outcome (F = 0.52; df = 1; p = 0.472). At the end-point evaluation comorbid BDZ patients with severe dependence reported a better social adjustment (76.93 ± 6.8) than patients without severe comorbid BDZ dependence (70.35 ± 9.3). Time effect (F = 310.43; df = 1; p = 0.000), time-group effect (F = 5.25; df = 1; p = 0.025) and time-outcome effect (F = 5.88; df = 1; p = 0.018) were significant. Time-group differences were not related to the outcome (F = 0.09; df = 1; p = 0.756).

Sixty-three patients without comorbid severe BDZ dependence and 14 with it were observed for 1 year; 35 without severe comorbid BDZ dependence and 13 with it for 2 years; 28 without severe comorbid BDZ dependence and 9 with it for 3 years; 22 without severe comorbid BDZ dependence and 18 with it for 4 years; 17 without severe comorbid BDZ dependence and 7 with it for 5 years; 15 without severe comorbid BDZ dependence and 6 with it for 6 years; 13 without severe comorbid BDZ dependence and 6 with it for 7 years and 10 without severe comorbid BDZ dependence and 6 with it for 8 years. Twenty-four patients (38.0%) without severe comorbid BDZ dependence and 1 (7.0%) with it failed to achieve the stabilization phase in 1 year; 4 (11.4%) without severe comorbid BDZ dependence and 4 (30.7%) relapsed during the second year of treatment; 1 (3.5%) without severe comorbid BDZ dependence relapsed during the third year; and 3 (13.6%) without severe comorbid BDZ dependence and 1 (12.5%) with it during the fourth. Neither patients with nor those without severe comorbid BDZ dependence relapsed into addictive behaviour after 4 years of treatment. The cumulative proportion of patients without severe comorbid BDZ dependence surviving at the end of the observational period was 0.44. The proportion for patients with severe comorbid BDZ dependence was 0.58. The higher, but not statistically significant (p = 0.082) survival rate for patients with severe comorbid BDZ dependence was due to the greater number of subjects who stayed in treatment rather than to a difference in the number of patients who left the programme with a positive outcome (detoxified after a period of MMT or referred, once stabilized, to other programmes), as the latter parameter was not modified by the presence or absence of severe comorbid BDZ dependence (Fig. 3.1). Females (0.52) and males (0.44) showed similar retention rates (Wilcoxon statistics = 0.04; df = 1; p = 0.837). Males with (0.38) and without (0.46) severe comorbid BDZ dependence showed no significant differences between their respective retention rates (Wilcoxon statistics = 0.77; df = 1; p = 0.379). Females showed a full retention rate (1.00) compared with participants showing a lack of severe comorbid BDZ dependence (0.39). This difference was statistically significant (Wilcoxon statistics = 3.87; df = 1; p = 0.049).

On average, patients with severe comorbid BDZ dependence needed a higher methadone dosage in the stabilization phase (190.73 ± 103.4 mg/day) than those without severe comorbid BDZ dependence (105.73 ± 40.7 mg/day). This difference was statistically significant ($F = 9.52$; $p = 0.000$). No differences were observed according to the outcome ($F = 0.12$; $p = 0.724$) or according to the group-outcome effect ($F = 2.41$; $p = 0.124$). In the comorbid group, BDZ dependence was treated systematically, according to the following procedure, which is very similar to an agonist substitution approach. We started switching patients from the use of BDZ to a slow-onset, long-acting, high-potency BDZ agonist (clonazepam). As the dosage of the used BDZ was progressively lowered, clonazepam dosage was progressively raised until the substitution was complete. In this way, the patient stopped his/her primary use of BDZ without any switch from intoxication to withdrawal states. Patients then passed through four successive phases: induction, stabilization, maintenance and, whenever possible, medication withdrawal. This methodology was recently set out by Liebrenz et al. in BDZ-dependent patients [511]. For more information on this procedure, see Maremmani et al. [401].

When the toxicological examination performed at the time of enrolment in the programme (which was required to be positive) was eliminated from the analysis, 11,002 urine samples were analysed in all: 2422 for 16 patients dismissed with a positive outcome, 1776 for 38 patients with a negative outcome and 6805 for 23 patients who stayed in treatment throughout the observation period. A total of 8056 samples taken from patients without severe comorbid BDZ dependence were examined, and a further 6805 from those with severe comorbid BDZ dependence. On average, 76.0% of these samples tested negative for morphine. No patient provided positive samples for the entire duration of treatment. No patient provided exclusively negative samples. In patients who left the programme with a positive outcome, the urinalysis index was 91.00 ± 4.3; in patients with a negative outcome, it was 62.13 ± 9.2; in patients still in treatment, it was 88.65 ± 4.6. These differences were statistically significant ($F = 73.67$; df = 2; $p = 0.000$) when comparing positive and negative outcomes, but not between patients who left the programme with a positive outcome and those still in treatment ($p = 0.342$). No differences were observed between patients without and with severe comorbid BDZ dependence ($F = 0.44$; $p = 0.509$). The group-outcome interaction was not significant either ($F = 0.18$; $p = 0.813$). The index in long-term-treated patients revealed differences ($F = 53.31$; df = 2; $p = 0.000$) between different outcomes: positive (0.36 ± 0.2), negative (0.07 ± 0.0) and still in treatment (0.67 ± 0.2). Differences were also observed between patients with (0.47 ± 0.3) and those without (0.28 ± 0.3) severe comorbid BDZ dependence ($F = 13.81$; df = 1; $p = 0.000$). The group-outcome interaction was not significant ($F = 2.44$; df = 2; $p = 0.094$). In summary, differences were found regarding urinalyses for morphine between patients with and without severe comorbid BDZ dependence only when we considered a long-term result index.

In conclusion, we can now observe that:

- Groups differed at baseline in terms of number of altered mental status areas, frequency of unsatisfactory social and leisure time, time lapse from initial heroin use to initial treatment, severity of illness (heroin addiction) and concomitant use of cannabinoids.

These data agree with the observations of Drake et al. [486] regarding the possibility that MMT patients with BDZ dependence may belong to a dysfunctional group. The differences found by us did not, however, appear to be related to the better retention or better outcome of patients with severe concomitant BDZ dependence.

Patients with severe concomitant BDZ dependence were retained in treatment for longer, especially if women; they showed no differences in rates of opioid-negative urine specimens and, when using a long-term result index, they showed better outcomes; they required higher doses of methadone than patients without severe comorbid BDZ dependence.

The outcome and the retention rate in the application of therapy to our treatment-resistant patients with or without severe comorbid BDZ dependence did not differ from that of long-term standard MMT programmes [491–496]. The main difference between our programme and the standard Italian MMT lies in the amount of methadone administered during the stabilization phase; this ranges from 80 to 400 mg/day in our protocols and from 40 to 100 mg/day in standard protocols. A possible explanation for the need for these relatively higher doses in patients who have previously been unresponsive to standard treatments may be related to a pharmacokinetic and/or pharmacodynamic mechanism. Methadone is metabolized in the liver by the P450 cytochrome system and, more specifically, by the CYP3A4 isoform, which is involved in the metabolism of over 50% of the medical agents [497, 498]. The wide inter-individual variability [499–504] recorded and the fact that CYP3A4 can be induced by several active principles [505, 506] may explain why a number of patients are under-medicated if a standard dose of methadone is used.

Unfortunately, we did not measure plasma methadone levels in our patients during the stabilization phase, so we cannot determine whether the doses used were necessary to maintain a proper therapeutic window or to control an underlying underestimated psychopathology.

In selecting our patients, only axis I psychiatric disorders were taken into consideration, and the existence of a minor form of psychopathology in the other patients hidden under the main addictive symptoms cannot be excluded. There is significant overlapping between behaviours in some types of psychiatric disorders and drug-related behaviours: maladaptive behaviours, such as those commonly displayed by drug addicts, may sometimes be due to, or exacerbated by, concurrent psychiatric disorders. Thus, a low degree of compliance with therapies is a common symptom of drug addiction and of several forms of psychiatric disorders [194, 507–509]. However, patients were followed up for 3 years on average, and diagnoses were subject to revision whenever further clinical evidence or retrospective information was gathered—a factor that reduces the likelihood of false absence of DD patients. Moreover, the duration of addiction was such as to make it improbable that subjects assessed as being without dual disorder had a silent psychiatric history. The availability of significant others was itself extremely helpful in increasing the level of diagnostic accuracy. In addition, we found that the outcome of MMT patients with or without dual disorder is the same in the short [55] and long term [56].

The fact that females with severe comorbid BDZ dependence stayed longer in treatment that peers without such dependence is an important gender-specific difference. Gender and racial/ethnic differences have been found in addiction severity, HIV risk and quality of life among adult HUD patients [512]. Our findings may indicate the need to require separate gender-oriented therapeutic interventions in heroin addiction.

The high GAF score values recorded for our patients with comorbid BDZ severe dependence and without hospitalizations throughout the treatment period showed that these subjects were simultaneously compliant both with MMT requirements and with the specific BDZ therapy adopted.

Additional medication (clonazepam was used systematically by us) for the treatment of BDZ use—a medication not completely changed by the need to treat addiction—may partly explain the more positive outcomes obtained in our comorbid patients, which cannot be attributed exclusively to the effects of methadone. A lack, whether of appropriately flexible methadone doses and/or of specific medications given in association with methadone treatment for these patients, could have been responsible for the conflicting results obtained by other researchers, who reported that BDZ and alcohol use were linked to worse treatment outcomes (retention in treatment) [479–483]. In addition, psychotherapeutic support provided by our team and the high therapeutic pressure of our programme could have been responsible for better results [510].

In any case, the incisiveness of our study was limited by several factors, such as the observational nature of the protocol, the impossibility of evaluating a follow-up in the case of the patients who dropped out, the multiple interference caused by inter-individual variability (personality traits and their neurobiological correlates), the clinical setting and the temporary use of adjunctive medications.

The main conclusions to be drawn from our results were:

- In the presence of problematic non-compliant patients with a comorbid BDZ severe dependence, a flexible dosing regimen that permits the administration of higher doses may lead to higher retention rates. The relevance of the present data becomes clearer when we consider that 35% of patients entering methadone treatment are 'regular/problem users' [478].
- Patients with comorbid BDZ severe dependence, treated with higher dosages of methadone and co-treated with CMT, may have outcomes that are as satisfactory as those without comorbid BDZ dependence, as long as they are maintained on their medication in the long term.

3.4   Proposal

The following strategies, which are derived from the clinical practice of our research group, are proposed as guidelines to the treatment of patients with DD (HUD and anxiety disorders):

- Restrict the medical use of BDZs to acute episodes of anxiety (excluding panic attacks) or to states of psychomotor agitation, especially in psychotic patients.
- Always keep in mind the addictive potential of BDZs.
- Never give BDZs to opioid use patients during the withdrawal syndrome, especially if they are BDZ 'naïve', as BDZs have strong rewarding power in tolerant withdrawal subjects and there is a risk of inducing a BDZ addiction.
- Do not detoxify HUD patients using BDZs.
- Do not use BDZs in opioid-intoxicated patients or in treatment with buprenorphine and methadone, if their tolerance to opioids is not yet known; otherwise, these patients will run the risk of narcosis and respiratory arrest.
- Do not use BDZs for agitation (otherwise infrequent) or insomnia in patients treated with opioid agonists. Central anti-histamine medications are to be preferred.
- Do not use BDZs to treat anxiety in HUD patients. Use the anxiolytic properties of certain SSRIs, such as paroxetine or fluvoxamine, always considering the effects of these drugs on the opioid system.
- Use the anxiolytic properties, already present at low doses, of long-half-life opioid drugs. Prefer buprenorphine.
- Associate BDZs with methadone and buprenorphine only in patients with double addiction. Craving for BDZs cannot be fully controlled by therapeutic opioids.
- Associate BDZs with therapeutic opioids only in BDZ-tolerant patients. In the case of BDZ withdrawal syndrome, that syndrome is initially masked by the onset of opioid therapy.
- Prefer BDZs that are not metabolized by the liver and that have low addictive power (i.e. those with high intrinsic power, delayed initial action and long-acting), such as clonazepam.

4.1 Vulnerability, Neurotransmitter Pathway and Clinical Presentations of Psychosis in Substance Use Disorder Patients

The presence of psychotic symptoms is widespread in psychiatric disorders. Delusions and hallucinations, which are among the main symptoms of psychosis, belong to the schizophrenic spectrum. In the bipolar disorder, manic or depressive episodes, as well as mixed states, are frequently marked by psychotic symptoms. Moreover, psychosis may set in after SUD, often intervening with the effect of making the clinical picture indistinguishable from that of a primary psychosis. Psychosis induced by the non-medical use of substances is most commonly developed by cannabinoids [23, 24, 150, 513–516], stimulants [517–520], hallucinogens [521, 522], alcohol [523–525] and poly-use [526]. Among SUD users, it has not yet been ascertained whether opioids exert a psychotic effect, but some authors have supported the view that opioids have antidepressant, antipanic and antipsychotic effects [158, 527, 528]. We investigated the relationship between SUD and psychosis using as variables of interest (a) vulnerability to psychosis, (b) the development of psychosis during an intoxication or withdrawal state, (c) the clinical presentation, (d) the role of gender and (e) the neurotransmitter pathway involved [51]. More specifically, we intended to shed light on the various correlations between opioids and other substances of use in developing or acting against psychosis. Table 4.1 reports the main characteristics of substance-induced psychosis.

4.1.1 Alcohol and Psychosis

Only a few epidemiological findings on alcohol-induced psychotic disorder and delirium (alcohol-induced psychotic syndrome, AIPS) are currently available. In one inquiry on a sample of 8028 subjects drawn from the general population of

I. Maremmani et al., *Dual Disorder Heroin Addicts*,
https://doi.org/10.1007/978-3-031-30093-6_4

Table 4.1 Substance use disorder and psychosis

	Cannabis	Amphetamines	Cocaine	Hallucinogens	Inhalants	Alcohol	Opioids
Clinical presentation	Violence	Violence	Paranoia	Unusual experience	Bizarre delusion	Jealousy, delirium tremens, hallucinosis	Not clearly described
Intoxication or withdrawal psychosis?	Intoxication	Intoxication withdrawal	Intoxication withdrawal	Intoxication withdrawal	Intoxication withdrawal	Intoxication withdrawal	Withdrawal
Gender	M = F (M > F?)	M = F	M = F	?	?	M ≠ F	?
Vulnerability	Schizotypical genes	Family history of mental illness	Paranoicism during cocaine use	Family history of psychotic illness	Family history of mental illness	Presence of psychopathology	Presence of psychopathology
Neurotransmitter pathway involved	Endocannabinoid system	Dopaminergic system	Dopaminergic system	Glutamatergic system	Glutamatergic system	GABA system	Opioidergic system

Finland, the topics chosen for investigation were the epidemiology of AIPS, the risk factors for developing AIPS among people with alcohol dependence and mortality associated with AUD, with or without AIPS. The lifetime prevalence was 0.5% for AIPS and was highest (1.8%) in men of working age. Younger age at the onset of AUD, low socioeconomic status, problems with father's mental health or alcohol use and multiple hospital treatments were associated with an increased risk of AIPS. Participants with a history of AIPS reported a considerable level of medical comorbidity [523]. Some studies have shown that the major differences observed between AUD patients and controls, in terms of psychopathology, and represented by symptoms pertaining to mood, anxiety and externalizing disorder domains, fall below the diagnostic threshold [529, 530]. AIPD seems to be a discrete clinical entity that can be differentiated from schizophrenia and uncomplicated AUD; its reported features are a significantly lower educational level, later onset of psychosis, higher levels of depressive and anxiety symptoms, fewer negative and disorganized symptoms, better insight and judgement and less functional impairment compared with patients with schizophrenia [525]. Proneness to alcohol use has been studied at the temperamental level, where AUD patients turned out to differ significantly from controls in terms of cyclothymic traits, including a depressive component [77, 531].

There is good evidence for a direct involvement of the cortical gamma-aminobutyric acid (GABAergic) system in the long-term administration of alcohol. An indirect genetic link between the GABA-A receptor and schizophrenia or other psychoses has been reported. One important implication of considering GABA interneurons as playing a pivotal role in psychotic disorders like schizophrenia is the potential excitotoxicity which GABA inhibition might generate through increased glutamate transmission to the cortex. The profound and enduring memory impairments and the progressive enlargement of lateral ventricles that accompany chronic schizophrenia may be a consequence of GABA imbalance, which is not necessarily reversed by the antipsychotic drugs that act on the dopamine and serotonin systems [532].

The psychotic manifestations of physical and psychiatric disorders in cases of alcoholism have been well documented; however, the distinctions between the various disorders remain less well defined. Individuals often have comorbid elements belonging to several disorders, and the psychotic phenomena are often differentiated. Psychotic manifestations of alcohol withdrawal include delirium tremens [533–535], alcohol hallucinosis, Wernicke-Korsakoff psychosis, alcohol pellagra and hepatic encephalopathy, Marchiafava-Bignami disease, central pontine myelinolysis and alcohol dementia [524]. This sindrome is characterized by an acute change in cognition and a disturbance of consciousness that is usually related to alcohol withdrawal, but that may also be associated with the presence of a hallucinatory state [533, 534, 536–538]. One striking case reported was of palinacousis during alcohol hallucinosis after remission from the acoustic hallucinations that are typical of the disorder [539]. About 30% of chronic AUD patients seem to suffer from morbid jealousy, which takes various forms. Some of the examined patients expressed it only when intoxicated, others even when sober; in some, their jealousy took the form of a delusional disorder. One conclusion to be drawn is that alcoholism appears to have an aetiological role in the development of morbid jealousy [540, 541].

Psychotic symptoms during alcohol use may be associated either with continuous use or with a withdrawal state. Psychotic manifestations of continuous use could lead to a jealousy delusion [540, 541], while delirium tremens and hallucinosis were involved in alcohol withdrawal psychosis [524, 533–535].

Women had a longer duration of illness before treatment and exhibited a greater number of affective symptoms, while men were more socially isolated and had a greater number of negative symptoms. Alcohol and drug use appeared significantly more frequently among men. Women received comparatively more heavily medicated treatments than men [542].

4.1.2 Cannabis and Psychosis

Gender did not seem to be involved in the onset of psychosis; this highlights the finding that cannabis is a dangerous, unspecific drug in young people at risk of developing psychosis [514, 515, 543]. It must, however, be pointed out that men who consume cannabis run a higher risk of developing psychosis than women. In a 3-year study, the researchers assessed a total of 535 people with a cannabis-induced psychosis, and the rate for developing schizophrenia was 47.6% in males vs. 29.8% in women [544].

Converging lines of evidence suggest that cannabinoids can produce a full range of transient schizophrenia-like positive, negative and cognitive symptoms in some healthy individuals. It is also clear that in individuals with an established psychotic disorder, cannabinoids can exacerbate symptoms, trigger relapse and have negative consequences on the course of the illness. The mechanisms by which cannabinoids produce transient psychotic symptoms, while still unclear, may involve dopamine, GABA and glutamate neurotransmission. A variety of factors have been proposed to mediate an individual's vulnerability to the harmful effects of the drug, one of which is their proneness to psychosis. Smoking cannabis in a naturalistic setting reliably induced marked increases in psychotomimetic symptoms. Highly psychosis-prone individuals experienced enhanced psychotomimetic states following acute cannabis use, which suggests that an individual's response to acute cannabis use and his/her psychosis-proneness scores are related and that both may be markers of vulnerability to this drug's harmful effects [545].

Schizotypy, for instance, was associated with more frequent psychosis-like experiences and their after-effects, and high-scoring schizotypy patients reported more pleasurable experiences when smoking cannabis, so suggesting that cannabis use may reveal an underlying vulnerability to psychosis in those with high-scoring schizotypal traits [546, 547]. Looking now at the relationship between cannabis use and psychosis, the role of affective disorders is often undervalued. Bipolar I resembles the schizoaffective disorder, in its schizovariant, and SUD is rather common in bipolar subjects, especially those with a chronic relapsing course, so that chronic psychosis may be an artefact of enduring substance use. The proneness to use shown by bipolar subjects across the whole bipolar spectrum may be a crucial link with atypical bipolar pictures involving chronic psychotic symptoms. On this view, a trait-dependent behaviour of taking psychotogenic drugs may justify the independent chronicity of bipolar 1 subjects with comorbidity for SUD; if correct, this perspective would tend to assign schizoaffective disorders to the bipolar spectrum, as an extreme, atypical variant [548]. In schizophrenic patients, the risk of developing cannabis use disorder is six times what it is in the general population. Despite this, only a very small proportion of the general population exposed to cannabinoids develop a psychotic illness. It is likely that cannabis exposure is a 'component cause' that interacts with other factors to 'cause' schizophrenia or a psychotic disorder, without this being either necessary or sufficient by itself to induce this result [549]. In the absence of known causes of schizophrenia, the role of component causes remains important and warrants further study. Dose, duration of exposure and age at first exposure to cannabinoid along with genetic factors that interact with exposure to cannabinoids to moderate or amplify the risk of a psychotic disorder, are all beginning to be elucidated [550, 551]. Debates on the real chronology of the appearance of psychiatric disorders and addictive cannabis behaviour are on-going, and cannabis continues to appear as a risk factor for psychotic disorders, because it interacts with a pre-existing vulnerability [552].

While the epidemiological signal between cannabis and psychosis has gained considerable attention, the biological mechanism through which cannabis increases the risk of psychosis remains poorly understood. The endocannabinoid system plays an important role in fundamental brain developmental processes such as neuronal cell proliferation, migration and differentiation. As a result, changes in endocannabinoid activity during this specific developmental phase, induced by the psychoactive component of marijuana, THC, might lead to subtle but lasting neurobiological changes that may affect brain functions and behaviour, so increasing the risk of contracting certain neuropsychiatric diseases such as schizophrenia [553]. Animal research that has been focused on the psychotomimetic effects of cannabis [554] suggests that THC increases dopamine levels in several regions of the brain, including the striatal and prefrontal areas. On the other hand, cannabidiol (CBD), the main non-psychotropic component of the *Cannabis sativa* plant, has shown therapeutic potential in several neuropsychiatric disorders [555, 556]. Different types of cannabis (i.e. marijuana and hashish) have distinctive proportions of THC and CBD. In a sample of subjects who had used the same type of cannabis on most occasions, an inverse relationship was found between CBD content and self-reported positive symptoms, but not with negative symptoms or depression; the use of cannabis with a high CBD content was associated with a significantly lower incidence of psychotic symptoms, so providing further support for the hypothesis of the antipsychotic potential of cannabidiol [557].

Cannabis-induced psychoses were distinguished by unusual thought content, excitement, hallucinatory behaviour and uncooperativeness. The least common symptoms were anxiety, guilt feelings, depressive mood, motor retardation and blunted affect. Cognitive dysfunctions were described, too. Those with cannabis-related psychosis presented with a predominantly affective psychosis and prominent thought disorder, excitement and violence and later presented with an improvement in symptoms if there had been abstinence from cannabis [558]. Another study similarly reported the presence of less blunted affect, more clastic aggression and violence towards others, with respect to functional psychosis [516].

The relationship found in some patients between cannabis use and an earlier onset of psychotic illness can now be more clearly understood [23–25, 513, 543, 559–561]. A significant gradual reduction in age at the onset of psychosis was found as dependence on cannabis increased, consisting in a progressive fall in the number of years for users, misusers and dependents, with respect to non-users. For psychotic symptoms, a dose-related effect of cannabis use was seen, with vulnerable groups including individuals who used cannabis during adolescence, those who had previously experienced psychotic symptoms and those running a high genetic risk of developing schizophrenia. Cannabis seems to be an independent risk factor, both for psychosis and for the development of psychotic symptoms [549]. In addition, studies on sibling pairs have provided further support for the hypothesis that early cannabis use is a risk-modifying factor for psychosis-related outcomes in young adults [562].

4.1.3 Amphetamines and Psychosis

There were no significant differences between men and women with regard to age, ethnicity, years of use, route of administration or amount used in the most recent period before the onset of psychosis. During drug use periods, women were more likely than men to report delusions of grandeur, paranoia and tactile hallucinations, while in non-use periods, women were significantly more likely than men to report the feeling that something was wrong with the way a part of their body looked, olfactory hallucinations and dressing inappropriately [563]. In reviewing the general picture, women seem more dependent on and committed to meta-amphetamines (MA), but show diminished (amphetamine-stimulated) dopamine responses and a less severe degree of toxicity, as indicated by a lower incidence of emergency department-related deaths involving MA [564].

Patients who have already developed psychosis are probably more inclined to experiment again with the use of amphetamines. Moreover, Ecstasy is frequently used by youngsters, in whom psychopathological symptoms will inevitably occur regardless of whether they continue to use it. The presence of a personal or family history of psychiatric disorders is important in determining the onset of psychosis [565, 566], although some authors have reported cases of psychosis that occurred in individuals who had no history of psychiatric disorders or positive precedents in their family [567, 568]. It must therefore be concluded that the relationship between ecstasy use and psychosis onset has not yet been clearly established. Ecstasy could directly induce psychotic symptoms or act as a trigger on susceptible individuals.

The severity of psychotic symptoms, including negative ones, observed in psychotic and in schizophrenic patients taking Ecstasy is very similar [517].

MA psychosis, with rapid onset and poor prognosis, seems to be related to genetic variants of the D2 but not the D3 or D4 dopamine receptor gene [569]. As previously mentioned, amphetamine use is related to higher levels of aggression, but the underlying processes or mechanisms remain somewhat elusive. The neurotoxic pharmacological effects of amphetamine on the dopaminergic and serotonergic systems are related to aggressive, hostile behaviour in both animal and human studies. Of particular interest is the converging evidence that amphetamine use is related to the impairment of executive functions (including self-control) that are regulated by the prefrontal cortex. Taken together, these findings suggest that amphetamine users may have an impaired capacity to control or inhibit aggressive impulses. In addition, high levels of impulsivity related to amphetamine use may also play a role [570].

Aggressiveness and violent behaviour are the most common effects related to the use of Ecstasy, and these issues have been explored in some inquiries [571, 572]. A higher level of violence seems to be present not only in active Ecstasy users, but in abstinent users, too [573]. MA use is associated with hostility, aggression and positive psychotic symptoms. This pattern of findings suggests that MA use leads to greater hostility by increasing positive psychotic symptoms that contribute to a perception of the environment as a hostile, threatening place as well as by increasing impulsivity. Those who had high scores for positive symptoms and impulsivity were the most hostile [574]. Regrettably, these studies often fail to reveal whether patients only used Ecstasy. Acute psychotic users showed 'less blunted affect' and more 'clastic aggression' and 'violence towards others' than psychotic non-users, while 'verbal aggression' and 'self-harm behaviour (SHB)' were present with equal frequency. Despite the fact that Ecstasy users take the substance in view of its supposed empathetic/entactogenic effects and to achieve a heightened sense of closeness with other people, in asymptomatic patients Ecstasy causes an opposite effect to that being sought, by increasing impulsive and violent behaviours [575]. Lastly, amphetamine use is associated with increased positive symptoms of psychosis, particularly paranoia, which contributes to a perception of the environment as a hostile, threatening place [570].

Psychotic symptoms attributable to an intensive use of Ecstasy have been widely documented [518, 568, 576–582] and persecutory delusions are the most common presentation [565, 583]. Psychological complications following the use of ecstasy are rare, but, when they do occur, they are really severe [584]. In some cases, there is the persistence of psychopathology, even when the substance is no longer being taken [567, 585–587]. Persistent psychosis is a common finding in heavy, chronic users of Ecstasy, but some authors have documented cases in which psychotic symptoms occur after a single recreational dose of Ecstasy [584, 588].

4.1.4   Cocaine and Psychosis

Among cocaine users, there were no significant differences between men and women with regard to ethnicity, years of use, route of administration and amount used in the past week, though they differed significantly in terms of age. During a period of non-use, women were significantly more likely than men to report experiencing auditory hallucinations and tactile hallucinations, whereas men were more likely to report delusions of grandeur. During a period of drug use, women were significantly more likely than men to report delusions of grandeur, tactile hallucinations and olfactory ones [563]. In a study that examined subjective and physiological responses to cocaine smoking, those who reported feeling paranoid/suspicious were more likely to be elderly and male [589].

Experiencing transient paranoia in heavy cocaine users during intoxication could be the highest risk factor for developing psychosis; this danger does not exist with cocaine users who do not experience paranoia [590]. Factors underlying the development and severity of cocaine-induced psychosis (CIP) are still poorly understood [591]. To date, it has been reported that an early age of initiation of regular cocaine use occurring during vulnerable periods of brain development may lead to the increased severity of these paranoic events [520, 592]. Of course, an onset of cannabis use during adolescence can increase the risk of CIP in cocaine-dependent individuals [593]—a risk that may be present in cases of the antisocial personality disorder too [594].

Amount and duration of use are related to the development of psychosis, in which a kindling model of cocaine-induced psychosis seems to be implicated [595]. The fact that paranoia became more severe and developed more rapidly with continued drug use is consistent with a sensitization model of cocaine-induced paranoia [596, 597]. In vulnerable individuals, limbic sensitization may underlie its expression, but the hypothesis of localization in a specific brain region is still speculative [590].

In a clinical setting, it may be difficult to differentiate a cocaine-induced psychotic group from a schizophrenic one; both of these groups feel fear that individuals or organized groups may harm them in some way, but the delusions of paranoid schizophrenic subjects are more often bizarre than those of cocaine use subjects. 'Cocaine bugs' (parasitosis) were a perception more often found in cocaine use subjects. Command hallucinations were found in both groups, but in the schizophrenic group the commands perceived were more often related to harming or killing others. Cocaine users had a more frequent sensation of visual hallucinations, distinguished by shadows, flashing lights ('snow lights'), objects moving and bugs crawling on their arms. The most distinctive characteristics were identity delusions, possession delusions, grandiosity delusions (besides those involving identities and possessions) and delusions in which 'family members' were impostors (Capgras syndrome) reported by paranoid schizophrenics. Cocaine users did not report any such delusions [598].

Psychotic symptoms and experiences of paranoia and suspiciousness are reported during the use and withdrawal of cocaine. Furthermore, although psychotic symptoms were found to be common among substance users, there was also a risk of a chronic psychotic disorder developing [518].

4.1.5   Hallucinogens and Psychosis

Few studies have been dedicated to the role of gender in hallucinogen use. Some studies have shown that female rats tended to self-administer ketamine more rapidly and took more of the drug than male rats [599, 600].

In some individuals who have affected family members, psychosis may be predictable, but the specific symptom profile may not be. A placebo-controlled study on healthy individuals investigated whether individual variability in baseline physiology, as assessed using functional magnetic resonance imaging, permitted the psychosis elicited by the psychotomimetic drug ketamine to be predicted. Brain responses to cognitive task demands after a placebo had been taken predict the expression of psychotic phenomena after drug administration. Front-thalamic responses to a working memory task were associated with the tendency of subjects to experience negative symptoms when taking ketamine. Similarly, bilateral frontal responses to an attention task were predictive of negative symptoms. Frontotemporal activations during language processing tasks were predictive of thought disorders and illusory auditory experiences. A sub-psychotic dose of ketamine administered during a second scanning session resulted in increased basal ganglia and thalamic activation during the working memory task, in parallel with previous reports on schizophrenic patients [601]. A personal or a family history of psychotic disorders and other severe psychiatric disorders is considered to be a risk factor for the development of psychotic symptoms during the use of ketamine [602].

The psychosis-inducing effect of ketamine provides important evidence in support of the glutamate hypothesis of schizophrenia [603–605]. The discriminative stimulus effects of LSD (lysergic acid diethylamide) in rats occur in two temporal phases, with the initial effects mediated by the activation of 5-HT2A receptors and the later temporal phase mediated by dopamine D2-like receptors [521]. This behavioural effect is not blocked by haloperidol—a finding which supports the idea of mediation through the N-methyl-D-aspartic acid (NMDA) receptor [606]. Glutamatergic neurons are the major excitatory pathways linking the cortex, the limbic system and thalamus, regions that have been implicated in schizophrenia. The NMDA subtype of glutamate receptor may be particularly important in enacting a blockade of this receptor by the dissociative anaesthetics that reproduce in normal subjects the symptomatic manifestations of schizophrenia, including negative symptoms and cognitive impairments, while dopamine release increases in the mesolimbic system [603].

Phencyclidine (PCP)-induced psychosis incorporates both positive (e.g. hallucinations and paranoia) and negative (e.g. emotional withdrawal and motor retardation) schizophrenic symptoms. PCP-induced psychosis also uniquely incorporates the formal thought disorder and neuropsychological deficits associated with schizophrenia. Hallucinogens are capable of producing florid psychotic states in individuals who have misused them, and it should also be noted that, when given to healthy volunteers, drug-induced paranoia, perceptual changes and a wide range of other symptoms occur including disorganization of thought, negativism, apathy, withdrawal, poverty of speech, perseveration and catatonic posturing [607]. In stable schizophrenic volunteers, ketamine is able to induce a dose-dependent, short-lived increase in psychotic symptoms, often reminiscent of their own acute symptoms. With regard to functional psychosis, patients taking ketamine seem to have a significantly shorter stay in hospital, and were treated more aggressively with conventional antipsychotics [522]. Comparing these kinds of symptoms with stimulant-induced psychosis, PCP-induced psychoses were less strongly associated with suspiciousness and more strongly associated with delusions of physical power, altered sensations and unusual experiences (e.g. out-of-body experiences and experiencing religious figures or events directly, as in a patient's report of being 'with Noah at the time of the Ark') [608]. On some occasions, acute PCP-induced psychosis in normal persons is indistinguishable from an acute episode of schizophrenia [609].

Ketamine appeared to have four main effects:

- a general depressant and/or intoxicating effect on the central nervous system;
- perceptual alterations often referred to as 'dissociative', but not hallucinations;
- referential ideas or delusions, plus other subjective changes in thinking; and
- negative-type symptoms [610].

Even in healthy volunteers, ketamine induced psychotic symptoms [607]. There is a close relationship between PCP and psychosis. Low doses of PCP produce symptoms of inebriation and mild stimulation, while at higher doses it causes perceptual alteration, depersonalization and disturbances in cognition [611, 612]. The psychotropic effects of ketamine range from dissociation to psychotic experiences and include a sensation of feeling light, body distortion, absence of any sense of time, novel experiences of cosmic oneness and out-of-body experiences. Use of ketamine has typically been reported in individuals who use multiple drugs, and it seems to activate significant tolerance to the substance without prominent withdrawal symptoms [613]. The most likely risk of ketamine consumption is overwhelming distress during drug action (a 'bad trip'), which could lead to potentially dangerous behaviour. Prolonged psychoses triggered by hallucinogens are less common, and, even if rare, persistent adverse reactions can occur as well [602, 614].

4.1.6   Inhalants and Psychosis

No data pertinent to gender were found by us in the relationship between solvents and psychosis. A family history of psychiatric disorders seems to be a risk factor in the development of psychosis due to inhalants. In any case, fewer than 10% of these SUD patients had a family history of schizophrenia, and the development of inhalant-induced psychosis appeared after about 6 years of continuous use. These considerations suggest that chronic psychiatric symptoms are caused not only by inhalant use, but also by each patient's genetic factors, which may predispose him/her to psychosis [615].

The neuropharmacological effects of these solvents do not appear to be limited to modulation of the GABA receptor. Drug-discrimination studies using laboratory animals [616] have shown that toluene can induce subjective effects similar to those of the psychedelic anaesthetic PCP, suggesting that toluene, like PCP, may block the NMDA receptor. It should be noted, however, that toluene failed to induce subjective effects similar to those of dizocilpine, another selective NMDA receptor blocker, in a similar drug-discrimination study [617]. Exposure to toluene increases dopamine levels in the rat's prefrontal cortex and striatum and increases neuronal firing in the ventral tegmental area in a manner similar to that of other drugs of use—effects that could be intrinsic to the rewarding effects of toluene [618, 619].

The long-standing use of inhalants may evolve into severe psychosis resembling schizophrenia. Clinical presentations may be marked by serious disturbances, such as delusions of persecution, a bizarre delusion (e.g. that of having a five-headed snake inside one's body) and auditory hallucinations [620]. This clinical condition was shown in a young man who had no family history of schizophrenia; it was observed in the sober period when he was not under the influence of the thinner. Thus, it was difficult to diagnose this case as schizophrenia or as a flashback phenomenon due to thinner dependence [621, 622]. The symptomatological characteristics of solvent-induced psychosis and schizophrenia have been studied comparatively. The two conditions did not show any differences in age of onset or family history. These clinical observations lead to a very complex psychopathology, but they seem to stress the fact that the 'amotivational syndrome' may be a characteristic feature of patients suffering from solvent-induced psychosis and suggest that 'solvent psychosis' should be recognized as a discernible syndrome, to be distinguished from psychotic symptoms of typical schizophrenia [623]. To better understand the effects and the damage done by inhalants, animal models have been used. Exposure to toluene in adolescence leads to social deficits and cognitive impairment in adulthood, as well as neurochemical dysfunctions in mice, which correlate with the symptoms observed in patients suffering from solvent-induced psychosis [624]. Inhalant users with or without an inhalant use disorder (IUD), according to *DSM-IV*/*DSM-5* criteria, had greater levels of suicidal ideation and substance use problems than non-users. Youngsters with IUDs have personal histories marked out by high levels of trauma, suicidality, psychiatric distress, antisocial behaviour and substance-related problems. A monotonic relationship between inhalant use and dependence is known to lead to serious adverse outcomes [625].

Solvent-induced psychosis has been clinically identified among patients suffering from dependence on volatile solvents and those in a psychotic state as a result of chronic solvent use. Positive symptoms of schizophrenia have been reported, especially first rank symptoms, such as auditory hallucinations, and delusional perceptions, but not negative ones. Even if not in an intoxication phase, psychotic symptoms have also been observed in a period of abstinence, in the form of a flashback phenomenon [621, 622]. Besides this, by studying the symptomatological differences between solvent-induced psychosis and schizophrenia, it seems possible to recognize 'solvent psychosis' as a discernible syndrome to be distinguished from the psychotic symptoms of typical schizophrenia [623].

4.1.7   Opioids and Psychosis

In studies relying on the current research methodology, no data pertinent to gender were found in the relationship between opioids and psychosis.

In several studies, the prevalence of psychotic symptoms associated with opioids, covering a spectrum going from users with no diagnosis to those with severe dependence, ranges between 6.7% and 52.2% [526, 626]. One of our studies on 574 patients with DD showed a diagnosis of chronic psychosis in 15.5% of HUD patients [627]. Premorbid conditions such as temperamental assets, hyperactivity, impulsiveness, sensation-seeking, subthreshold and/or full-blown mental disorders related to mood, anxiety and impulse-control dimensions could increase vulnerability to substance use and/or progression to addiction [36]. Temperamental profile seems to play a crucial role at the beginning of substance use. Cyclothymic, and to a lesser extent irritable traits (the 'dark side'), may represent the temperamental profile of HUD, largely irrespective of comorbidity, and tend to cohere with previous conceptualizations that hypothesize 'sensation-seeking' (and 'novelty-seeking') as the main personality characteristics of addiction [78].

A dose of morphine blocks dopamine receptors and stimulates prolactin secretion, creating a significant elevation in basal serum prolactin [165, 628]. Opioid agonists are known to induce acute neuroleptic-like effects on the endocrine system, such as hyperprolactinaemia and the suppression of adrenal activity. Sedation may also take place when the tolerance threshold is exceeded during the induction phase of AOT [628, 629]. On neurochemical grounds, typical antipsychotics and opioids both act on the same neuronal targets and interfere with dopaminergic transmission, though they move along different molecular pathways [241]. Buprenorphine has shown it is active against hallucinations and delusions over a time-span of 4 h in a small group of heterogeneous psychotic patients [630]. Selective k-agonist receptors (such as pentazocine), on the other hand, have psychotomimetic properties [631, 632]: this toxicological property is in line with the finding that the levels of the endogenous selective k-agonist dynorphins are related to the severity of symptoms in schizophrenic subjects [633]. Opioid antagonism was also considered in relation to psychotic symptoms. For instance, naloxone administration did produce an improvement of symptoms in selected schizophrenic patients, but the results were not homogenous [634]. Subjects who were suffering from independent psychotic disorders were more likely to drop out of NTX treatment by the end of the first year [44].

Ultrarapid opioid detoxification is a procedure that uses high doses of opioid antagonists to precipitate rapid opioid withdrawal and could develop into a psychotic episode [635]. Even if uncommon, psychosis occurring after the discontinuation of buprenorphine has been described. The clinical presentation was characterized by mystical and paranoid delusions and intense auditory hallucinations [636].

The initial hypotheses formulated on a causal link between chronic morphine intake and the onset of psychosis [637, 638] were not confirmed by later studies [639, 640], and most studies on the epidemiology of DD have shown the low frequency of psychotic spectrum disorders in HUD patients and those in methadone treatment programmes. To the best of our knowledge, no studies have been published on psychosis due to opioid intoxication. On the other hand, there have been reports in the literature on psychotic episodes related to opioid withdrawal [635]. The gradual elimination of methadone in subjects affected by previous psychotic episodes was followed by psychotic relapses [427, 641]. Even if uncommon, psychosis occurring after the discontinuation of buprenorphine or other opioids has been described [636]; it usually disappeared after buprenorphine reintroduction [642].

4.2   Psychotic Chronicity and Schizoaffective Pictures

The pathogenesis of schizoaffective disorders is a controversial issue. On grounds of prognosis, premorbid status and familial history, schizoaffective disorders occupy an intermediate position between affective and non-affective psychoses [643]. Some authors hypothesized that affective disorders, coupled with genetic disposition, rather than affective disturbance or psychosis, result in either bipolar psychosis or schizoaffective disorder, respectively [644]. According to that model, inter-episodic psychotic symptoms may be combined with minor affective alterations, on the basis of a psychotic diathesis possibly expressed as a schizotypal personality picture [645]. A major limitation to further acknowledgements about schizoaffective pictures is that the two *DSM-IV* subtypes (schizoid-bipolar and schizoid-depressive) are often investigated as a unique entity and often grouped together with schizophrenia or schizophreniform disorder. In other studies, small schizoaffective samples are considered together with larger samples of schizophrenics [646–654]. In fact, the schizoid-bipolar form of illness, unlike the schizoid-depressive one, may otherwise belong primarily to the family of bipolar disorders [655], in line with a Kraepelinian view. On the other hand, studies based on RDC (research diagnostic criteria) [656] do not account for longitudinal differences, but focus on the presence of what are sometimes called 'schizophrenic symptoms', which do not seem to discriminate as far as outcome and longitudinal diagnosis are concerned.

The issue of independent psychotic chronicity has not been clarified satisfactorily on pathophysiological grounds, especially as far as concurrent substance use behaviour patterns are concerned.

Although the theoretical definition of schizoaffective disorder requires that a causal relationship between symptoms and substance use is ruled out, such a criterion has been dropped, for example, in the conception of the bipolar spectrum according to Akiskal and Pinto [84]: substance- or drug-induced mania can be viewed as a subtype of bipolar disorder and does not fall into a different category. Substance use and misuse may either induce stable psychotic syndromes or else psychotic symptoms may be maintained due to enduring substance self-administration. Used substances may just produce or favour neuronal activities that may otherwise happen spontaneously, through the same neurochemical processes and pathways, without any actual difference as to symptoms or pathophysiology.

4.3   Substance Use and the Chronic Course of Psychotic Symptoms

Studies focusing on substance-related acute episodes provide us with little help in clarifying the nature of substance-related chronic psychotic pictures, and no causal link between chronic substance use and chronic psychosis can be ascertained. On the other hand, the body of longitudinal studies investigating the impact of substance use on the incidence of psychotic disorders is quite limited, and the major study focuses on schizophrenia [657, 658]. Other authors suggest the resemblance of cannabis-related psychosis to schizophrenic pictures misusing such terms as schizophreniform or schizophrenic-like, which should be referred to as longitudinal patterns rather than acute episodes.

Subjects may become hypersensitive to the psychotic effects of certain drugs: as a consequence, the emergence and course of psychotic symptoms may start as a sharply SUD phenomenon, whereas later relapses may require lower charges of substances, possibly developing into a completely spontaneous chronic relapsing pattern.

As many as 8–11% of SUD patients do, in fact, develop a chronic psychotic disorder persisting months after the discontinuation of substance use [253, 659–661], especially as far as delusions are concerned [590, 662, 663]. Those subjects experience relapses after self-administering the same drugs again, although in single or smaller doses [664–669].

The clinical picture is distinguished by a lower prevalence rate of negative symptoms as measured by the Scale for Assessment of Negative Symptoms (SANS) [565, 670]. Although classic hallucinogenic drugs tend to be used transiently before addiction is established, substances commonly used by SUD patients (cocaine, cannabis and alcohol) are likely to induce psychotic symptoms when self-administered on a chronic basis. In a group of HUD (Maremmani, unpublished data), with a high rate of poly-use, screened by means of SCL90, paranoia and psychoticism as dimensions proved to be dominant in 10.0% and 10.4% of the patients tested, respectively. Such rates are far higher than those to be expected for schizophrenia or schizoaffective disorders [150, 157, 162, 640, 671]. This suggests that current or past SUD may relate to psychotic symptoms through a diagnostic cluster separate from schizophrenia and broader than schizoaffective disorders, such as bipolar psychosis. Chronic psychotic symptoms may therefore occur combined with diagnoses other than schizophrenia on the basis of the on-going use of psychotogenic drugs.

In populations of SUD patients, psychotic symptoms are more likely to be autonomous when used substances show weak psychotogenic properties. In the history of chronic psychotics, heroin use and dependence on it are rather infrequent, despite the presence of the high addictive potential of heroin itself and consistently with the psychotogenic effects of other substances commonly used by this population, such as cannabis, stimulants and alcohol [672]. On the other hand, non-affective psychotic disorders are the least common type of DD in methadone-maintained subjects [162]. Lastly, a 6-year follow-up of heroin users revealed no risk of developing any psychotic disorder [672].

4.4   Proneness to SUD and Proneness to Psychosis: Is There a Bipolar Connection?

The prevalence rate of lifetime and current SUD in patients with schizoaffective disorders seems to be higher than in schizophrenics and bipolars [673]. Schizoaffective disorder has a stronger lifetime link with SUD than with either bipolar disorder or schizophrenia and a current link similar to that of bipolar disorders. Though they derive from a smaller sample, such data suggest that substance use may have a precipitating effect on affective episodes of either disorder to a similar extent. As the number of hospitalizations was similar, substance use in the past seems to underlie a schizoaffective pattern more often than a bipolar or schizophrenic one.

Schizoaffective disorder, at least its bipolar subtype, may be quite close to bipolar disorder with psychotic symptoms, chronic substance use accounting for the autonomous persistence or recurrence of psychotic symptoms occurring independently of major affective episodes. Otherwise, schizophrenia fits the model of a spontaneously chronic psychosis in which SUD merely plays the role of an exacerbating factor.

Suggestive data emerge from the analysis of 111 psychotic subjects admitted for in-patient treatment, all of whom had used cannabis shortly before the onset of psychotic symptoms or had been using cannabis continuously for periods of variable length until admission. All of them had started using cannabis before their first psychotic episode, and psychotic symptoms had shown chronic-persistent or chronic-relapsing features up to the time of the index episode. Most of them were diagnosed as affected by bipolar 1 disorder; schizoaffective disorder came second, and schizophrenia was far less frequent. A diagnosis of bipolar disorder was more likely among current cannabis users (THC+), whereas schizophrenia was more frequent among past cannabis users (THC–). Moreover, bipolars have a higher likelihood of continuing their use of cannabis after discharge, whereas the extinction of cannabis use is a characteristic almost peculiar to schizophrenics [516]. It has been proved that SUD are linked to impulsiveness and sensation-seeking rather than to anhedonia [646]. Although the schizoaffective subsample was a tiny minority, the two explored dimensions may be interpreted as links either to the affective or the schizophrenic prototype, respectively. Thus, the affectivity of psychotic subjects, through an impulsive disposition, appears to condition the likelihood of SUD as a chronic trait, even in the absence of any major affective disturbance.

Therefore, a bipolar status, in a bipolar-spectrum-wide view, may justify the disposition to enduring or relapsing substance use, despite the unfavourable clinical course. Chronic use of psychotogenic substances and autonomous chronicity of psychotic symptoms may root in a bipolar substrate: mood instability may lead to frequent substance use, and the peculiar effects of used substances may result in autonomous clinical dimensions with corresponding symptoms.

In other words, on-going substance use may produce chronic paranoid, schizotypal or, less probably, schizoid pictures with symptoms of fluctuating intensity. Sensitization to the psychotic effects of substances, coupled with a proneness to continuous or recurrent use by bipolar subjects, would then result in complex longitudinal patterns distinguished by enduring psychoticism and intermittent affective episodes [548].

Homeless individuals are an extremely vulnerable and underserved population characterized by overlapping problems of mental illness and substance use. Given the fact that mood disorders are frequently associated with SUDs, in one of our studies [164], our aim was to further highlight the role of excitement in SUD. Patterns of SUD among homeless subjects suffering from unipolar and bipolar depression were compared. The 'self-medication hypothesis', which leads to the prediction of no significant differences in substance preference between unipolar (UP)- and bipolar (BP)-depressed homeless individuals, was tested (Fig. 4.1).

Homeless individuals from the 'Vancouver At Home/Chez Soi study' were selected for lifetime UP and lifetime BP depression and patterns of substance use in the previous 12 months were identified by applying the Mini-International Neuropsychiatric Interview. Differences in substance use between BP-depressed homeless patients and UP-depressed ones were tested at univariate and multivariate levels. No significant differences were observed between UP and BP homeless demographics. The bipolar-depressed homeless (BDH) group displayed a higher percentage of CNS stimulants and opioids as compared with the unipolar-depressed

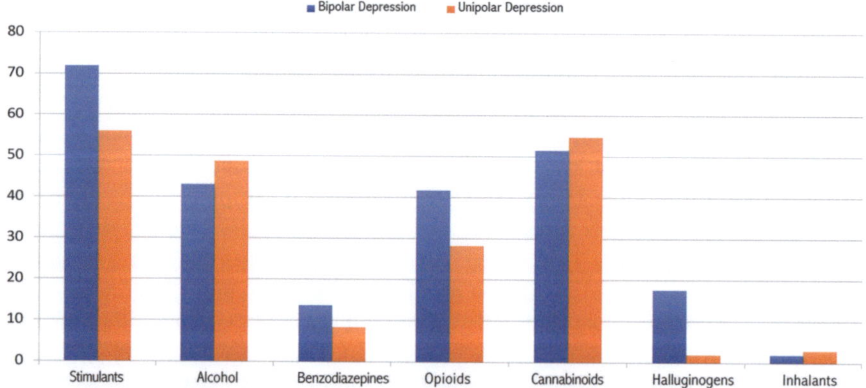

Fig. 4.1 Affective symptoms and substance use in homeless SUD patients

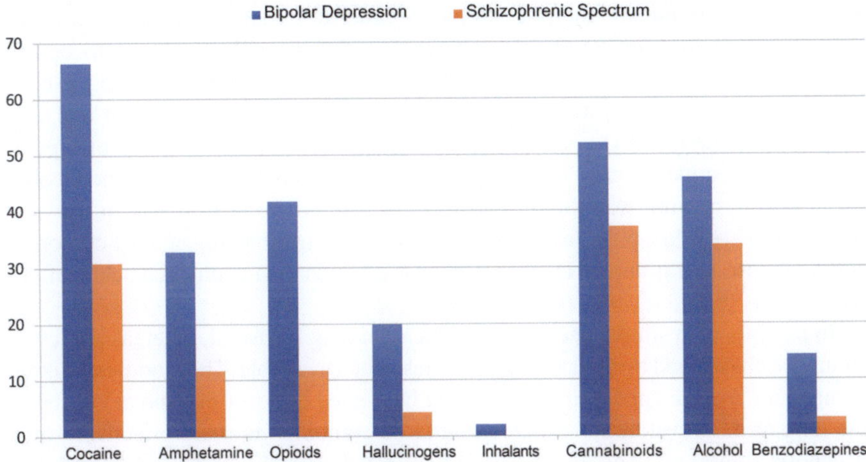

Fig. 4.2   Substance use in psychotic and bipolar homeless

homeless (UDH) group. The CSN stimulant was the only predictor within the BDH group. In another study [163], we compared substance use patterns between homeless individuals diagnosed with the schizophrenia spectrum and with bipolar disorders using the Mini-International Neuropsychiatric Interview. From a sample of 497 subjects drawn from Vancouver, Canada, who participated in the At Home/ Chez Soi study, 146 and 94 homeless individuals were identified as BP and S-S (schizophrenic spectrum), respectively. In the previous 12 months, a greater proportion of BP homeless subjects reported greater use of cocaine, amphetamines, opioids, hallucinogens, cannabinoids and tranquillizers compared with S-S patients (Fig. 4.2).

Cocaine and opioids were significantly associated with BP homeless individuals. These studies illustrated the relationship between substance use and BP in a vulnerable urban population of homeless subjects affected by adverse psychosocial factors and severe psychiatric conditions and further supported the hypothesis that beyond the self-medication hypothesis, bipolarity—not psychosis—is strictly correlated with SUDs.

4.4.1   Therapeutic Implications

In spontaneous psychoses, antipsychotics are the logical choice as a long-term strategy. As far as DD is concerned, it is advisable to employ agents that do not heavily affect dopamine metabolism in an inhibitory way, since the effectiveness upon psychotic symptoms is hampered by the exacerbation of use. Substance users, even if not addicted, may resort to known substances in order to reverse the negative symptoms induced by neuroleptics. On the other hand, when the tie with substances is stronger, their use may amplify as a direct consequence of dopamine antagonism, as a compensatory mechanism effective throughout the reward pathway. Psychotic symptoms would thus be the price to pay in order to obtain a satisfactory level of reward and arousal, on a subjective basis. Novel antipsychotics seem to permit equivalent effectiveness on psychotic symptoms without promoting drug use, at least to the same extent, and might have anticraving properties. Brown and colleagues tried the novel D2-partial agonist aripiprazole on a small group of bipolar and schizoaffective patients, reporting improvements in both symptoms and alcohol use. Cocaine craving was diminished too, but no consistent decrease in use was recorded [674]. Clozapine has shown its value as an agent acting against comorbid substance use in a group of chronic psychoses, which also comprised schizoaffective patients [675].

In patients with simple use, psycho-education may be useful, whereas addiction should be challenged by anticraving therapies, when available. The mood-stabilizing component and the anticraving one should be treated as a priority and enhanced in the long term. Novel antipsychotics should be combined to more effectively treat psychotic symptoms. The chronic use of antipsychotics should be considered as a long-term strategy when psychotic symptoms are proven to persist despite abstinence from psychotogenic substances. Chronic substance use may account for the independent course of psychotic symptoms in bipolar-type schizoaffective disorders. On the other hand, the incidence of actual schizophrenia is higher for psychotomimetic-using subjects, but the course of treatment seems to be independent of on-going SUD. On epidemiological grounds, the increasing rates of comorbidity between affective disorders and SUD may be responsible for a higher prevalence of schizoaffective disorders. Such pictures result from the psychotic properties possessed by certain substances, when used on a regular pattern by bipolar subjects. Proneness to use shown by bipolar subjects, across the whole bipolar spectrum, may be a crucial link with atypical bipolar pictures that comprise chronic psychotic symptoms.

4.5   Substance Use in Psychotic Patients

The prevalence of substance use among psychotic patients varies over a wide range, between 10% and 70% [676, 677], but it appears that 47% of schizophrenics, on average, display lifetime alcohol or substance-related disorders; these data imply a relative risk as much as 4.6 times greater than that of the general population, where SUD occurs as often as 16% [678, 679]. Over 70% of schizophrenic patients are heavy tobacco smokers [57, 678]. Young age, male gender, low educational level [677] and a family history of substance use are predictive of a higher risk of addiction [676]. Schizophrenic patients with a history of substance use stand out in displaying an earlier age of onset, better premorbid global functioning and adaptation, higher occurrence of positive symptoms, frequent need for medical intervention due to intoxication or psychiatric symptoms, shorter overall symptom-free time, and a worse response to typical antipsychotic drugs [676, 680]. Up to 50% of subjects admitted to in-patient treatment who subsequently proved to be unresponsive to standard treatments also reported concurrent substance use [681]. On the other hand, drug users who also suffer from mental illness are those most likely to be offered treatment facilities [681, 682]. As regards the occurrence of complications and psychosocial adjustment, substance-using schizophrenics show less compliance with treatment programmes, a higher risk of medical events (including HIV-related issues) and a higher frequency of suicidal acts [680, 683]. The destructive influence of substance use is also significant for these patients in terms of a sharp fall in their level of social functioning and a sharp rise in levels of poverty, wandering and homelessness, violence and familial maladjustment [683]. However, when interventions succeed in keeping substance use under control, substance-using schizophrenics follow a more favourable disease course than that of their non-using peers [684].

Various hypotheses have been formulated to explain the relationship between substance use and schizophrenia. According to the 'liability' model, in particular, non-psychotic users may become schizophrenic as a result of the toxic action of used psychotropic substances on their brain functioning. A higher incidence of schizophrenia among non-psychotic users than in the general population goes to support this hypothesis [684]. Another theory hypothesizes that schizophrenics tend to resort to substances as a result of their condition itself, or their exposure to neuroleptic medication, as a form of self-medication against disease-related or treatment-related negative symptomatology [143, 685–687]. The high occurrence rate of drug use might alternatively be a consequence of a cognitive impairment typical of schizophrenia, which consists in an incapacity to anticipate the consequences of one's choices [688]. This interpretative model does not fit the fact that drug-using chronic psychotics display higher levels of psychosocial functioning or the observation that their involvement in sensation-seeking behaviours suggests an absence of major cognitive impairment [676, 689].

Comorbid mood or anxiety disorders are common among schizophrenics, and antidepressant treatments are effective on them [690, 691]. Dysphoria is a major, though not the only, drive towards substance use among schizophrenic patients. Substance use among schizophrenics cannot, in fact, always be justified in terms of dysphoria: some authors provide evidence that the number of depressive symptoms exerts only a minor influence on the risk rate for alcohol, cannabinoid use or polyuse [692, 693]. Conversely, others have reported the association between depressive and anxiety disorders to be quite strong. In drug users, depression can develop during a period of using practice or may simply be a response to the interruption of drug use. It is, however, not uncommon to find that depression among schizophrenic patients, when it is responsive to antidepressants, develops into an alcohol-free condition [690]. Pharmacotherapies for the control of dysphoric mood may be as useful in treating drug-using schizophrenic patients as they have proved to be with non-psychotic cannabis and cocaine users [691]. Other medications, such as BDZs, high-dose glycine or anticonvulsants, may likewise be useful in treating comorbid anxiety in schizophrenics. Despite this, the administration of BDZs in DD patients should always be pondered carefully, because of their intrinsic addictive potential. Novel antipsychotics may contribute to the reduction of dysphoria in DD patients. Studies on olanzapine, risperidone, quetiapine and clozapine agree in suggesting a significant anxiolytic effect [694, 695].

Drug-using schizophrenics do not have a drug of choice, and the pattern of their choices among the various available substances is similar to that in the general population [676, 696]. In other words, no specific relationship is likely to stand between schizophrenic symptomatology and the choice of used substances; but this choice does tend to reflect the rate of consumption of that substance in these subjects' environment. The use of at least one substance is quite likely (three times more likely for alcohol than for other substances), and the less addictive a substance is in the general population, the more likely it is to induce addiction among chronic psychotics (relative risk is as high as six times that in the general population for psychostimulants and hallucinogenic drugs). When changes in the popularity of a substance coincide with changes among the same cohort of psychotics, this is mostly due to a change in its availability. On the whole, chronic psychosis does favour the onset of addiction to various different classes of psychotropics, with no particular selectivity, thus making what are normally fewer addictive substances as addictive to these psychotics as other substances. Schizophrenia does not differ from other psychiatric diseases in the typology of used substances or the quality of experienced effects, whether positive or negative [679, 697, 698]. As regards the subjective evaluation of the drives to use substances, surveys on the question of the reason patients give for resorting to substances suggest no peculiarity: schizophrenics use substances for the same reasons as other subjects, that is, to 'be high' or to avoid 'feeling down', to 'feel better', to 'enjoy' and 'to buffer depression' [699]. Polydrug use is the most frequent substance use pattern among schizophrenic users. Alcohol is the most used (37%), and a lifetime diagnosis of alcohol use disorder is frequent too (22–47%). Cannabinoids come second (23%), followed by stimulants and hallucinogenic agents (13%) [700]. Other substances, such as opioids or sedative hypnotics, are far less common [57, 684]. The Epidemiologic Catchment Area (ECA) study did not report any relationship between the typologies of used substances and psychiatric diagnoses [701].

4.6   Impact of Comorbid Psychosis on the Natural Course of Heroin Use Disorder

4.6.1   Natural History of Addiction in Psychotic Heroin-Addicted Patients at Their First Agonist Opioid Treatment

To date, considering all the foregoing, the relationship between opioids and psychosis is far from having been elucidated. The literature is unable to resolve the question of whether the use of heroin could somehow induce a psychotic state, in either the intoxication or withdrawal stage, or whether psychotic SUD patients who use heroin are actually looking for the antipsychotic properties of opioids. In one of our studies [702], we aimed to shed light on this question. We therefore compared the clinical characteristics and the natural history of HUD between psychotic and non-DD/PSY-HUD patients at their first agonist opioid treatment. We supposed that DD/PSY-HUD patients, compared with their non-psychotic peers, showed a more severe psychopathological condition and a shorter, less severe drug addiction history at treatment entry. If borne out, this interpretation would support a 'self-medication' approach to heroin use in DD/PSY-HUD patients. The research study was implemented using the PISA-DATASET: a database including anonymous individual information originally collected for clinical research purposes [40, 83, 703].

We selected patients who had already requested their first AOT. The sample consisted of 23 HUD patients who, after psychiatric screening, had received an additional diagnosis of chronic psychosis. Of these, 56.6% were males and 43.4% females. The average age was 31 ± 8 years (full range: 19–45). Most of the patients were single (60.9%), with less than 8 years of education (56.5%), and were unemployed (39.1%). No differences were observed between males and females with respect to demographic data. As our control group, we selected 209 patients who underwent psychiatric screening and showed the absence of any psychiatric disorder; 76.6% were males and 23.4% were females. The mean age was 30 ± 8 years (full range: 16–51). These two groups were then compared for sociodemographic, toxicological, psychopathological and treatment-related variables. With respect to sociodemographic data, no differences were observed regarding age, marital status (single), education (<8 years), occupation (student, white collar, blue collar and unemployed), income (poor) and living situation (alone). DD/PSY-HUD and non-DD/PSY-HUD patients significantly differed in their gender and welfare benefits; 56.6% of DD/PSY-HUD patients and 74.6% of controls were males; 8.7% of DD/PSY-HUD patients and 1.4% of controls received welfare benefits.

Considering clinical aspects and addiction history, no differences were observed as regards the presence of somatic comorbidities, major work problems, major household problems (conjugal/partner relationships), loving major problems, social and leisure major problems and legal problems. Compared with controls, DD/PSY-HUD patients showed a lower frequency for major household problems (parental relationships, parental role) and a higher frequency for poly-use and again for combined treatment (comprehensive treatments with psychopharmacology). Obviously, DD/PSY-HUD patients showed a more endangered mental status (number of disturbed areas). Comparing the variables that are featured in drug addiction history, no differences were found regarding age at heroin first contact, age at onset of continuous heroin use and age at first treatment. Psychotic HUD patients presented a lower duration of dependence.

With reference to self-reported lifetime concomitant SUD at treatment entry, DD/PSY-HUD patients showed a significantly greater frequency in their use of alcohol, illegal methadone, BDZs, hypnotics, amphetamines, hallucinogens and cannabinoids. The concomitant use of other opioids such as painkillers, inhalants and cocaine was a topic where no significant differences emerged.

Considering the differences between DD/PSY-HUD patients and controls with reference to use modalities, DD/PSY-HUD patients more frequently showed the following characteristics: multi-daily heroin intake and less stable modalities of heroin use; they typically belong to stage 2 (intermediate or 'dose-increasing' phase) of the illness, including its psychopathological antecedents. They show less frequent attempts at periodic self-detoxification. By contrast, non-DD/PSY-HUD

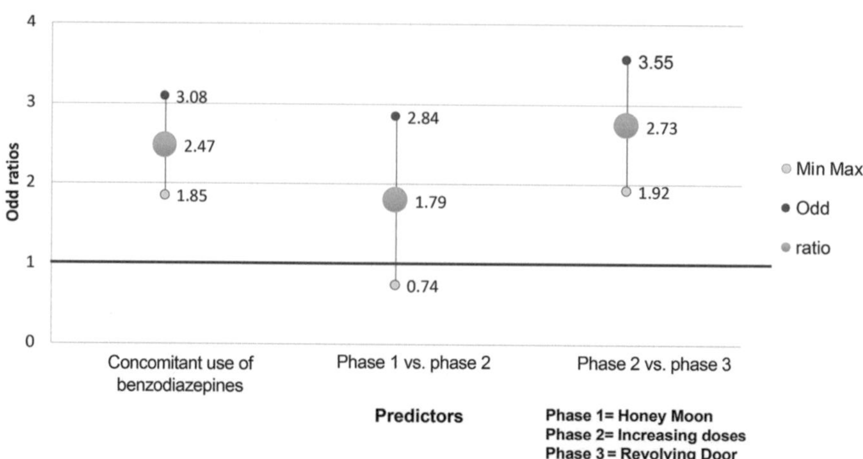

Fig. 4.3 Clinical aspects of DD/PSY-HUD patients at their first methadone treatment

patients showed the following characteristics: daily heroin use, stable modalities of use and periodic self-detoxification; they typically belonged to stage 3 (the 'revolving door' phase) of the illness, without any psychosocial or psychopathological antecedents (Fig. 4.3).

Finding the most discriminant traits of DD/PSY-HUD patients, the odds of being a DD/PSY-HUD patient were significantly higher in the case of patients who had a concomitant use of BDZ (OR 2.47) and in patients who were in stage 1 (the 'honeymoon' stage) vs. stage 3 ('revolving door' stage; OR 1.79) and, similarly, in stage 2 (dose-increasing stage) vs. stage 3 (revolving door stage) (OR 2.73).

Psychotic HUD patients are more likely to be females, to be receiving welfare benefits, to have a higher number of disturbed mental status areas, to have a duration of dependence that is lower, to be poly-users (of: alcohol, BDZs, hypnotics, amphetamines, hallucinogens, cannabinoids and illegal methadone) and to be undergoing treatment with additional psychopharmacology. They show a multi-daily heroin intake and less stable modalities of heroin use. They are in stage 2 (the intermediate or dose-increasing phase) of the illness and report psychopathological antecedents (type 2). They less frequently report major household problems and periodic self-detoxification. Non-DD/PSY-HUD patients showed the following features: daily heroin use, stable modalities of use and periodic self-detoxification; they belong to stage 3 (the 'revolving door' phase) of the illness and report no psychosocial or psychopathological antecedents. The fact of being in stage 2 of the illness and the use of BDZs at the moment of treatment entry are the two features that most clearly distinguish between psychotic and non-DD/PSY-HUD patients. Psychotic HUD patients seem to reach their first AOT with a shorter, less severe addiction history (setting aside poly-use) and a more severe psychopathology than their non-psychotic peers. These results support the hypothesis that, in requesting treatment, DD/PSY-HUD patients are looking for the antipsychotic properties of agonist opioid medications. This is in line with the reports in the literature that strengthen the view that opioids possess antipsychotic, anxiolytic, antipanic and mood stabilizer effects [158, 436, 527, 528, 704, 705]. Methadone and buprenorphine have shown their beneficial effects on the psychopathology of HUD and DD patients [43, 50, 55, 56, 706–709].

In further support of our hypothesis, we wish to note that our psychotic patients are using illegal methadone (street methadone). We have found that street methadone, at least in Italy, can be considered as a self-medication treatment—in practice, a prelude to treatment entry [85]. Moreover, our patients reported psychopathological antecedents to heroin use and we have recently found that DD/PSY-HUD patients could suffer from a primary psychiatric disorder and respond by using opioids in an attempt at self-medication [627]. In line with these arguments, it appears that the use of heroin could itself represent a sort of self-medication. Khantzian's self-medication hypothesis states that the psychotropic effects of used substances interact with abnormal mental states, the outcome being that these substances become compulsively necessary to susceptible subjects [143]. In other words, patients appear to select substances that they expect to have a 'healing' effect. In this way, we can understand the frequency of poly-use and the use of BDZs (on account of their anxiolytic and sedative properties), as well as illegal methadone at treatment entry [75].

The last consideration is about the pharmacokinetics of heroin and of methadone or buprenorphine. Heroin is a short-acting opioid, while methadone and buprenorphine are long-acting opioids. A short-acting opioid is useless in any long-term administration. As a result, it is only logical that psychotic patients can use heroin to treat their psychosis for a long period without experiencing the side effects that accompany heroin use (tolerance, withdrawal and craving). At this point, either illegal methadone or straightforward methadone treatment could be viewed by them as an attractive choice.

In summary, DD/PSY-HUD patients presented for AOT with more severe psychopathological aspects and a shorter, less severe addiction history (setting aside poly-use) than their non-psychotic peers. The fact that our psychotic patients requested AOT earlier and with a less severe addiction history suggests that these patients are likely to benefit from an opioid medication more on account of the improvement it will bring to their psychopathology than for its alleviation of their HUD. These data indirectly speak in favour of the antipsychotic effects of opioids and Khantzian's self-medication hypothesis for DD/PSY-HUD patients.

4.6.2   Primary or Secondary Nature of Comorbid Psychotic Disorders in Relation to HUD

The high comorbidity rate of SUD with other mental health disorders has been highlighted in a number of trials conducted in clinical samples and in the general population [237, 452, 701, 710–712]. All of these studies have suggested that anxiety disorders, passive-aggressive disorder, behavioural disorders and attention deficit hyperactivity disorder may generally precede SUDs, while mood disorders are generally secondary to SUDs [234]. However, there is still a lack of conclusive data able to explain these temporal relationships. The existence of a common factor that predisposes to both drug and mental health problems cannot be excluded. Furthermore, there is a dearth of European data available describing the issue of co-existing mental health problems and their relationship with illicit drug dependence.

In one of our studies [627], the primary aim was to document the presence of DD in a large sample of Italian HUD outpatients at treatment entry. From our viewpoint a patient could be considered to demonstrate a DD (so qualifying as belonging to the category of DD patients) in cases where an independent psychiatric disorder was concomitant with a SUD disorder. A description was then provided of individual DD patients to explore the temporal relationship between these diagnoses based on age at onset. When the onset of SUD was at least 1 year prior to the associated mental disorder, the patient was described as 'primarily' (PR) affected by 'SUD'— (SUD-PR). In contrast, when the onset of mental disorder had happened at least 1 year prior to the associated mental disorder the patient was described as 'primarily' (PR) affected by 'mental disorder' (PSY)—(PSY-PR). If there was less than 1 year between the diagnoses of either condition, then the patient was not assigned to either category. A secondary objective of the study was to compare the presenting characteristics of the DD patients belonging to the two different categories—those assessed as, primarily, drug addicted (SUD-PR) and those evaluated as, 'primarily', mentally ill (PSY-PR).

The study was a retrospective, observational study of patients requesting treatment at the PISA-V.P. Dole Research Group between 1994 and 2005, inclusive. Data were drawn from standardized data recorded in the client database and associated case notes. Positive decisions on the presence of DD were determined by consensus between three independent researchers; only cases in which a consensus was reached as to the diagnosis and chronology of illness were included in the analyses. Compliance with the assessment protocol over a long time-span was ensured by the supervision of a senior psychiatrist (I. Maremmani), who continued to work at the PISA-V.P. Dole Research Group for as long as the research lasted and now is retired. Once the diagnosis and chronology of illness had been confirmed, we divided patients into three groups: SUD-PR, PSY-PR and NDD/HUD, and compared their demographic and clinical characteristics.

A total of 1090 HUD outpatients were enrolled in the study. All patients satisfied the *DSM* diagnostic criteria for opioid dependence. Mean age ± SD was 29 ± 6 years (ranging from 16 to 51 years). A majority of these patients were male (76.2%), had never married (64.4%), reported an educational experience lasting less than 9 years (70.7%); 39.6% were unemployed at the time of clinical assessment, and 363 (33.8%) were beginning treatment for the first time. Patients commonly reported polydrug use, with 62.8% choosing cannabinoids, 44.6% stimulants, 33.9% alcohol, 28.5% hallucinogens, 27.6% unprescribed BDZs and 4.1% inhalants. All patients were Italians and were included only once in the analyses. A total of 574 (52.7%) patients met the criteria for a DD. The mean age of these patients was 29 ± 6 years (ranging from 17 to 50). Most of these patients were male (72.9%) and had never married (63.8%); 48.2% were not employed and 65.8% reported less than 9 years of education. In terms of the diagnoses, 89 patients (15.5%) had chronic psychosis, 263 (45.8%) had recurrent depression, 148 (25.8%) satisfied the criteria for bipolar spectrum disorders according to Akiskal's criteria and 74 (12.9%) had anxiety disorders. There was no relationship between these diagnostic groups and gender or age (when considering two age groups under and over the mean age of 29 years. A total of 339 (31.1%) were NDD/HUD patients. Their mean age was 30 ± 6 years (ranging from 16 to 51) and a clear majority of 266 (78.5%) were male. Consensus as to the presence of DD was not reached in 177 patients (16.2%)—the reason why these subjects were excluded from subsequent analyses.

The temporal order of the initial diagnosis could not be determined for 68 patients (11.8%). These patients were excluded from further analyses. Of the 574 patients who had DD at treatment entry, a clear majority, 362 (63.1%), presented with initial diagnoses of drug addiction (SUD-PR). Of these, 265 (73.2%) were male and 97 (26.8%) female. The mean age was 30 ± 6 years (ranging from 18 to 45). On the other hand, 144 (25.1%) patients were diagnosed as primarily affected by a mental disorder other than SUD (PSY-PR). Of this second group, 111 (77.1%) were male and 33 (22.9%) female. Mean age was 29 ± 6 years (ranging from 17 to 45). The category of illness was not related to gender. It is worth noting that 84 (58.3%) of PSY-PR patients had a lower age than the sample mean (29 years) and were relatively younger at the time of treatment entry.

There were no significant differences between DD and NDD patients as to age, gender, marital status, type of accommodation or working activity. NDD patients had had a significantly shorter educational experience than DD-patients, independent of the chronology of illness. However, an extremely compromised economic status was present in a limited number of HUD patients, more so in SUD-PR patients. Regarding addiction history, only familial difficulties showed no significant differences between the groups. Mental state at treatment entry, substance poly-use and number of associated treatments were graded as more severe in DD patients, independent of illness chronology, than those without a DD. Conversely, DD patients presented fewer sentimental/sexual difficulties and leisure time issues. The NDD/HUD patients used significantly fewer drugs but had been dependent upon heroin for a significantly longer time. SUD-PR patients presented with significantly more physical complications, more working difficulties and legal issues. These subjects reported more previous therapeutic failures, followed by PSY-PR and NDD patients. DD patients, independent of the chronology of illness, were less frequently able to autonomously suspend heroin consumption and presented for treatment with less frequent heroin intake, but in a less stable manner. 'Stable' opioid-dependent patients espouse conventional values, hold legitimate jobs, are generally law-abiding and do not associate with other SUD patients [713]. These subjects will often seek treatment at an earlier stage of dependence. Moreover, the time-span from the beginning of addiction until the first treatment (latency to treatment) was inferior. PSY-PR patients as well as NDD patients were more likely to be found seeking treatment for the first time, were older and the duration of their addiction was shorter when compared with SUD-PR. They had dependence length lower than that of NDD patients. In summary, drug use severity was lower in PSY-PR patients, followed by NDD patients, and proved to be highest in SUD-PR patients. Chronic psychotic and anxious subjects were more prevalent within the group of PSY-PR patients, whereas HUD patients with recurrent depression and bipolar spectrum disorders were mainly represented in the SUD-PR group. More precisely, the diagnosis of recurrent depression and bipolar spectrum disorders, associated physical complications and a history of treatment failures were the strongest predictors of belonging to the SUD-PR patient group. Diagnoses of chronic psychosis and anxiety disorders were significant predictors of belonging to the PSY-PR patient group. In summary, our study reported the prevalence of DD among a large representative sample of Italian heroin users seeking treatment. It was found that approximately 52% of patients met the criteria for a DD; of these, approximately 63% had progressed from SUD to mental disorders (classified as SUD-PR), while 25% had progressed from a mental disorder to drug addiction (classified as PSY-PR). Compared with PSY-PR, SUD-PR patients were more frequently affected by mood disorders and had a more severe clinical presentation. PSY-PR patients were more frequently diagnosed as psychotic or affected by anxiety disorders. These data permit epidemiological, diagnostic and therapeutic considerations.

From the epidemiological point of view, more than 50% of our sample of treatment-seeking HUD patients met the criteria for a DD; of these, approximately 46% presented with depression, 16% were bipolar, 13% showed anxiety disorders and 16% presented with chronic psychosis. Unfortunately, there are no recent records of the prevalence of these disorders among the general Italian community. The prevalence of these disorders was, however, comparable with previous studies from elsewhere. According to the ECA study [701], in the general population, among those who had ever received a diagnosis of a mental disorder, as many as 15% had a history of a SUD, while approximately 29% reported alcohol and other types of SUD. Similar findings were reported in the National Comorbidity Study (NCS) [452, 710]. NCS respondents with a lifetime alcohol or drug use disorder also met the criteria for at least one lifetime mental disorder in 51.4% of cases, while past alcohol or drug use or dependence was present in 50.9% of the NCS respondents with a lifetime mental disorder [452, 701, 710]. Our study was consistent with these previous studies and confirmed that 50% of those addicted to substances (heroin in this case) may present for treatment with a mental disorder. One possible explanation for our results is the setting in which the sample was recruited. The Psychiatric Clinic of the University of Pisa, is, in fact, one of the few Italian University psychiatric clinics in which patients can receive MMTP (for details see Maremmani et al. [56]). It could, therefore, attract a greater number of HUD patients with DD.

From the diagnostic point of view, consistent with the diagnostic criteria of *DSM-IV*, approximately 15% of our HUD patients displayed comorbidity with chronic psychosis. The incidence of comorbidity associated with mood disorders is approximately 46%, and with anxiety disorders about 12%. The co-diagnosis of bipolar disorder spectrum according to the formulation of Akiskal and Mallya is about 26%. Considering depressive and bipolar disorders, this accounts for 72.5% of our sample. Mood disorders proved to be the best represented diagnostic cluster in our sample. Our data on the lifetime prevalence of patients in methadone show a range of values reported by other studies, which detected a prevalence of 70–90% [128, 129, 131]. It should, however, be added that the previously reported prevalence at treatment entry has a range of 34–54% [130],—much lower than the percentage detected in our sample. Mood disorders may persist during MMT among those who continue to experience the opioid withdrawal syndrome despite a high methadone dosage [714], which demonstrates the clinical importance of mood disorders in the successful treatment of HUD. The ratio between bipolar disorder and recurrent depression is 0.56, much higher than that reported in other studies [157, 159, 222]; it could, after all, constitute a unique feature of this population. Our data are in agreement with commonly reported results regarding the prevalence of chronic psychosis in HUD patients, which ranges from 11% to 19% [155]. Anxiety disorders are uncommon in HUD patients when not due to an abstinence syndrome [448, 450]. Our data are in accordance with the literature, which reports the presence of anxiety disorders in around 10% [157] of patients. Our data from Italian HUD treatment seekers differ from previous findings, as we have detected a higher percentage of mood disorders, with a higher frequency of non-bipolar disorder than bipolar disorder, but with an odds ratio indicative of the higher presence of bipolar disorder. The high presence of bipolar disorders may be due to the classification system used in this study (bipolar spectrum according to Akiskal and Mallya) [84, 170, 176, 177, 715]. Justifications for the use of this diagnostic system in SUD patients are reported in detail in Maremmani et al. [49].

Switching our focus now to the chronology of illness, approximately two-thirds of our DD patients developed a mental disorder subsequent to drug addiction. This finding differs from the review of the available literature by Kessler, who reported that, in a majority of patients with DD, mental disorders generally precede drug use [234–237, 716, 717]. One difference is that our study was restricted to those with a primary diagnosis of HUD. Our patients, however, presented with a high rate of poly-SUD, so that we may safely assume that the observed progression from SUD to mental disorder was not dependent on heroin use alone. Our data suggest that patients affected by chronic psychosis and anxiety disorders tend to progress from a psychiatric disorder to SUD, while patients with mood disorders are initially affected with drug addiction. The most important predictors of progression from SUD to psychiatric comorbidity were a diagnosis of mood disorders, repeated treatment failures and physical complications, which is consistent with the previous literature [238, 239].

Psychiatric symptoms can represent the pharmacological effects (intoxication or withdrawal) of drugs of use [714]. When considering psychosis, there is certainly a correlation between the use of psychostimulant agents and psychotic symptoms [590, 718–721], without necessarily having an inherited psychiatric vulnerability [722]. Such a correlation can be induced experimentally [723–728]. In any case, drug-induced symptoms are often short-lasting, whereas longer-lasting psychosis usually manifests with manic features [729–735]. The same is true of cannabinoids, where depersonalization and de-realization are frequent features [736] and are often found associated with hallucinations and delusions [258, 737–739]. There is no conclusive evidence as to the role of cannabinoids in determining the onset of schizophrenia [740–744]. Data emerging from our study do, however, suggest that psychosis is more likely to be a prevalent diagnosis in primarily (earlier) mentally ill dual-diagnosis patients. This supports Khantzian's self-medication theory [143, 745]. Our primarily psychotic patients might find heroin to be a substance that can, initially, ease psychotic symptoms and fragmentation anxiety [240, 241, 746, 747]. The continued use of heroin would then lead to a state of dependence (DD). Khantzian's hypothesis is confirmed by the low percentage of psychotic patients detected in study samples receiving methadone, which could mask the existence of a psychosis [683, 748–751]. Other evidence supporting Khantzian's theory is the observation that depressed HUD patients treated with antidepressants (doxepin) report a significant reduction of the craving [752], besides the fact that individuals addicted to stimulants, sedatives and opioids have phobic and depressive clinical presentations. Rounsaville and colleagues [137] were the first to report data confirming Khantzian's [143, 745] and Wurmser's [455] theories. The same theory can be used for our anxious patients [99]. SUD has, in fact, been repeatedly documented in anxious subjects as producing relief in the symptoms of anxiety [753–755]. It must, however, be recognized that this problem is still unresolved [756]. Conversely, we observed progression, in our sample, from SUD to mood disorders. In this regard, we cannot rule out that emotional dysregulation may be a factor that predisposes to drug addiction [49, 79, 186, 757]. As a separate issue, it has been reported that changes in mood may be secondary to pathological conditions such as drug intoxication or withdrawal states [315, 317, 758–764]. Most bipolar patients use substances such as alcohol, stimulants and cannabis [54, 199, 701] that may contribute to worsening the severity of the disease [197, 765–767]. In any case, the frequent association of substance-induced excitement with the presence of a specific predisposition to bipolar disorder makes it difficult to distinguish between spontaneous and induced hypomania [170]. As a result, doubts remain about the validity of the *DSM* criteria for 'substance-induced mood disorders' [84, 182]. In our study, mood disorders were more common in dual disorder HUD patients in whom drug dependence was diagnosed first. Self-medication theory should not, therefore, be applied to patients with mood disorders. We can speculate that in these subjects the presence of a premorbid state (such as cyclothymia, anxiety or impulse decontrol) alongside poly-SUD could destabilize their psychopathological condition, so creating a predisposition to the onset of diagnosable mood disorder [36, 49].

The chronology of illness in DD patients has important clinical implications. A commonly held view supposes that a majority of DD patients present primarily with a mental disorder that complicates over time as a result of drug dependence [234]. This would suggest that treating the psychiatric disorder may prevent the onset of drug dependence. Moreover, treating the psychiatric condition as a priority, even in the presence of concomitant drug dependence, may resolve the addiction when the psychiatric condition is effectively controlled. Our data, however, confirm this view only partially. First, the majority of our patients demonstrated a progression from drug dependence to a psychiatric disorder. In these cases, the treatment of the comorbid psychiatric condition would not be sufficient to prevent drug dependence. What is more, our data suggest that the theory of Khantzian can be applied to the treatment of patients affected by psychosis or anxiety disorders but is difficult to extend to patients affected by mood disorders. We suggest, therefore, that in all cases where DD is present, drug dependence should be treated first [49]. Further studies are necessary in order to verify if this approach is also valid for dependence on substances of use other than heroin.

In our study 52.7% of the patients presented for treatment with a DD. Approximately two-thirds of the sample demonstrated a progression from drug addiction to a mental disorder. These were the patients most frequently affected by mood disorders, and the same group turned out to be those who had the most severe clinical presentation. Conversely, primarily mentally ill dual-diagnosed patients were more frequently diagnosed as psychotic or as affected by anxiety disorders. The data emerging from this study do not support the common view reported in the literature as to the progression from mental disorder to drug addiction, which, in fact, confirms the self-medication theory only for schizophrenic and anxiety disorders, but not for patients affected by mood disorders. In conclusion, when treating patients with dual diagnoses, clinicians should pay at least the same attention to the treatment of drug dependence as they do to the treatment of any comorbid psychiatric condition.

4.6.3   Clinical Aspects of DD/PSY-HUD Patients Compared with Bipolar Ones at Time of AOT Entry

The presence of aggressive, self-harming behaviours is common in HUD patients, but these frequent co-occurrences have been poorly investigated. Given the fact that self-harm may be seen both as a clear addictive behaviour, with its opioid theory, and as part of psychiatric illness, such as psychosis and bipolar spectrum disorders, in one of our studies [248] our aim was to investigate which of the two models is more consistent.

Self-harm behaviour, otherwise called 'deliberate self-harm' (DSH) or 'non-suicidal self-injury' (NSSI), has been defined as 'the deliberate, direct destruction or alteration of body tissue without conscious suicidal intent, but resulting in injury severe enough for tissue damage to occur' [768]. DSH can be divided into three categories: major, stereotypic and moderate/superficial. Moderate/superficial self-injury (M/SSI) is the form that has received most attention in the literature and consists of acts leading to little damage, such as skin cutting, burning, scratching and tearing [768]. Although most often self-harm is not a suicidal gesture, it is statistically associated with suicide and can result in unanticipated severe harm or fatality [769]. Some authors estimate that as many as 4% of the general population have been through a self-harm experience [770], while the prevalence reported among students ranges from 12% to 35% [768, 771]. Some studies indicate rates of DSH among SUD patients ranging from 29% to 52% [772], thus at levels higher than those found among other groups at risk for DSH, such as high school students (14–35%) [773] and patients with eating disorders (23–25%) [774].

Together with social and psychological explanations, self-harm has also been described as an addictive behaviour. According to the 'addiction hypothesis' [775], the endogenous opioid system, which regulates both pain perception and levels of endogenous endorphins, is chronically over-stimulated by frequent self-harm behaviours that aim to attenuate dysphoria and negative emotional states. The subject develops a tolerance for the endogenous opioids, suffers a cyclical withdrawal reaction and is driven to further opioid stimulation by means of impulsive self-harm behaviours. The increase in negative emotions prior to DSH is analogous to the aversive withdrawal symptoms experienced by SUD individuals [776], and people who engage in DSH frequently experience strong urges to self-harm, similar to craving in addiction [777]. Nixon and colleagues [778] investigated the addictive qualities of DSH in adolescent psychiatric patients, by using a self-reported evaluation of the addictive aspects of self-harm based on the *DSM-IV* criteria for substance dependence. These authors observed that a high percentage of the participants (78.6%) reported almost daily urges to self-injury, and 81% of them endorsed more than five criteria out of seven. One important difference does, however, separate self-harm from addictive behaviours: while substance addiction is maintained by both positive and negative reinforcement, DSH appears to be almost exclusively motivated by negative reinforcement, such as frustration and sadness [779]. The finding that opioid antagonists attenuate self-harm behaviours is the strongest evidence found so far for the opioid hypothesis [780]. Opioid antagonists demonstrated their effectiveness in animals [781, 782] and humans with and without mental retardation [780, 783–788].

Impulsiveness and emotional dysregulation have been reported both in DSH and SUD [789]. Self-mutilation behaviours are often present in disorders, which have a strong component of impulsiveness and risk behaviours [790]. The link between DSH and impulsiveness can be seen on a number of levels: self-harm has a pattern of urges to cut, there is tension or arousal before cutting takes place, and a momentary sense of pleasure and relief after the act, similar to what is seen in drug addiction [791].

On psychopathological grounds, HUD itself may be considered a chronic and severe form of impulse control disorder [391]. Furthermore, cyclothymic temperamental disposition is associated with personality dysfunction, with anxiety and impulsiveness [189], and has been shown to be a characteristic temperamental profile in HUD patients [78]. All these similarities, and the frequent comorbidity between bipolar spectrum disorders, personality disorders, self-harm and addiction, favour the hypothesis that emotional dysregulation, impulsiveness and a cyclothymic temperamental disposition may constitute the common substrate which can be recognized as an important risk factor for the development of both self-harm and HUD.

We compared the clinical characteristics of HUD patients, after dividing them according to the absence or presence of moderate/superficial self-harm behaviours in the month before treatment was sought. If self-harm is a form of addiction, we would expect no differences between HUD patients with and without DD; conversely, if self-harm is influenced or moderated by psychiatric comorbidities, it will be more frequent in the group of DD patients. We considered a data set of 1090 HUD patients, who had requested treatment during the years 1994–2005 at the PISA-V.P. Dole Research Group in Pisa, Italy. For details see Maremmani et al. [83]. We selected patients with:

- No lifetime self-harm or assault episodes
- At least one moderate/superficial self-harm episode in the last month before requesting treatment
- At least one assault episode in the previous month

In our clinical practice, the month before entering treatment allows us to distinguish, temporally, what is remote from patients' recent history. Of the patients reviewed for possible selection in the study sample, 90 did not have this information in their clinical records and were therefore excluded. The sample comprised 1000 HUD patients. Mean age was 29 ± 6 (range: 16–51). Of the study sample, 23.2% were female; 71.0% had had less than 8 years of education; 73.7% were single; 37.6% were unemployed; 17.0% earned a low income; 2.6% were receiving welfare benefits; 13.3% were living alone. More specifically, 3.0% of these patients showed at least one moderate/superficial self-harm episode in the last month before requesting treatment. Of these, 33.3% were female; mean age was 29 ± 4 (range: 16–37). As many as 16.2% of the patients showed at least one assault episode in the previous month. Of these, 29.0% were female; mean age was 29 ± 6 (range: 16–50); in addition, as many as 80.8% of the patients did not show lifetime self-harm or assault episodes. Of these, 175 (21.7) were female. Mean age was 30 ± 6 (range: 16–51). The three groups did not show statistically significant differences when compared on the basis of available demographic data.

Aggressive HUD patients were marked out by having been diagnosed as DD patients, especially with chronic psychosis and bipolar spectrum, as defined by Akiskal and Mallya. Patients without aggressive behaviour at treatment entry less frequently showed somatic complications, altered mental status, legal problems, poly-use (especially alcohol, BDZs, stimulants and hallucinogens). Their heroin use modality was less 'unstable'. In other words, they were HUD patients who had adopted conventional values, had legitimate jobs, were generally law-abiding and did not associate with other HUD patients. They had taken heroin for the first time when they were older than their aggressive peers; their age at the onset of dependence was higher; their age at first treatment was higher, too. The presence of a bipolar spectrum diagnosis proved to be the most prominent risk factor for the presence of aggressive behaviour in the month prior to the request for treatment. Concomitant high-risk factors were an unstable modality of heroin use, the presence of a chronic psychosis diagnosis and the simultaneous use of CNS stimulants or depressants. Conversely, the presence of depressive (non-bipolar) or anxiety disorders and a greater age at first contact with heroin corresponded to a lower risk of aggressive behaviour, whether self-harm or aggression. The most prominent risk factor for the presence of moderate/superficial self-harm, as opposed to aggressive behaviour, was a chronic psychosis DD, whereas the factor of receiving the first treatment lowered that risk.

If self-harm behaviours are consistent with the 'addiction hypothesis', in HUD patients the endogenous opioid system should be balanced by the chronic use of heroin and we would expect to find fewer episodes of self-injury, or at least no DSH withdrawal symptoms during toxicomanic practices. Moreover, at the time of treatment entry HUD patients should show frequent self-harm behaviours or at least a high number of episodes, as a result of the dysphoric state they are experiencing. In fact, even if patients did not undergo detoxification prior to treatment entry, withdrawal symptoms are frequent in patients looking for AOT [83]. Conversely, our data show that at the time of treatment entry self-harm behaviours were infrequent, as they appeared in only 30 (3.0%) out of 808 HUD patients. In particular, when DSH occurs, it seems to be linked with the presence of a DD, especially psychosis, rather than with the gravity of a patient's toxicomanic history. Deliberate self-harm is frequently found among psychotic patients, in which, due to delusions and hallucinations, the most severe forms of DSH may occur, including eye enucleation and genital castration [792]. A study conducted on a sample of 87 patients with chronic psychosis found that 59 (68%) of them reported past self-harm behaviours, and those involved in self-injury were significantly more likely to report depression, impulsiveness, premorbid intelligence quotient (IQ) and poly-SUD [793]. To the best of our knowledge, no previous studies have investigated the importance of DD in predicting self- or hetero-aggressive behaviour in HUD patients presenting at treatment entry. Our data suggest that

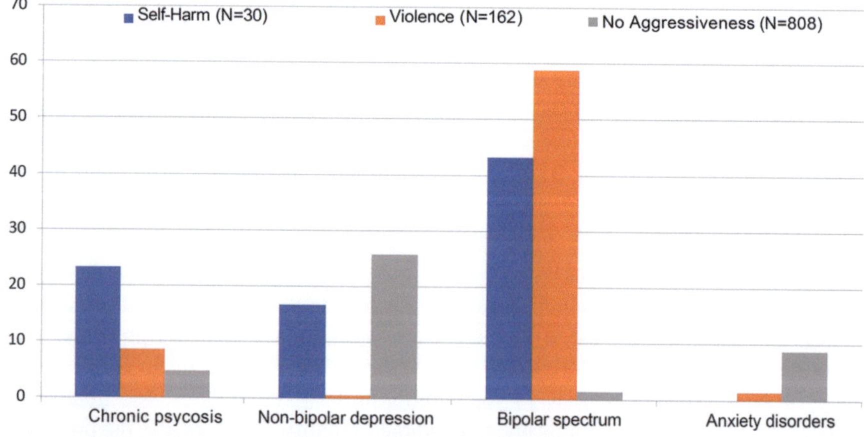

Fig. 4.4 Self-harm and violence in dual disorder HUD patients

moderate/superficial self-harm behaviours could be linked with the presence of a DD, without being influenced by heroin abstinence at the time of treatment entry in decompensated HUD patients. In particular, bipolar spectrum disorders seem to be responsible for the aggressive and physically violent behaviours of HUD patients, while moderate/superficial self-harm appears to be strongly supported by psychotic disorders. As a limitation, we can say that, although (lifetime) self-harm as well as assault are frequent traits in SUDs, an overwhelming majority of our patients did not show lifetime self-harm or assault episodes. Regrettably, we were only able to gather information on lifetime self-harm and/or assault by self-report (Fig. 4.4).

In summary, in our clinical experience a co-occurrence of aggression and bipolar spectrum disorder in HUD patients, which is manifested as violence, is often present. On the other hand, self-injurious behaviour appears to be strongly correlated with psychotic disorders. Bipolar spectrum disorder is a risk factor for aggressive behaviour (violence), and psychotic disorders are a risk factor for self-harm. Thus, in HUD patients before entry into treatment, aggressive behaviour appears to be correlated with DD rather than with a natural history of HUD.

4.7   Negative Symptoms in SUD Patients

Negative psychiatric symptoms were originally conceptualized as part of one of the two major psychoses, schizophrenia. That cluster of features corresponds to the loss of normal arousal, drive and affective liveliness. In other words, they make clear what the patient is lacking, and thus stand in opposition to positive symptoms, which loom as something in excess, or in addition to normal functions, both as regards perceptions (hallucinations) and thought (delusions). On the whole, negative symptoms can be summed up as a state of detachment and disengagement from the environment. The development of negative symptoms starts early in the course of schizophrenia, proceeds gradually and is often associated with typical depressive symptoms that may result in a state of affective numbing and flattening of emotions that gives a poor response to pharmacological treatment [794].

Later on, negative symptoms have been conceptualized as a dimension appearing in various different disorders. As a result, interest rose in the evaluation of negative symptoms within the clinical picture of bipolar disorders and obsessive-compulsive disorders, and also in degenerative neurological disorders such as dementia, Parkinson's disease and vascular-related damage (stroke) [795, 796]. Moreover, researchers have been looking further into the difference between negative symptoms and concurrent features of cognitive impairment, so that the concept of 'negative' functioning has been extended to include negative affections and cognitive deficiencies [797, 798]. Several authors have pointed out that some symptoms, such as apathy, abulia, anhedonia and social isolation are shared by depression and schizophrenia [799, 800]: this overlap between two major psychotic conditions suggests that negative symptoms are an expression of a general psychotic process rather than a specific feature of either clinical picture [801, 802]. In any case, negative symptoms show a different response to pharmacological treatment: the introduction of antidepressant treatment following the discontinuation of neuroleptic medication is followed by a sharper reduction of negative symptoms in depression affecting schizophrenic patients [803].

In major depression, which, in comparison with other mood disorders, mostly features negative symptoms, those symptoms weigh as negative prognostic factors, especially as regards affective indifference, the sensation of an empty brain (thought-lessness) and lack of drive (abulia) [804]. Negative symptoms and cognitive impairment have also been reported in pictures of pathological grief, which, on clinical grounds, stands half-way between depression and post-traumatic stress disorder, but is classified as an autonomous disorder [805]. Pathological grief can follow the loss of a significant other through the dynamics of attachment [806]; it also features avoidance and mumbling as a consequence of a lower ability to elaborate the body of information that is associated with the loss that has been experienced [807, 808]. As far as negative symptoms are concerned, pathological grief is characterized by social and job-related impairment [809]. In particular, the weakening of memory is greater in pathological grief than in depression or post-traumatic stress disorder [810]. Memory impairment has also been described in the obsessive-compulsive disorder, together with the disturbance of procedural functioning that is surely implied by that condition. Memory appears to be hampered as a consequence of the abnormal arrangement and the encoding of information at an output level. The most common cognitive features of this type are the prolonged latency of answers, the perseverance of wrong reactions to stimuli and the awkwardness of adaptation to change on the basis of registered feedbacks [811]. Such abnormalities were mapped as pertinent to the function of the frontal lobes and basal ganglia [812].

In the field of SUD, an interesting analogy stands out between classic negative symptoms and the amotivational syndrome displayed as an expression of chronic cannabis intoxication. We will now mainly focus on the amotivational syndrome (AS) and its links with the RDS, which was originally described as a consequence of chronic alcohol and stimulant use. These two latter conditions are closely related too to the PWS described by Martin and colleagues as an enduring pathological state in abstinent detoxified HUD patients [220, 355, 356]. Bearing in mind the amotivational syndrome model, it may be hypothesized that some of its prominent negative symptoms constitute a common endpoint of late clinical pictures linked to chronic intoxication by various substances of use. AS is one major complication of chronic exposure to cannabis and combines the flattening of affects with elements of cognitive impairment similar to those displayed in schizophrenia and depression. It is characterized by gradual detachment from the outer world and loss of emotional reactivity, drives and aims. Responsiveness to outer stimuli is blunted, and subjects are unable to experience or anticipate any pleasure except by using cannabis. Memory and attention are hampered [316]. AS-affected subjects have a poor level of school-related functioning, are less satisfied by their educational activities and easily enter into conflict with scholastic authorities. Both cannabis consumption itself and a cannabis-related environment are thought to contribute to the cognitive profile of AS [813]. A body of research has shown that the acute administration of

THC increases metabolism in the ventral tegmental area by a CB1-mediated input, so causing an increase in dopamine release to the shell area of the nucleus accumbens [814–816]. This phenomenon has recently been confirmed in vivo in the human striatum by studies of functional neuroimaging that apply the positron emission tomography (PET) technique [817]. Marijuana use increases blood-oxygen level dependence (BOLD) [818], which is related to a magnetic measurement of changes in the level of blood oxygen and corresponds to various states of metabolic activation of specific brain areas engaged in the production of certain feelings or outputs. Two different cannabinoid receptors have been described in the human body. The CB1 type [819] is widespread in basal ganglia, the cerebellum and the hippocampus, and modulates the activity of the GABAergic, glutamatergic and dopaminergic systems, all of which are influenced by exposure to cannabis. By contrast, the CB2 type is expressed in the immune system [820].

Both in the animal model and in man, continued exposure to cannabis causes a change in neuronal functioning [816, 821, 822]. The acute increase in dopaminergic release is followed by a reduction of dopamine in the same areas of the reward-system. This phenomenon is likely to be linked both to the down-regulation and the desensitization of CB1 receptors [816, 823–825]. On clinical grounds, these changes appear to be related to the development of anhedonia and a loss of sensitivity to previously pleasant stimuli [826, 827]. The application of 'functional magnetic resonance Imaging' (fMRI) succeeded in linking chronic exposure to cannabis to an alteration in reward sensitivity [823]. Although dopamine is by far the most studied neurotransmitter in terms of the issue of reward and motivation, it should be recalled that dopaminergic pathways are influenced by other receptor systems and intermingle with both opioid and cannabinoid systems [828–833]. On the whole, the amotivational syndrome, or cannabis-related reward-deficiency syndrome, may be directly related to a change in dopaminergic function, in this case through a cannabis-induced modulation of the cannabinoid receptor activity.

4.7.1   Substance Use and Reward-System Acquired Abnormalities

A well-known paradigm of acquired reward pathology is the natural history of heroin addiction. The course of heroin addiction develops in three stages [834]: the first stage is pleasant involvement in substance use (the 'honeymoon' stage). In healthy, non-tolerant subjects, acute opioid administration produces a marked state of euphoria, coupling serenity and peacefulness with actual mood elation and reward. At this stage, substance use does not take place on a regular basis, and people express confidence that they can break the habit at any time if so wished. No full-blown addictive behaviour is displayed, the substance is self-administered at stable doses and the desire to use it is not very urgent or compelling. In most cases, withdrawal has not yet been experienced. The possible risks are underrated both by the person and the surrounding environment, although the first signs of mood instability and a lowered threshold for affective distress can be detected. The second stage follows the 'honeymoon' one and corresponds to the phenomenon of self-administration at increasing dosages: the transition to regular substance use leads to the development of tolerance, so that the euphoric effects dwindle, while the opposite, withdrawal-related feature starts to recur and becomes ever more prominent. In order to restore the balance and reproduce drug-related euphoria, these subjects automatically increase substance dosages, but in so doing they pave the way for heavier rebound symptoms. The desire to self-administer the substance has now become urgent and overwhelming, despite the reduced persistence, intensity and frequency of satisfactory drug-induced euphoric states. Eventually, subjects swing away from a state of normal liability concomitant with recurrent states of withdrawal or discomfort on account of the absence of drug-induced euphoria. By this stage, the subject could be defined as a drug addict, because of his/her incapacity to change behaviour so as to reverse this undesirable condition and prevent relapses into it. Depending on a variety of factors, but especially as a result of the level most likely along the grade of addiction severity itself (craving, withdrawal), people get fully engaged in substance-seeking, by any available resource and by any means, no matter how hazardous or illegal it may be. The third stage is a series of stereotypically repeating cycles (the 'revolving door' stage) featuring detoxification, temporary suspension of use with possible psychosocial recovery, addictive relapse and rapid impairment. At this stage, due to the increased difficulty of finding regular and consistent amounts of the substance, and to react to feelings of desperation about the individual's general condition, SUD patients resort to treatment facilities. What can be noted at this point is the 'clean' part of the revolving door cycle, from an addictive viewpoint, in a way that is able to reverse tolerance and so cut down on drug-related expenses. At this juncture, a new cycle is ready to begin, contrary to the subject's expectation of being able to handle drug use from a condition in which craving is reset. Occasionally, deadly events interrupt the cycle, and this becomes more and more likely as cycles go by. Notably, the 'clean', non-tolerant periods bear the highest risk of overdose-related deaths, especially when they are spent in artificial environments [3].

Within the framework of these three stages, the hedonistic-euphoric dimension, which was prominent at the beginning, is gradually replaced by a counterpolar state, distinguished by anhedonia and hypophoria (lack of drive, motivation and reactivity with respect to what the person in question regards as being satisfactory). From a withdrawal-related point of view, through each detoxification cycle the patient passes from the acute withdrawal state (counterpolar to intoxication) to a later and enduring drug-free state featuring symptoms of hypophoria, looming as an acquired feeling of discomfort related to the absence of drug-related stimulation. Hypophoria includes somatic, vegetative and mental symptoms such as susceptible or irritable mood, amplified pain perception, inability to perform simple tasks and make normal efforts and inability to experience reward in any way other than resorting to substance use. This syndrome closely resembles the subthreshold symptoms of dysthymia and the residual symptoms of chronic bipolar disorder [361].

In conclusion, the natural history of heroin addiction displays three stages, eventually leading to a chronic state of hypophoria, possibly interrupted by relapses,

Table 4.2   Clinical characteristics of reward impairment in substance use disorder

Post-withdrawal syndrome	Reward-deficiency syndrome	Amotivational syndrome
Feelings of hypophoria	Gradual detachment from the outer world	Social withdrawal
Dysphoria	Loss of emotional reactivity, drives and aims	Loss of impulse and motivation
Extreme sensitivity to pain	Blunted responsiveness to outer stimuli	Emotional detachment
Inability to complete even simple tasks	Inability to experience or anticipate any pleasure	Detachment from reality
Inability to experience pleasure through recreational or natural stimuli	Hampered memory and attention	Reduction in attention and memory

which recalls the features of the reward-deficiency syndrome described as a sequel of alcohol and stimulant chronic use [834] (Table 4.2).

From a neurophysiological point of view, a variety of substances are involved in the dynamics of experiencing pleasure and reward, among which dopamine, GABA and opioids are the best known. Anatomic sites where feelings of pleasure and reward-seeking originate seem to correspond to brain areas known as the ventral tegmental area, the nucleus accumbens, caudate and substantia nigra. Dopaminergic activity is concentrated in the accumbens, caudate and ventral tegmental area, which are referred to as the afferent arm of reward circuitry. GABAergic activity, which has been shown to be considerable in the ventral tegmental area, and opioidergic activity in the substantia nigra and accumbens also contribute to reward dynamics. Basic neurochemical events that correspond to reinforcement and reward take place in the brain areas just named [835–837].

Substances of use act on specific receptors placed on neuronal cells, often mimicking the effect of endogenous equivalents. Thus, substance-inducing acute effects can be described as the stimulation of neuronal circuits corresponding to their endogenous equivalent. A number of studies (resorting to pharmacological parameters, neuroimaging and micro-dialysis) have agreed on the fact that the acute administration of rewarding drugs causes a release of dopamine due to the projection of neurons with a cell body located in the ventral tegmental onto the post-synaptic surfaces of the nucleus accumbens, especially at the *shell* part level [838–840]. This process normally takes place when people are exposed to salient stimuli and underlies the dynamics of adaptation and selection of available sources of euphoric self-stimulation in one's natural environment. An increased availability of dopamine in the pre-synaptic *grasp* of the accumbens shell builds a memory of salience for certain stimuli, which are functionally related to survival, nutrition, reproduction or relief, through such feelings as sexual arousal, competition, appetite or discomfort [841–843]. In other words, salience is a basic way to bookmark rewarding stimuli as crucial to attaining one's aims sooner or to getting spatially closer to craved objects. As far as substance use is concerned, salience is the crucial node between the acute experience of substance-related effects and expected rewards from new episodes of consumption. Pleasant side effects, environments and situations which happen to be associated with substance availability are remembered as conditioning stimuli, so that they can cause reflected withdrawal and automatic drug-seeking behaviours, even in the absence of a direct craving for drug-related effects [213].

This learning process corresponds to changes in the structure of the brain (gene expression, neuronal structure and morphology) due to the mechanisms of neuronal plasticity, particularly in memory-related areas [844–847]. Experimental research consistently indicates how such changes persist in the long term [331, 848–850]. These areas become sensitized to the presentation of drug-related stimuli, both in the animal model and in man, and they maintain that acquired sensitivity long after the latest exposure to the drug [848, 850, 851]. Although dopamine release in the accumbens shell plays a crucial role in associative learning, other brain areas too are involved in the development of addiction starting from substance use. In particular, the anterior cingulated and orbitofrontal cortices at a prefrontal level mediate behavioural outputs produced by drug-related cues [852–855]. Neuroimaging studies have clearly mapped the metabolic changes in specific areas associated with subjective craving and drug-related cueing: the extent of metabolic changes in the orbitofrontal and anterior cingulated cortex areas is directly related to the intensity of cue-induced craving [275, 854, 856–860]. On the other hand, neuroimaging studies on the brains of abstinent individuals with a history of chronic addictive use reveal reduced level of baseline metabolism in the same areas [275, 860–865]. Such metabolic 'depression' also includes responses to normal biologically relevant stimuli, such as food-related or sexual cues [853] and to decision-making challenges in certain experimental settings [866, 867]. In the striatum, both a lower level of available dopamine and a reduced number of D2 receptors have been documented [868–872]. To sum up, chronically exposed individuals who have developed drug addiction show they are hypersensitive to drug-related stimuli, while they are less responsive to other sources of direct stimulation or cueing.

Other systems have an impact on addiction biology, such as the hypophysis-pituitary-adrenal axis (HPA) which mediates response to stress. Substances of use stimulate the HPA axis, which can itself become involved in the process of reward and reinforcement of self-administration [873, 874]. Moreover, substance use and withdrawal are linked to the production and release of the corticotropin releasing factor (CRF) by extra-hypothalamic sites [339, 340, 875, 876]. Stressful stimuli may increase extra-hypothalamic CRF-producing activity, so amplifying the reinforcing effects of drugs, appetition for them and addictive behaviours [338, 877]. It has also been documented that CRF-like factors are related to acute and long-term withdrawal, and to relapse proneness, along with the well-known clinical link between the low threshold to subjective stress and relapses in abstinent SUD patients [340, 878–880].

On the whole, the dopaminergic system plays a crucial role in substance use and addiction. A number of research papers have indicated how cannabis, as well as other substances of use, share a dopamine-releasing action in the nucleus accumbens (the main node of the dopaminergic mesolimbic pathway) [816, 838,

881–885]. Likewise, THC and other drugs (amphetamines, cocaine, alcohol, nicotine and heroin) share the property of selectively increasing dopamine release in the shell part of the accumbens, rather than its core [816, 828, 839, 886, 887]. Alcohol has proved to increase dopaminergic pulsatility and a generalized increase in arousal and sensitivity to reward [860]. Chronic cocaine use is also responsible for reducing dopaminergic release in the accumbens [888].

Since all these different substances seem to share a common mechanism of action, they may be thought to share the feature of eventual damage too. Bowirrat and colleagues argue that dopamine is the main neurotransmitter responsible for both the reward cascade common to all substances of use and the amotivational syndrome: reduced dopaminergic activity underlies all conditions of chronic alcohol or drug administration, which correspond to reduced sensitivity to reward and a lower ability to cope with stress [889]. Different substances own one specific neurochemical property linked to their direct molecular target (i.e. the cannabinoid system, GABAergic receptors for alcohol and BDZs, the opioidergic system, cholinergic receptors for nicotine) and a common eventual effect on the dopaminergic system, especially with respect to the reward pathway circuitry [889]. There is therefore no justification for using the concept of the amotivational syndrome or reward deficiency syndrome to indicate one specific condition (e.g. chronic cannabis use), but a common clinical ground for all kinds of chronic use.

One could also hypothesize that the rewards of drug users are already impaired before drug use, on the basis of genetic dispositions to drug use, possibly involving the polymorphism of DRD2 receptors, which are a key element in the reward cascade [890]. Blum and colleagues have suggested that cannabis users may be distinguished by a primary abnormality of the reward-system, with a lower level of dopaminergic activity, which becomes normalized through exposure to cannabis [316, 891]. This view recalls the self-medication hypothesis of addictive disorders originally formulated by Khantzian with respect to the addictive use of opioids and cocaine: in that case, specific emotional distress and mental disorders were hypothesized as the basis for involvement in regular drug use with a self-medicating purpose [143].

4.7.2   Therapeutic Implications

On therapeutic grounds, AS, RDS and PWS, all developing as late consequences of intensive drug use, achieve stability through a reduced dopaminergic metabolism in the reward-system circuitry, and require the employment of specific types of agonist drugs (opioidergic, cholinergic, GABAergic) and counter-indicate the employment of functional antagonists of the reward-related dopaminergic system, for the purpose of reward rebalance. In other words, therapeutic medications should interact with the same targets as those of used drugs, at a neurochemical level, in order to replace damaged physiological functions.

In the case of heroin addiction, for instance, methadone treatment can be seen as providing a general paradigm: methadone does replace impaired functions and prevents the PWS, does not impede the reprise of the dopaminergic metabolism and prevents further damage by the mechanism of narcotic blockade. Drugs like vareni-cline (cholinergic agonist) [892] and bupropion (cholinergic antagonist, but dopamine agonist) [893, 894] have been tried with some success in the treatment of nicotine withdrawal and nicotine dependence. Unlike varenicline, bupropion is not specific to nicotine, but acts upon the common reward pathway: its dopaminergic and noradrenergic actions are responsible for nicotine withdrawal symptoms and favour detachment from nicotine, although bupropion is not effective in keeping craving under control in the longer term. At least at tolerated dosages, bupropion looms as the paradigm of dopaminergic agents and is capable of producing positive effects in drug use, regardless of a specific anticraving action, because of its action on the shared ground of a reduced dopamine-related function.

By contrast, the use of neuroleptic drugs should be applied with great caution in patients with a history of reward impairment, since they fulfil a sharp dopamine-antagonist action. Atypical antipsychotics, despite their different profile of neuro-chemical action, may elicit or worsen reward impairment, though to a lesser extent, or interfere with dopamine metabolism by different pathways [895]. Even if their use is recommended with respect to acute psychosis, those with low affinity and specificity (fast-off interaction dynamics from dopamine receptors) are prefera-ble [896].

4.7.3   Final Remarks

A variety of substances of use, despite their different mechanisms of action, con-verge on a common pathway centring on the circuitry of reward. The eventual dam-age produced by all substances involves dopaminergic dysfunction, mirroring the initial dopaminergic stimulation corresponding to euphoria and increased reward. In the case of cannabis, this picture has been described as the amotivational syndrome. Adopting a longitudinal view, the course of addiction starts from the experience of hyperstimulation, which develops by overcoming dysphoria and the loss of motiva-tion. Basic changes in brain function and microscopic structure underlie these clini-cal grounds and correspond to the concept of addiction as a unique metabolic disease, regardless of the meaning and clinical picture of earlier phases. The abnor-mal dopaminergic metabolism of the addictive brain implies the impairment of gen-eral reward capacity, again involving the same substance responsible for addiction, together with the ability to cope with stress and the lack of continuous stimulation.

We have tried to give a comprehensive description of the cannabis-related amo-tivational syndrome, the alcohol/cocaine-related reward deficiency syndrome and the opioid-related post-withdrawal syndrome. These three clinical pictures, which originally referred to three different classes of substances, share the feature of moti-vational loss, which looms as the specific acquired functional leak affecting the addict's brain. On therapeutic grounds, pro-dopaminergic drugs are to be regarded as useful, because of their positive impact on the hypo-trophic dopaminergic sys-tem, while antidopaminergic drugs are to be avoided if possible, especially in long-term regimens [357]. What we have just said is of great importance when dealing with the treatment of psychosis in HUD patients.

4.8   The Therapeutic Aspects of Psychotic Disorders in Addicted Patients, with Special Reference to HUD

The relationship between SUD and psychosis is far from having been completely clarified. Even if there is evidence of causal correlations between substance use and psychosis onset for most substances of use, this connection is less clear for opioids. Some authors have hypothesized a direct involvement of opioid neuropeptides in the pathophysiology of psychotic disorders [897]. The antipsychotic effectiveness of opioid agonists [528, 704, 748, 898] is supported by the fact that MMT is responsible for the prevention of psychotic relapses in individuals who have a history of psychotic episodes. In these same subjects, the gradual elimination of methadone was followed by psychotic relapses [427, 635]. This therapeutic finding is in line with the antidopaminergic activity of methadone, as documented by the increase in serum prolactin after its administration [165, 628]. Moreover, the low frequency of any recurrence of psychotic episodes makes it hard to recognize schizophrenic disorders, possibly related to SUDs, in patients who are receiving methadone treatment [104, 683, 750, 751, 899]. The use of methadone has been proposed as a treatment in cases of schizophrenia that have turned out to be resistant to traditional medications, and again in cases of the early development of dyskinesia [451]. In addition, when combined with methadone, low dosages of antipsychotics such as chlorpromazine, fluphenazine and haloperidol are needed to control psychotic symptoms [82, 241, 408]. In HUD patients admitted to hospital for an acute psychotic episode, either an increase in methadone dosage or the actual initiation of methadone treatment was effective in achieving control of psychotic symptoms by prescribing lower treatment dosages of antipsychotics and antimanic drugs, even when the period spent in hospital was the same [82]. The profile of DD/PSY-HUD patients at their first treatment attempt displays a higher level of global symptom severity, even when coupled with less severe addictive symptoms and a shorter duration of addictive history than their non-psychotic peers. We may speculate that the presence of a psychotic background underlying opioid use leads to an early worsening of global mental status through fast-acting opioid use, so that these patients may benefit from opioid stabilization by agonist treatment. Apart from the resolution of the withdrawal-related exacerbation of psychotic symptoms, the positive impact of opioid agonism, which may have been the reason for the transition to regular heroin use, may be recovered by slow-acting, stable dose agonist treatment, but in a restabilizing form rather than a destabilizing one [344]. In other words, the long-term use of opioid agonists may be effective in treating psychotic symptoms in former psychotic patients who later became classifiable as HUD through a self-medication habit [143, 344]. Psychotic HUD may be included among those who resort to street methadone as a regular practice before entering treatment, and this decision should be regarded as a self-harm-reducing behaviour rather than a poly-use pattern. Those patients may, in fact, have an independent motivation to look for treatment earlier and stay in treatment longer, which may overcome addictive ambivalence and improve compliance [85]. In the evaluation of a psychiatric diagnosis of patients entering treatment, we have tried to distinguish between patients who had started heroin use after the onset of psychiatric disorders and those who had suffered from psychiatric disorders after the onset of their drug-using habit. Among the former, psychotic disorders and anxiety disorders were those best represented, and they were linked with a trend towards less severe addictive symptoms. The latter group mostly comprised patients suffering from mood disorders, who have more severe addictive symptoms. This time sequence does not stand as a definite proof of self-medication dynamics, but it is broadly consistent with the idea that some disorders, rather than others, may lead to heroin use in a self-medication manner [627]. The same patients would then suffer from the early worsening of their psychiatric disorders, due to acquired opioid imbalance, when the severity of their addictive disease is still lower; and they will benefit more directly from the opioid-balancing effect of agonist treatment [54]. Through the recent use of an exploratory factor analysis of the 90 items in the SCL90, a five-factor solution was identified for 1055 HUD patients who answered the SCL90 questionnaire at treatment entry. These factors were named on the basis of items that showed the highest loadings. W/BT, SS, S/P, PA and V/S were the five dimensions that were extracted. On the basis of the highest z-scores obtained on the five SCL90 factors (allowing the identification of a number of dominant SCL90 factors), subjects could be assigned to one of five mutually exclusive groups. These five groups were sufficiently distinct and have failed to reveal any significant overlap [40]. As to current knowledge, a variety of opioid medications seem to be capable of a specific action on psychopathological symptoms. Using the SCL90 five-factor solution, HUD patients with prominently psychopathological S/P characteristics showed a better level of retention in treatment when treated with methadone [43]. Methadone dosage would partly work as a psychotropic stabilizer, regardless of addictive symptoms, so that the eventual stabilization dosage would be higher than in non-DD/PSY-HUD. Once both psychopathological grounds (addictive and psychotic) have been neutralized, DD/PSY-HUD may reach a positive outcome, unlike what could be expected in the absence of treatment [900, 901].

In summary, considering these results, effects of substances can be divided into those that are pro-psychotic and those that are antipsychotic. Psychoses correlated with SUD prove to be more common in cases involving cannabinoids, stimulants, hallucinogens, alcohol and poly-use. By contrast, opioids are the only sedative drugs that are marked by an antipsychotic effect. The addictive process is the same for all substances of use, but that sameness does not apply to their relationship with psychosis. Thus, poly-use can be considered as taking the initial form of a use of stimulants that leads to the onset of a psychosis that, at a later stage, is complicated by opioids into an attempt to take advantage of their antipsychotic effects. We therefore suggest that opioid agonists deserve reconsideration, not only because of their anticraving capability, but also because of their effectiveness on the psychopathological level, which makes them a perfect tool, even in the task of curing mental illness.

4.8.1   Antipsychotic Agents

Both typical and atypical antipsychotics have been evaluated in dual disorder psychotics. If it is to be comprehensive, any evaluation of antipsychotics must consider their impact on drug-related issues: on one hand, used substances may have psychotomimetic properties; on the other, the persistence of, or relapses into, drug taking are both predictive of an unfavourable course.

Typical antipsychotics (TAs) offer little help to DD psychotics [676, 681, 682, 695, 902, 903]. Substance use is common among schizophrenics treated with TAs, and it shows no reduction during treatment; in fact, a tendency towards an increase in consumption during treatment has emerged for some substances, such as nicotine [904, 905]. Psychotic patients who are also drug users show a less favourable response to TAs, presumably due to the pro-psychotic effects of persistently used substances, which limit the incisiveness of that treatment. When substance use foreruns a psychotic outburst, agents such as haloperidol or perphenazine can be expected to prove less effective than would otherwise be the case.

Since both TAs and use substances act on the CNS dopaminergic system, it can be hypothesized that special phenomena may intervene in the relationship between the pharmacodynamics of the specific agent and its impact on the course of psychoses, when substance use co-occurs [695, 902]. At clinically effective dosages, it has been shown that TAs turn off the mesolimbic dopaminergic firing, which is the known substrate for the reinforcing effects elicited by many used substances, such as cocaine. Cocaine itself and alcohol are the two most frequently used drugs among psychotics. Several addictive substances induce an increase in the levels of homovanillic acid (OVA), an index of dopaminergic activity, and enhance the release of dopamine in the nucleus accumbens which is the terminal of the dopaminergic mesolimbic pathway [906]. On this basis, it is plausible that the use of substances is effective in reversing the dopaminergic blockade induced by TAs. On one hand, this is consistent with the relapse-provoking role of drug use; on the other, it suggests that treated psychotics may resort to substances to counter the blunting effect on emotional life brought about by the mesolimbic antagonism of TAs. In a highly tolerant mesolimbic system, like that of drug users, which is more sensitive to the lack of stimulation than that of normal individuals, the administering of TAs is likely to elicit an intense and intolerable hypophoria, followed by compensatory behavioural activation towards sources of reward. For individuals who have already learned to achieve rewards by substance use before treatment, resorting to available substances would automatically ensure compensation. The use-enhancing effect of TAs would be directly related to the antidopaminergic potency of the specific compound. Consistently with that, the use of desimipramine as adjunct to a TA for cocaine-using psychotics has been reported to reduce cocaine use, which does not happen with the same agent among non-psychotic cocaine users. In other words,

TAs appear to enhance drug use in a way that is reversible by desimipramine, which is effective on drug use to the extent to which it counteracts the mesolimbic dopaminergic antagonism achieved by TA.

Clozapine, which possesses low specificity on dopaminergic receptors, showed a poor capacity to reduce dopaminergic transmission in animal models, when compared with TAs. Again, in animal models, clozapine, unlike other antipsychotics, has been shown to decrease cocaine consumption, when a fixed dose schedule is used, and to lengthen cocaine-free periods, when an increasing dose schedule is used. On clinical grounds, clozapine has revealed anticraving properties. First, the responsiveness of psychotic patients to clozapine is independent of concurrent substance use, in a way that is not attainable with TAs, which, as a rule, prove to be less incisive in substance-using individuals. Some authors have even suggested that substance-using psychotics may display a better response to clozapine than non-users [907, 908].

In DD schizophrenics, clozapine treatment reduces nicotine use. Switching from haloperidol to clozapine did, in fact, lower nicotine consumption, whereas haloperidol had caused it to increase. The clozapine-related reduction in nicotine use is dose-related [905]. AUD patients treated with clozapine are likely to have stayed abstinent (50%) throughout the first year after discharge from hospital. Two psychotics with alcohol dependence, after treatment with 500 mg/day clozapine, were shown to have stayed abstinent in the long term [909, 910].

The interpretation of clozapine's effects on drug and alcohol use is not altogether clear, though: in some contexts, a primary anticraving effect seems to loom, whereas in others it seems plausible that drug use leads to a reduction because in its case there is no need for self-medication brought about by an antidopaminergic blockade, such as that which has to be dealt with in the case of TAs [143, 911]. Drug-using schizophrenics, in fact, report 'negative symptoms'—anxiety and mood especially—to a lesser extent, whereas counteraction by dopaminergic substances ends up by exacerbating psychotic symptoms, so unfavourably affecting the course of the illness and impairing the efficacy of antidopaminergic antipsychotics (i.e. TAs). A vicious circle is set up, first comprising negative symptoms and treatment by TAs, then the use of dopaminergic substances, including psychotic relapses, and lastly the potentiation of TA treatment to achieve a wider antipsychotic defence spectrum.

In DD patients, TA-induced hypophoria could be the key to an explanation of the dynamics between antipsychotic treatment and the course of concurrent substance use. The frequency of depressed mood symptoms among TA-treated psychotics and their partial reversal following drug-taking are consistent with this explanatory model. The novelty-seeking dimension of Cloninger's Tridimensional Personality Questionnaire, which implies a higher risk for substance-related behaviours, has recently been associated with the D4 receptor subtype. Agents acting as D4 antagonists may reduce drug-seeking behaviour, whereas D2 antagonists (such as TAs) appear to increase them, especially in individuals who are highly positive to D4. In reality, clozapine's profile is distinguished by its higher specificity for D4 receptors

Table 4.3 Drug interactions and methadone dosages in the experience of the PISA-V.P. Dole Research Group in HUD patients with chronic psychosis and violent behaviour

	Dosage (mg/day)	
	Mode	Range
Methadone (stabilization dose)	140	30–290
Typical antipsychotics (haloperidol equivalent)	7	3–9
Clozapine	100	100–300
Olanzapine	10	10–20
Risperidone	3	2–6
Quetiapine	200	100–300
Aripiprazole	15	5–20
Asenapine	20	5–20
Lurasidone	40	15–80

Pay attention during the AOT induction phase for the increase in plasma concentration of both methadone and antidopaminergic drugs. Reassess the dosage if the patient is already on treatment. Consider the QTc prolongation action of anti-D2 drugs

(higher D4/D2 ratio) [684]. Risperidone, which has the highest specificity for D4 receptors, has not yet been evaluated on this issue.

4.8.2   Methadone and Antipsychotics

The concurrent use of antipsychotics in methadone-maintained psychotics can be considered acceptable and helpful [912, 913]. When combined with methadone, low dosages of TAs such as chlorpromazine, fluphenazine and haloperidol are needed to control psychotic symptoms [408]. One problem is that antipsychotics are quite likely to be poorly tolerated by HUD patients. Usually, TAs are not used, but if they are, patients should be urged to comply. Depot preparations make it possible to skip the limitations posed by non-compliance, and concurrent methadone treatment seems to act as a shield against extrapyramidal side effects. Table 4.3 shows the methadone and antipsychotic dosages needed for DD/PSY-HUD patients.

Clinicians should be particularly careful during the induction phase, in order to minimize the narcotic mutual potentiation of antipsychotics and opioids, especially when TAs are used. As a rule, the recommendation is to avoid administering antipsychotics until the steady state has been reached with methadone. In the meantime, the sedative action of methadone itself can be resorted to. In addition, the use of BDZs cannot be recommended. In cases of severe psychomotor excitement requiring neuroleptic administration, limited amounts of neuroleptics can be used, as long as they are under medical control, and as long as neuroleptic doses are not taken late in the evening. Antihistaminic agents are a valid and suitable alternative option for achieving sedation in DD/PSY-HUD patients.

4.8.3 Dopaminergic Partial Agonist Medications

Third-generation antipsychotics are distinguished by a partial agonist action on the D2 receptor (or various subtypes of the D2-like group, as well as D3), combined with the action on the serotonin system via 5-HT2A. The third generation represents an interesting novelty in terms of anticraving therapies. The most certain fact about the relationship between antipsychotics and substance use is, in fact, the inverse correlation between D2 antagonism and the tendency to use substances. This happens at least in chronic psychosis or for therapies that are still protracted.

In DD psychotic patients, it is necessary to bear in mind:

- The characteristics of the acute phase of psychosis and its short-term course, when studying the effect on acute phases brought about by the substance
- The characteristics of the rehabilitation course when the main aim is to establish, beyond the objective use of substances, the specific action of the antipsychotic medication on functional recovery or the preservation of residual functions
- The characteristics of the course in the natural environment, in terms of the use of substances, with or without simultaneous major psychotic relapse, in case the driving aim of a study is to establish the objective anticraving effect

With regard to the third-generation antipsychotics currently available, the most consistent data, with clinical evidence, concern aripiprazole, a partial agonist at 30% of D2s that is also active on D3, with a close relationship (Ki < 1).

In terms of anticraving activity, partial agonists do not seem to be capable of acting decisively. Dopaminergic agonism that includes D2 receptors (or D2-like ones) has been the rationale for numerous studies on drugs with various indications (antidepressants, endocrine, antiparkinsonians), with no appreciable results. Often these results are not assessable, because of the small sample and poor retention in treatment. These are typically studying about cocaine addiction. The hypothesis is that the increase in dopaminergic tone should compensate for the reduced metabolism that results from chronic cocaine intoxication. In this way the imbalance between decrease in dopaminergic metabolism and the presence of craving would be compensated. However, an increase in dopaminergic metabolism in certain key areas of the reward-system induces the appearance of appetitive behaviours, or their amplification. In other words, beyond a certain limit, the increase in dopaminergic metabolism (in general) will produce an increase in behavioural output, according to a reverberating pattern; on the other hand, the reduction below a certain level will produce a deficit model, which is reversible according to a compensatory dynamic.

At the receptor level, D2 antagonist medications tend to worsen the attachment towards the used substances in psychotic subjects. Among antipsychotics, clozapine is the only medication that seems to have anticraving properties, or otherwise improves attachment developed through the effects of a powerful D2-blockade. A partial agonist, in this case, produces an effect that is "pro-dopaminergic" on a low-dopaminergic brain (depression, stimulant intoxication or, in general, from euphoric substances) and "antidopaminergic" on a high-tone brain (mania, psychosis).

Some D2 blockers, in preclinical models, show antagonistic properties on addictive behaviours, i.e. a reduction of the craving effect, understood as a boost to the search for and consumption of a substance. This fact, however, depends on several factors, one of which is D2 antagonism. In addition, some anti-D2 antipsychotics, especially at minimal doses, can act on pre-synaptic D2 receptors, facilitating the release of dopamine. According to this model, if the dopaminergic signal 'entering' the reward circuit (mesolimbic pathway) is very small, craving tends to rise. If the outgoing dopaminergic signal is very low, the craving is blocked. Depending on the D2/D4 ratio, the outcome may be equilibrium states (no craving) under low conditions (as in depressive/negative/deficit syndromes) or high dopaminergic tone (euthymia, hyperthymia). Euphoria, whether at the hypomanic or manic level, is, instead, connected with a dopaminergic tone such as to generate an output signal that is, in any case, sufficient to feed the craving.

The ideal medication to control craving, by acting on the dopamine metabolism, should therefore be a 'partial' agonist of D2 or, instead, an antagonist of D4 receptors, at a level not inhibiting personal initiative. A powerful D2 antagonism generates amotivational, abulic and slowed-down blocking just as a powerful D4 antagonism can generate 'outgoing' hyper-control on the propensity to take initiatives.

Pre-treatment with aripiprazole attenuates the effects of D-amphetamine [914, 915] and methamphetamine [914, 916] in recreational users, but in drug addicts the positive effect of methamphetamine [917] and of cocaine [918] increases, only buffering the negative effects. Pre-treatment with aripiprazole does not change the dynamics of cocaine self-administration in humans in a laboratory context [919]; it increases its use and decreases liking for the self-administered substance [920], that is, it worsens the type of imbalance characteristic of addiction. The effect seems to decay over time [918] and is most evident at higher doses of cocaine [921].

During cocaine withdrawal, aripiprazole increases craving, with no impact on behaviour [919]. The initial effect in amphetamine addicts seems similar (worse than placebo in the first weeks of treatment, whereas methylphenidate is already better than placebo) [922].

In abstinent cocaine addicts, treatment with aripiprazole is shown to be undatable (regarding relapsing into cocaine use) because the relapse exceeds 50% even before the end of the study [919]. An Italian study of a small sample confirms the same amount of dropouts in the first few weeks [923]. A double-blind study on methamphetamine addiction failed [924].

Aripiprazole reduces the potential for alcohol use [925]. The effect on alcoholism is neutral [926], although in a laboratory context alcohol use seems to be reduced by aripiprazole in subjects with greater impulsivity [927]. A randomized double-blind study has identified the possible indicators of aripiprazole efficacy, such as the fall in the severity of addiction, while not acting on all the parameters of alcoholism [928]. Similarly, in the comparison with NTX, there is only a greater latency, but not less frequency, of relapse [929].

Efficacy in DD patients has been proved more thoroughly. In a group of schizophrenics (open-label), aripiprazole reduces psychotic symptoms and craving for alcohol (misuse) and cocaine (addiction), reducing cocaine use after 2 months, with a dropout rate of 40% [930]. These data have not been confirmed to be specific to aripiprazole in a double-blind study comparing it with perphenazine [931], which was used to treat schizophrenic subjects with anamnestic substance use, even if they were not using in the last few days before the study.

In subjects with acute psychosis and methamphetamine use disorder, aripiprazole does not produce use reduction in 8 weeks, as shown in a study comparing subjects already in treatment for 2 weeks with aripiprazole and divided into two groups—the first treated with aripiprazole, the second (as a control sample) with placebo [932]. From a longer term perspective, injectable aripiprazole is associated with a 6-month effect on schizophrenics, but this effect is not easily interpretable. A minority of cocaine and alcohol patients ceased its use, but of those—a majority—who continued its use, only a subgroup experienced a reduction in illness severity [933].

In a group of depressed patients with alcohol addiction, the effect on craving has also been reported for the effects of adding aripiprazole to escitalopram. This happened in a controlled neuroimaging study evaluating the left anterior cingulate activity, considering the resumption of function in this brain sector as a sign of craving reduction [934]. Antidepressant response and reduction of substance use were reported by adding open-label bupropion to aripiprazole and valproate after 4 weeks of treatment. These cocaine addicts, however, showed variable frameworks and an unknown current use status, with a self-report measurement of substance use [935].

A particular open-label study in HUD patients with schizoaffective disorder, who were treated with aripiprazole and topiramate while taking methadone at an average of 80 mg/day, showed a good improvement in psychopathology, at least in the short term [936]. The rationale of the study hypothesized a generic anticraving activity of mood stabilizers and atypical antipsychotics when a well-referenced anticraving therapy (methadone) was already under way. The prospect, in the case of a reduction in psychiatric symptoms, was to proceed with a rapid subtraction of methadone therapy for reasons that were no better defined. The study provided objectively useful data on the use of aripiprazole in schizoaffective psychosis associated with opioid addiction, covering the full course of methadone treatment. None of the findings, however, indicated the same level of effectiveness after the removal of treatment for heroin addiction. This condition, whether favoured or not by the best psychopathological compensation, would lead patients to a new condition of non-treatment for their opioid addiction, with presumably negative results also affecting the control of psychosis and compliance with antipsychotic treatment. As for the idea that treatment can prevent heroin relapses, there is no concrete element to suggest or hypothesize this property, nor is there any evidence that the therapy in question makes it easier to up methadone therapy.

Our research team described three cases of psychotic bipolar subjects successfully treated with aripiprazole [937].

Apart from the effect on craving and psychosis, third-generation antipsychotic drugs represent an undoubted advantage over other antipsychotic drugs due to the lower action on the reward-deficit syndrome and drug-induced hypophoria, both of which in psychotic DD patients contribute to complicating the success of long-term treatments. Even drugs such as lurasidone that tend not to aggravate the negative symptoms of psychosis may have to be preferred to other antipsychotics for their supposedly less hypophoric action. Our research group has adopted anti-D2 drugs for psychosis in drug users only until the resolution of the acute phase, and if not responding to partial agonists. Among anti-D2 therapies, we prefer drugs that do not aggravate negative symptoms. For long-term treatment, where the prevention of psychotic relapses requires it, we prefer partial agonistic drugs even in depot formulation.

4.8.4   Disulfiram

Disulfiram counteracts alcohol consumption regardless of the presence of psychotic symptoms. The reduction of alcohol use is bound to have a positive impact on the course of psychosis itself, because alcohol is known to worsen psychotic symptoms. In subjects treated with high-dose disulfiram, however, psychotic symptoms have been reported to deteriorate [684, 700]. Schizophrenic AUD patients have been reported to benefit from disulfiram treatment to the same extent as non-psychotic AUD patients. In particular, alcohol use in schizophrenics seems to show an excellent response to the clozapine–disulfiram combination [700].

In conclusion, disulfiram is useful in psychotic AUD patients at a dosage of 250 mg/day: at this dosage, the likelihood of an iatrogenic worsening of psychotic effects carries less weight than the impact of on-going alcohol use in causing exacerbation and in harming the overall course of the illness.

Disulfiram has also been shown to be useful in treating cocaine dependence in methadone-maintained opioid addicts [938].

4.8.5   Desimipramine

Desimipramine has been used at doses of 100–150 mg/day in cocaine-addicted psychotics, as an adjunct to antipsychotic treatment. In these patients, that combination achieved a good level of control over cocaine craving. The same agent when tried on non-psychotic cocaine addicts failed to show any definite efficacy [939, 940]. Anticraving dopaminergic agents must be avoided during acute psychotic phases, because of the risk of exacerbating psychotic symptoms, as well as the uncertainty of their impact on substance use. In stabilized chronic psychotics, our anecdotal evidence suggests that ropinirole, up to 1.5 mg/day, can lead to a reduction in craving, with no concurrent psychopathological destabilization.

4.8.6   The Long-Term Outcome of Patients with Heroin Use Disorder/Dual Disorder (Chronic Psychosis) After Admission to Enhanced Methadone Maintenance

Opioid use disorder patients show a high rate of psychiatric comorbidities (anxiety, depression, sleep disorders) during AOT [941]. The presence of psychotic and affective symptoms is a common feature of psychiatric disorders, and their link with SUD has been widely demonstrated in the literature [701]. Regarding patients with HUD, according to our previous studies, the onset of psychosis generally occurs before substance use begins, whereas affective symptoms develop afterwards [233, 627]. The natural history of HUD differs between psychotic and bipolar HUD patients, so these two categories of patients often present different clinical pictures at the moment of admission to their first AOT. In HUD patients with chronic psychosis (DD/PSY-HUD), the progression of the addictive disease is limited, whereas DD/BIP1-HUD patients show a more severe substance (i.e. heroin) use illness [249]. In patients with PSY-HUD, a therapeutic use of heroin cannot be excluded, at least at the beginning of their clinical history. This kind of situation was not reported in the case of bipolar HUD patients [233]. During AOT, especially during methadone treatment, our patients with and without DD show extreme variability of the dose needed to prevent a relapse during treatment [67, 942]. In our patients, above-standard methadone doses are usually needed in the presence of high severity psychopathological symptomatology characterized by somatization, depression, paranoid ideation, and psychoticism [50]. Above-standard doses are likewise needed for DD patients [55]. Good outcomes were also related to methadone dosage in our previously studied DD/BIP1-HUD patients [52].

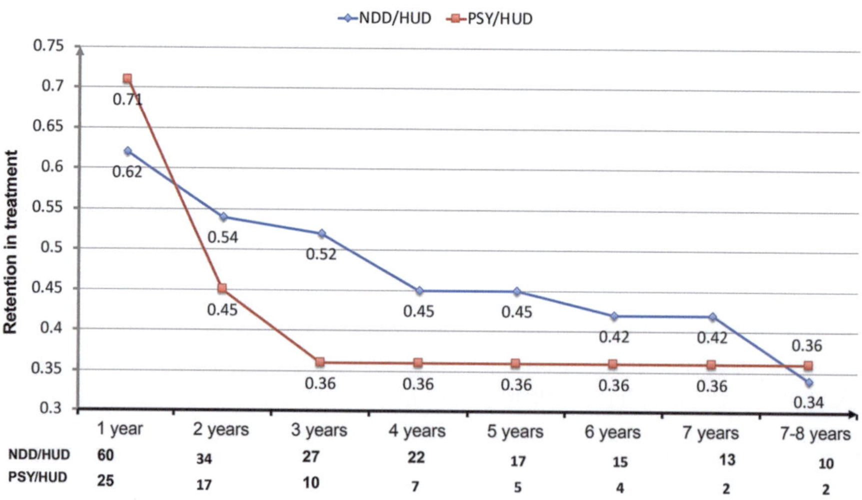

Fig. 4.5 Retention in treatment of dual disorder (chronic psychosis) HUD patients compared to NDD/HUD patients

In one of our studies [101], we aimed to compare the long-term outcomes of treatment-resistant DD/PSY-HUD with those of HUD patients without psychiatric comorbidity (Fig. 4.5).

We decided to evaluate whether chronic psychosis was able to influence methadone treatment outcomes in patients who had previously been non-responders in front-line, low-threshold treatment facilities when those patients were included in a high-threshold, maintenance-oriented, high-dose methadone programme. The study hypothesized that a diagnosis of chronic psychosis would not affect treatment outcomes if DD/PSY-HUD patients received individualized (above-standard) doses of methadone and that a good outcome would be related to long-term, on-going treatment (assessable through retention). To test this hypothesis, DD/PSY-HUD and HUD patients were followed in a naturalistic approach applied for up to 8 years in the context of the maintenance high-threshold, high-dose PISA-MMT program, using retention in treatment and rates of heroin use as the primary end-point parameters.

The discriminant demographic characteristics of DD/PSY-HUD patients were as follows. DD/PSY-HUD patients more frequently had education lasting less than 8 years, presented a lower level of social adjustment with a lower frequency of legal problems, and self-reported a lower severity of drug addiction history. More specifically, DD/PSY-HUD patients less frequently showed physical concerns and poly-substance use, talked about having experienced unsuccessful treatments or having received on-going psychosocial treatments at local units, declared 'daily or more' heroin intake before requesting treatment, and reached stage 3 of heroin addiction. Also, DD/PSY-HUD patients were older when they first started using heroin and when they began their continuous use of heroin. Lastly, the duration of their dependence was shorter. Cox regression analysis using the variables reported above—showing differences between DD/PSY-HUD and HUD patients—as predictors, and patients' poor outcome as a criterion, did not show significant correlations except for a low educational level.

Regarding the outcome of the patients, as related to chronic psychotic comorbidity, at the end of the observational period, 20% of the HUD patients and 32% of the DD/PSY-HUD patients completed their rehabilitation programme and either left the treatment or were referred to another programme as a 'stabilized patient'. About 53.3% of the HUD patients and 60.0% of the DD/PSY-HUD patients had not reached stabilization within a year or had relapsed into heroin use during the programme, so they were terminated and referred to their local treatment services; 26.7% of the HUD patients and 8.0% of the DD/PSY-HUD patients were considered 'stabilized' and were still in treatment at the end of the period of observation. These differences were not statistically significant. No patients left the treatment because of side effects; 6.6% of the HUD patients and none of the DD/PSY-HUD patients were dismissed for violence; none were imprisoned or re-hospitalized because of a psychotic episode. None of the DD/PSY-HUD patients relapsed into addictive behaviour (reusing heroin) after 3 years of treatment. In summary, according to the Kaplan–Meier methodology, the HUD patients' cumulative proportion retained (CPR) in treatment at the end of the observational period was 0.34. The proportion of DD/PSY-HUD patients was 0.36. These differences were not statistically significant. Males and females showed a similar retention rate. Males did not show a significantly different retention rate from HUD females. The same results were observed in comparing DD/PSY-HUD females.

When the toxicological examination performed at the time of enrolment *into* the programme (which was required to be positive) was eliminated from the analysis, no patient provided positive samples for the entire duration of treatment. No patient provided exclusively negative samples. In summary, no differences were found regarding urinalyses for morphine between DD/PSY-HUD and HUD patients during the observational period. The CGI severity of illness and the *DSM-IV* GAF showed the following significant trends in participants. At the end-point evaluation, good-outcome DD/PSY-HUD patients reported a lower severity of illness than good-outcome HUD patients. Time effect and group-time effect were significant. Interestingly, at baseline, the severity of illness was equal in the two groups. These differences were not related to the outcome. At the end-point evaluation, good-outcome DD/PSY-HUD patients reported a better level of social adjustment than good-outcome HUD patients. Time effect and group-time effect were both significant. These differences were not related to the outcome. On average, DD/PSY-HUD and HUD patients did not need statistically different methadone dosages in the stabilization phase. Differences between groups were not observed even when dosage was controlled by the outcome. DD/PSY-HUD patients needed less months to reach the stabilization dosages.

It is not easy to correlate low educational level with poor outcome. It is known that, in SUD patients, successful treatment was associated with several baseline characteristics including older age, white race, having more than a high school education, lower level of care, and not having a history of opioid use [943]. It is also true that, at first sight, control patients seem to be a more seriously ill control group. We assume, however, that only the drug-related history is less severe in DD/PSY-HUD patients. The overall clinical judgement expressed by CGI stresses the same severity of disease in both groups. In addition, there is no doubt that, from the psychopathological point of view, DD/PSY-HUD patients are more seriously ill than their peers without DD.

In our study, the outcome and the retention rate in the therapy of treatment-resistant participants did not differ from that of long-term standard methadone programmes designed according to the methodology of Dole and Nyswander [491, 493, 495]. Participants were stabilized using middle-to-high dosages, but not with the above-standard dosages we used to stabilize BIP1-HUD patients [52].

Anecdotal evidence has been reported about the beneficial effects of opioids in reducing psychotic symptoms. In a 39-year-old man requesting treatment for positive psychotic symptoms, a low-dose of quetiapine and 140 mg daily of methadone subsequently controlled his psychosis for years. After interrupting the use of antipsychotic medication and methadone due to complaints in the sexual area, he returned to a condition of presenting acute psychotic symptoms. After he started taking heroin regularly, treatment with methadone and quetiapine was resumed, and his symptoms subsided. A few months later, he again stopped using methadone, without relapsing into heroin use; his psychotic symptoms reappeared, even though he maintained the antipsychotic medication [944]. The use of high methadone dosage has been confirmed in a series of DD/PSY-HUD patients [945] and one patient responded to an increased dose of methadone [898]. Reports of the occurrence of a psychotic episode after methadone or buprenorphine discontinuation are, in the literature, a little bit more frequent [427, 641, 642].

Higher methadone doses have been used in DD/HUD [946], as an anti-anxiety, antidepressant and antipsychotic treatment [947].

In our study, a possible explanation for the need for these relatively higher doses in patients who had previously been unresponsive to standard treatments may be related to a wide inter-individual variability in the methadone metabolism [499, 500], which may explain why a number of patients are under-medicated, if a standard (middle-to-low) dose of methadone is used. Unfortunately, we did not measure plasma methadone levels in studying participants during the stabilization phase, so we cannot resolve this doubt.

In study participants, only axis I psychiatric disorders were taken into consideration, and the existence of a minor form of psychopathology in the other patients concealed under the main addictive symptoms cannot be excluded. We refer to the psychopathological symptoms of axis II psychiatric disorders and/or psychopathological symptoms related to the HUD [40]. Participants were, however, followed up for a long time (up to 8 years), and diagnoses were subject to revision whenever further clinical evidence or retrospective information was gathered—a factor that reduces the likelihood of false HUD. Moreover, the duration of addiction was such as to make it improbable that participants rated as HUD had a silent psychiatric history. The availability of significant others was itself extremely helpful in increasing the level of diagnostic accuracy and grouping.

The high GAF score values recorded for DD/PSY-HUD participants without hospitalizations throughout the treatment period showed that participants were simultaneously compliant both with MMT requirements and with the specific therapy adopted for their comorbid psychopathology. The use of new-generation antipsychotics for the treatment of psychiatric symptoms—medication not wholly changed by the need to treat addiction—may partly explain the positive outcomes obtained in psychotic participants. This effect cannot be attributed exclusively to the effects of pharmacotherapy. A lack whether of appropriately flexible methadone doses and/or of specific medications given in association with methadone treatment for DD/PSY-HUD patients could have been responsible for the conflicting results obtained by other researchers, who reported that psychiatric disorders were linked to worse treatment outcomes (such as drug use and criminal activities) [948–950]. Also, the high therapeutic pressure associated with our programme could have been responsible for better results [510].

In the present study, methadone is potentially useful in treating psychosis, at least in HUD patients. This is in line with a series of observations about the correlation between opioid use and psychosis [51].

We are aware that it is very difficult to find published papers about the dosages of AO medications in DD patients, to corroborate the results of the present study. Our present results do, however, look stronger in the light of our previous studies, with all the limitations that this fact entails. The concern is that we may be overinterpreting our previous research despite the fact that it consisted of single-site, small sample size, homogeneous population studies carried out in Europe (selected for patients who had failed to achieve results at lower levels of treatment). In the literature there are still insufficient data to generalize the present results to cover all HUD patients with comorbid non-affective psychotic disorders. We wonder, of course, if our findings would apply to other HUD sub-populations (e.g. adolescents, or psychiatric patients with HUD not seeking SUD treatment). In any case, our previous studies do allow us to present some afterthoughts on the results of our present study.

In HUD patients admitted to hospital for an acute psychotic episode, we found that an increase in methadone dosage or the initiation of methadone treatment proved to be potentially effective in achieving control of psychotic symptoms by prescribing lower treatment dosages of antipsychotics and mood-stabilizing drugs, even when the period spent in hospital was the same [82].

We also found that the profile of DD/PSY-HUD patients at their first treatment attempt displays a higher level of global symptom severity, even when coupled with less severe addictive symptoms and a shorter duration of addictive history than their non-psychotic peers [249].

Our DD/PSY-HUD patients may be included among those who resort to street methadone as a regular practice before entering treatment, and this decision should be regarded as a self-harm-reducing behaviour rather than a pattern of use. Our patients may, in fact, have an independent motivation to look for treatment earlier and stay in treatment longer—an advantage that may overcome addictive ambivalence and improve compliance [85].

We also found that there is a distinction to be made between patients who had started heroin use after the onset of psychiatric disorders and those who had suffered from psychiatric disorders after the onset of their drug habit. Among the former, psychotic disorders and anxiety disorders were those best represented, and they were linked with a trend towards less severe addictive symptoms. The latter group mostly comprised patients with mood disorders, who had more severe addictive symptoms. This time sequence does not stand as a definite proof of self-medication dynamics, but it is broadly consistent with the idea that some disorders, rather than others, may lead to heroin use in a self-medication manner [627]. The same patients would then suffer from early impairment of their psychiatric disorders, due to acquired opioid imbalance, when the severity of their addictive disease is still lower; and they will benefit more directly from the opioid-balancing effect of agonist treatment [951].

Through the recent use of an exploratory factor analysis of the 90 items in the SCL90, a five-factor solution was identified for HUD patients, namely, W/BT, SS, S/P, PA and V/S [40]. Using this SCL90 five-factor solution, our HUD patients with prominently psychopathological S/P characteristics showed a better level of retention in treatment when treated with methadone [43].

According to our research group, methadone dosage would partly work as a psychotropic stabilizer, regardless of addictive symptoms, so that the eventual stabilization dosage is higher than in non-DD/PSY-HUD patients. Once both psychopathological grounds (addictive and psychotic) have been neutralized, many HUD patients may achieve a positive outcome, reversing what might be expected in the absence of treatment [247, 952].

Lastly, in the present study, methadone should accelerate the stabilization process in DD/PSY-HUD patients through the early normalizing of the opioid system.

Generally, patients requiring high-dose methadone are polydrug SUD patients or patients with psychiatric comorbidities [953]. That result was confirmed by us in HUD bipolar 1 patients [52], but not in psychotic ones, in which standard doses seem to be potentially effective, too. We should, in fact, keep in mind that an overall improvement in the psychiatric status of HUD patients has been reported, independently of the dosages used [954], and that a very high prevalence of psychiatric comorbidity is present in HUD patients receiving AOT [941].

4.8.7   Proposal

The following strategies, derived from the experience of our research group, are proposed as guidelines derived from our clinical practice in the treatment of patients with DD (HUD and chronic psychosis).

- Long-acting opioids have antipsychotic properties.
- Use the best achievable compliance with antipsychotic treatment, during treatment with opioid agonists, to avoid psychotic relapses.
- Add small doses of typical or atypical antipsychotics, in conjunction with mood stabilizers, to increase plasma levels of methadone and antipsychotics.
- Prefer clozapine-like drugs, such as quetiapine, but also partial agonists of D2 receptors and anti-D2 not aggravating negative symptoms.
- Consider the possibility of opioid withdrawal psychosis and, if necessary, reintroduce treatment with opioid agonists.
- Use antipsychotics with caution in PSY/HUD patients treated with opioid agonists, if their tolerance to opioids is unknown, or during the induction phase of treatment with opioid agonists.
- Avoid low-potency antipsychotics during treatment with opioid agonists, as the need for a higher dose results in greater metabolic interference, with higher plasma levels of therapeutic opioids.
- Consider the use of central anti-histamines, even intramuscularly, in case of psychomotor agitation or stubborn insomnia.
- Use anti-D2 drugs for as little time as possible to avoid causing double harm: on the negative symptoms of psychosis, and on the hypophoria of drug addiction, especially in patients who are not treated with opioid agonists.

5.1 Introduction

The study of aggression is crucial in psychiatry and psychopathology because hostile behaviours are involved in various physical pathologies and because aggression has an essential role in the genesis of mental pathology. In addition to the importance of pharmacology, the role of psychosocial factors in favouring the onset and influencing the course of diseases, by expressing or controlling aggressive thrusts, has been enhanced.

Aggression refers to a wide range of human behaviours that can perform different functions in adapting man to the reality that surrounds him. The term aggression can describe adaptation to the environment in both a practical, creative, and available way, and harmful and destructive, socially deplorable behaviour. Apart from the difficulty of defining the term itself, there are various theoretical approaches to the study of the origins and causes of aggressive behaviour. From time to time, starting from Freud's conception and arriving at the ethological view, aggression was an aspect of libido, a desire for control over external reality, a tool for achieving gratification or overcoming frustration. On the other hand, aggression was often perceived as an autonomous death instinct, already detectable in the last writings of Freud [955] and taken up in a particular way by Klein [956]. However, some psychoanalysts, such as Adler [957] and later Fromm and Storr [958, 959], highlighted the constructive aspect of aggression that appears to express the thirst for the domination of the individual. Ethologists, especially Lorenz [960], stressed its importance for the survival of the individual and the whole species. In the behaviourist view, the contributions of Dollard et al. [961] of the Yale school were the most important. According to this perspective, interest is focused on defining the contingent modalities rather than the original causes of aggression, which are understood to be a consequence of a state of frustration. Berkowitz [962] introduced the concept of disposition favourable to aggressive acts represented by the emotional reaction produced by frustration and by aggressive clothes (indicative of readiness) acquired

I. Maremmani et al., *Dual Disorder Heroin Addicts*,
https://doi.org/10.1007/978-3-031-30093-6_5

previously. Bandura [963] argued that aggression is a class of responses that the individual learns by more or less direct imitation of models. Buss [964] emphasized, above all, the instrumentality of the aggression oriented to overcoming pathogenic noxae or the acquisition of benefits and investigated the typology and its acceptability from the social point of view.

In this chapter, we analyse the aggressive behaviours of our patients suffering from HUD, using the concepts of the behavioural school and the diagnostic criteria of the various *DSM* [171]. Referring to the many years of experience of the PISA-V.P. Dole Research Group at Santa Chiara University Hospital in Pisa, we first analysed the aggressive behaviours displayed by HUD patients at treatment entry and then compared them with those of subjects of the same social extraction who, by contrast, were not substance users. We then addressed the problem of aggression in patients with DD and suicidal risk in HUD patients. Finally, we studied the role of the V/S dimension we found in HUD patients [40] and the effects of opioid medications (methadone and buprenorphine) on aggression.

5.2   Assessment

As investigating tools, our research group used the Buss–Durkee questionnaire, in the Italian version curated by us; the Hostility factor of SCL90, which was obtained in psychiatric patients from Derogatis et al. [965]; and the V/S factor highlighted by our research group in patients suffering from (SUD).

5.2.1 Buss–Durkee Hostility Inventory

Buss–Durkee Hostility Inventory (BDHI) defines the subclasses of hostility that are typically delineated in everyday clinical situations [964]:

1. Assault: physical violence against others. This includes getting into fights with others, but not the destruction of objects.
2. Indirect hostility: both roundabout and undirected aggression. Roundabout behaviour like malicious gossip or practical jokes is indirect, in the sense that the hated person is not attacked directly but by devious means. Undirected aggression, such as temper tantrums and slamming doors, consists of a discharge of negative affect against no one in particular; it is a diffuse rage reaction without a target.
3. Irritability: a readiness to explode with negative affect at the slightest provocation. It includes quick temper, grouchiness, exasperation, and rudeness.
4. Negativism: oppositional behaviour, usually directed against authority. It involves a refusal to cooperate that may vary from passive non-compliance to open rebellion against rules or conventions.

5. Resentment: jealousy and hatred of others. It refers to a feeling of anger at the world over real or fantasized mistreatment.
6. Suspicion: projection of hostility onto others. It varies from merely being distrustful and wary of people to beliefs that others are being derogatory or are planning harm.
7. Verbal hostility: negative affect expressed in both the style and content of speech. This style includes arguing, shouting, and screaming; its content includes threats, curses, and being overcritical.

The variable of guilt was added because the relationship of guilt to the total score may be of clinical interest. Accordingly, items were compiled for a Guilt scale, with guilt being defined as feelings of being inadequate, having done wrong, or suffering pangs of conscience.

The items of BDHI have been translated into Italian (QTA version) and then translated into English by a translator who did not know the English version. The accuracy of the translation and its conformity with the original version have been checked by a bilingual English expert native speaker, who confirmed the original meaning of the items of the QTA [966]. QTA was standardized in the Italian population ($N = 861$) [967]; standardized T points were corrected by gender and age (≤ 31 vs. >31 years). Factor analysis revealed two dimensions: without (type 1) and with (type 2) physical contact. The first dimension is characterized by verbal hostility, irritability, negativism, and indirect hostility; the second dimension by suspicion, resentment, assault, and guilt. The ratio Guilt/Total BDHI clustered subjects into (1) ego-dystonic and (2) ego-syntonic aggression groups. Subjects obtaining T-BDHI scores higher than 50 were considered to display highly aggressive behaviour; subjects who had scores of less than 50 were considered to have a low level of aggressive behaviour with respect to the general population (standardization sample).

5.2.2 SCL90 Anger-Hostility Factor

Developed by Derogatis et al. [968], the SCL90 comprises 90 symptoms, each of which is divided into five levels of severity. Usually, these items can be grouped into nine factors: Somatic Symptoms, Obsessive-Compulsive Symptoms, Interpersonal Sensitivity, Depression, Anxiety, Anger and Hostility, Phobic Anxiety, Paranoid Ideation, and Psychoticism. The sum of all the symptoms represents the total of the scale; ancillary indices are the number of symptoms present at the time of examination and their severity, calculated by dividing the total score by the number of recorded symptoms. The stereotype of the Hostility factor identifies a subject who feels easily annoyed or irritated, has uncontrolled tantrums, often feels the urge to hit, hurt oneself or hurt others, feels the impulse to break objects, or engage in other frequent arguments, screams, and hurls objects.

5.2.3 SCL90 Violence/Suicidality Factor

Maremmani et al. have instead identified a 5-factor structure that seems to be specific to the SUD [40, 969]. The five factors were renamed on the basis of the symptoms carrying higher weight within the factors. The first factor is characterized by a W/BT depressive dimension, which represents approximately 30% of the total variance of the instrument. The second factor, which accounts for about 4% of the total variance, is represented by SS, in which somatic symptoms of opioid withdrawal appear. The third factor identifies a dimension of S/P, which represents about 3% of the total variance. Symptoms of panic and agoraphobia are present in the fourth dimension, named PA, which accounts for about 2% of the total variance. Lastly, the fifth dimension, with its 2% of the total variance, can be called V/S. These five factors taken together cover approximately 40% of the total variance of the instrument. Based on the highest z score obtained by the subjects in the dimensions, it is possible to typify the addicted subjects into five subgroups, mutually exclusive and distinguished by the symptoms mentioned earlier. About 14% of subjects can be classified as W/BT; 24% are distinguished by the presence of SS; 19% show predominantly S/P symptoms; 22% PA symptoms; and 19% a preponderance of V/S feelings.

The V/S dimension qualifies subjects with a tendency to scream and throw objects, to feel the impulse to break objects and be dyscontrolled. To be more accurate, this dimension is mainly marked out by aspects that, according to the standard factorization, belong to the hostility, depression, and anxiety factors (above all, verbal and indirect aggressiveness). Patients scream and throw objects, often feel the impulse to destroy things, feel uncontrolled anger, engage in frequent polemical discussions, and feel inclined to hit, hurt themselves, and hurt others. Death ideation and suicidal ideation are also included in this dimension. Note that ideas of death, in the standard version, do not fit into any factor (Table 5.1).

Table 5.1 SCL90 anger/hostility and violence/suicide dimensions

Anger/hostility	Violence/suicidality
11. Feeling easily annoyed or irritated	81. Shouting or throwing things
24. Temper outbursts that you could not control	67. Having urges to break or smash things
63. Having urges to beat, injure, or harm someone	24. Temper outbursts that you could not control
67. Having urges to break or smash things	63. Having urges to beat, injure, or harm someone
74. Getting into frequent arguments	74. Getting into frequent arguments
81. Shouting or throwing things	15. Thoughts of ending your life
	59. Thoughts of death or dying
	2. Nervousness or shakiness inside
	78. Feeling so restless you couldn't sit still

5.3 Clinical Aspects

5.3.1 Aggressive Behaviour in HUD Patients at Treatment Entry

Our group investigated the psychopathological dimension in a sample of 1055 HUD patients entering an opioid-agonist treatment (AOT). In particular, patients were asked to fill in the SCL90. On the basis of the scores obtained, all subjects were assigned to one of five mutually exclusive groups: W/BT (14.2%), SS (24.4%), S/P (19.4%), PA (22.3%), and V/S (19.7%). In particular, youngsters showed higher scores for the last three factors listed [40] (Fig. 5.1).

Subsequently, we evaluated aggressiveness in a sample of 252 heroin-addicted patients entering AOT treatment from 1994 to 2012 by means of the DAH-Q and the BDHI; 81.3% of the participants showed highly aggressive behaviour. Of these participants, 23.8% displayed a type 1 dominant profile of aggressive behaviour, consisting of verbal hostility, irritability, negativism, and indirect hostility (aggressive behaviour without physical contact), while 76.2% exhibited a type 2 dominant profile, including suspicion, resentment, assault, and guilt (aggressive behaviour with physical contact) (Fig. 5.2).

More than half of the patients perceived aggressive behaviour as being ego-dystonic (55.6%), whereas the remaining (44.4%) perceived it as ego-syntonic. On the whole, heroin-addicted patients showed higher scores in all factors of BDHI, compared with the general population, with type 2 emerging as the predominant profile. As to addiction history, type 2 patients showed altered mental status and unsatisfactory social leisure activity, while patients with a low level of aggressiveness displayed fewer legal problems and more frequent self-detoxifications [970].

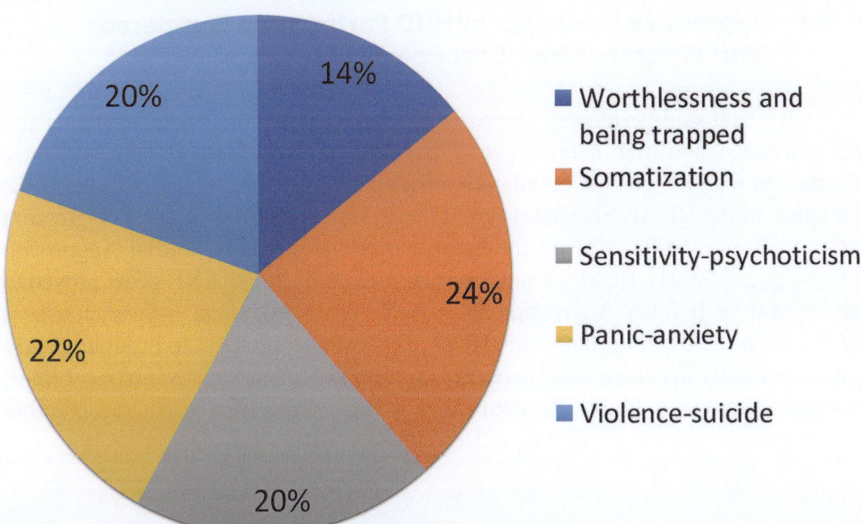

Fig. 5.1 Dominant groups in 1055 HUD patients at treatment entry

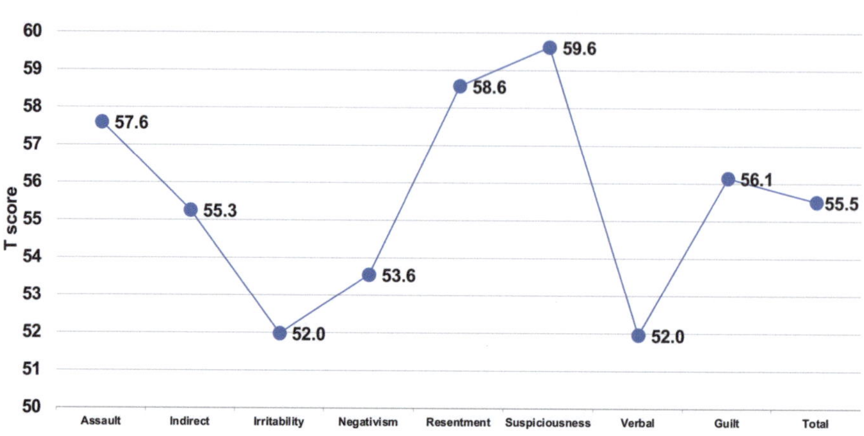

Fig. 5.2 BDHI dimensions in 252 HUD patients at treatment entry

During the treatment, Gerra et al. investigated aggressiveness in a sample of 18 abstinent HUD patients and 18 controls. SCL90 evaluated all participants, while BDHI and the Child Experience of Care and Abuse-Questionnaire (CECA-Q) were used to test the perception of parental neglect retrospectively. Oxytocin serum levels were measured too. Results revealed that SCL90, BDHI, and CECA-Q scores were significantly higher in probands than in controls. Furthermore, oxytocin serum levels were positively correlated with psychiatric symptoms, aggressiveness, and motherly neglect. By contrast, no correlation between oxytocin and extent of exposure to heroin, or heroin dosages, was reported [971].

5.3.2   Aggressive Behaviour of HUD Participants Compared with Substance Non-User Peers

A more recent study evaluated aggressiveness in a sample of 73 HUD patients and 45 substance non-user (SNU) peers, matched for sociodemographic features. Compared with the general population, HUD patients were deviant in all the items included in the BDHI: Suspiciousness ($T = 9.31$, $p < 0.001$), Indirect Aggression ($T = 8.59$, $p < 0.001$), 4-Negativism ($T = 6.80$, $p < 0.001$), Verbal Aggression ($T = 6.73$, $p < 0.001$), Resentment ($T = 6.38$, $p < 0.001$), while SNU peers proved to be deviant in Indirect Aggression ($T = 4.46$, $p < 0.001$) and 6-Suspiciousness ($T = 2.65$, $p < 0.011$). Furthermore, HUD participants turned out to be significantly more aggressive than their SNU peers in Assault ($F = 19.89$), Negativism ($F = 14.34$), Suspiciousness ($F = 14.34$), Resentment ($F = 7.82$), Guilt ($F = 6.26$), and 7-Verbal Aggression ($F = 6.10$) [972] (Fig. 5.3).

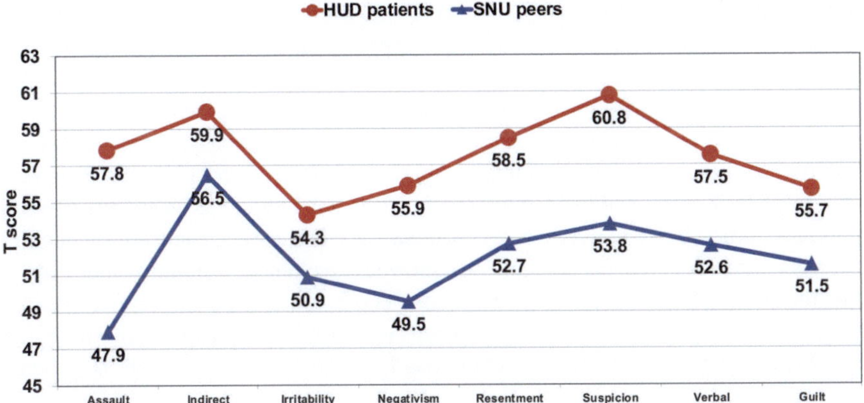

Fig. 5.3 BDHI dimensions in 73 HUD patients at treatment entry when compared with 45 non-user peers

5.3.3   Aggressive Behaviour in Dual Disorder HUD

In another study on 1090 HUD patients entering AOT, we focused on dual disorder. Patients were assessed using the DAH-Q and divided into three groups according to their degree of aggressiveness: no lifetime self-harm or assault episodes ($n = 808$), at least one moderate/superficial self-harm episode in the last month before requesting treatment ($n = 30$), and at least one assault episode in the previous month ($n = 162$). DAH-Q evaluated patients. Dual disorder, in particular, bipolar spectrum, resulted in being the most significant risk factor for aggressive behaviour. Other factors included unstable modality of heroin use, the chronic psychosis diagnosis, and the simultaneous use of central nervous system stimulants or depressants. Moderate/superficial self-harm was associated with chronic psychosis, while depressive (non-bipolar) or anxiety disorders and older age at first use of heroin were correlated with a lower risk of aggressive behaviour [248].

Subsequently, we assessed 1195 subjects entering TC. Of these, 25.9% ($n = 309$) were affected by one or more psychiatric disorders (DD/HUD), whereas 74.1% ($n = 886$) did not show any psychiatric comorbidities (NDD/HUD). SCL90 total and single domain scores turned out to be higher in DD/HUD patients than in NDD/HUD ones ($p = 0.000$, $p < 0.001$) [39].

Gerra et al. [973] also investigated the aggressive responses displayed in a sample of 20 HUD patients in AOT with methadone, comparing them with 20 healthy controls. Notably, 13 of the HUD patients showed psychiatric symptoms (anxiety, depression, and antisocial personality traits), while only 2 out of 20 met the diagnostic criteria for a psychiatric disorder (one with major depression and the other with the obsessive-compulsive disorder). Patients were evaluated using the Italian version of the BDHI and underwent the Point Subtraction Aggression Paradigm (PSAP), an experimental model to induce aggressiveness. As expected, aggressive responses were significantly higher in patients than in the control group ($p < 0.001$) and they were correlated with BDHI assault and irritability scores. By contrast, no correlation was found with methadone treatment [973]. Similarly, the same authors reported no impact of buprenorphine on aggressiveness. In particular, PSAP aggressive responses were evaluated in a sample of 30 HUD patients in treatment with buprenorphine (BUP, $n = 15$) or methadone (METH, $n = 15$) and in 15 healthy controls. Among HUD participants, 15 showed psychiatric symptoms, but only 7 met the criteria for an established diagnosis. As previously reported, aggressiveness was significantly higher in the HUD group, with no differences between the BUP and METH groups [973]. Both studies found that aggressiveness in HUD patients was correlated with personality traits and monoamine plasma levels, whereas no role of AOT emerged [973, 974].

5.4   Role of V/S Dimension on HUD Patients

Our group investigated suicidality in a sample of 616 HUD patients in AOT. Suicidal thoughts during the previous week were reported in less than one-third of the sample (29.1%); 2.8% of the patients displayed the highest severity of suicidal thoughts, according to the SCL90, while they were light or moderate in about one-fifth of the sample. Moreover, depression and hostility dimensions were correlated with suicidal thoughts. Concerning sociodemographic variables, a significant association between being unemployed, not receiving welfare benefits, living alone, belonging to blue-collar or unemployed families, and suicidality was found [303].

In 2008, Tremeau et al. reported significantly higher scores in the assault and irritability subscales of the BDHI in HUD with a personal history of suicidal attempts or family history of suicide. The latter also showed higher BDHI and Barratt-Impulsiveness Scale (BIS) total scores [975].

Some years later, Kazour et al. [976], investigated suicidality and other psychopathological dimensions in a sample of 61 HUD inpatients (vs. 61 controls) with the BIS-11, the Hamilton Depression Rating Scale (HAM-D), and the Beck Suicidal Ideation Scale (BSI). HUD patients showed significantly higher scores than controls on BIS-11 (82.11 vs. 45.74), HAM-D (14.7 vs. 2.43), and BSI (12.55 vs. 1.47). In line with the previously mentioned study, scores were higher in patients with a personal history of attempts at suicide when compared with those who had never attempted suicide (HAM-D, $p = 0.004$; BSI $p < 0.001$; BIS-11 $p = 0.014$). Furthermore, a positive correlation between HAM-D, BIS-11, and BSI scores and the number of lifetime suicidal attempts emerged (BSI, $r = 0.51, p < 0.001$; HAM-D, $r = 0.38, p = 0.002$; BIS-11, $r = 0.28; p < 0.03$) [976].

In a broad sample of 3949 HUD patients, the standardized mortality rate (SMR) for suicide was found to be fourfold higher than in the general population, with gender differences (3.7 higher for males compared with the general male population and 2.2 higher than females; 7.0 higher in females, compared with the general female population). Greater age was correlated with a higher risk of suicide, while no correlation was reported between male gender, living alone, and unemployment. By contrast, being at first AOT seemed to play a protective role [977].

Zhong et al. investigated NSSI in HUD. In HUD patients (n = 603) already in MMT, 13.8% of subjects reported NSSI during the previous month, while the most prevalent types of self-injury were burning (59%), cutting (19.3%), hitting (9.6%), and carving (6.0%). A positive correlation was found between NSSI and unemployment (OR = 2.54, p = 0.009), a short duration of MMT (OR = 1.04, p = 0.034), pain (OR = 2.3, p = 0.028), depression (OR = 4.32, p < 0.001), anxiety (OR = 3.74, p = 0.002), and loneliness (OR = 3.04, p = 0.012) [978]. According to a meta-analysis on Chinese HUD patients in compulsory or voluntary detoxification treatment (15 studies included, total sample n = 37,243), the pooled prevalence of NSSI was 4.4% (2.8–6.2%), including swallowing foreign objects, especially those designed for cutting, hitting, or burning, jumping from a height, cutting off fingers, apastia, attempts to break bones, knocking a nail into the head, and drug overdoses [978].

V/S typology is related to HUD natural history. Older patients were frequent in the W/BT group, while younger patients were frequent in S/P and V/P patients [313]. The sample consisted of 455 HUD patients (according to *DSM III/III-R/IV/ IV-R* criteria), of which 340 (74.9%) were males and 115 (25.3%) females. The average age was 28 ± 7 years old (range 16–50). Most of the patients were single (N = 295; 64.8%), had had less than 8 years of education (N = 346; 76.0%), and were unemployed (N = 212; 46.6%).

There is a significant association between V/S severity and the choice of AOT [35]. We investigated psychopathological features in a sample of 1195 patients entering a TC. Participants were clustered in the five groups: W/BT (16.7%), SS (17.3%), S/P (21.1%), PA (29.3%), and V/S (15.5%). In particular, V/S, as well as W/BT, SS, and PA, dimensions were more severe in AOT patients and females, compared with the TC group and TC group males, respectively. V/S was more severe for AOT vs. TC male patients but did not differ in TC vs. AOT females.

V/S was more severe in non-detoxified (NDTX) vs. detoxified (DTX) HUD patients, but typology did not differ [38]. In a sample of 1015 HUD patients, who underwent detoxification (DTX, n = 374) or not (NDTX, n = 641), SCL90 total scores, as well as V/S dimension, were significantly higher in NDTX patients, than in DTX ones [38].

V/S typology was less frequent in AUD vs. HUD and CUD patients [37]. According to the VOECT cohort study (Evaluation of Therapeutic Community Treatments and Outcomes), conducted in 2008–2009 on a sample of 2533 patients diagnosed with SUD (AUD, n = 449; cocaine use disorder, CUD, n = 670; HUD, n = 1195) admitted to a TC, the V/S dimension was higher in HUD and CUD patients than in those diagnosed with AUD. Furthermore, no differences were reported in V/S domain scores between HUD patients with CUD or AUD and patients without any other SUD.

V/S typology did not differ among HUD patients according to the secondary substance of use (alcohol, cocaine, or none) [37]. In the second part of the same study, the most frequent psychopathological dimension was PA for all the three groups of patients. The least frequent were V/S and S/P for the group of patients with alcohol as secondary used drug, V/S for the group of patients with no alcohol or cocaine as secondary drug, and W/BT for the group of patients with cocaine as secondary used drug. No statistically significant differences between the three groups were observed in any of the five SCL-based psychopathological dimensions.

V/S severity and typology did not differ in AUD, HUD, and CUD mono-users [312]. In one of our studies on 256 patients diagnosed with HUD, CUD, or AUD, with no other substances use comorbidities, no differences in the V/S dimension emerged among the three groups.

Traumatic life-events can also influence aggression in HUD patients. V/S severity was higher in heroin PTSD spectrum (H/PTSD-S) patients; conversely, V/S typology did not differ [979]. Concerning the role of life-events in patients with HUD, we found a higher V/S severity in those with H/PTSD-S symptoms. In particular, we investigated psychopathological and PTSD symptoms in a sample of 93 HUD patients, using the SCL90 and the Trauma and Loss Spectrum Questionnaire (TALS). Patients were divided into two groups according to their TALS scores and the presence or absence of H/PTSD-S (>32, presence, and <32, absence, respectively). H/PTSD-S HUD patients reported more severe scores in all the domains of SCL90, including V/S, compared with no H/PTSD-S subjects.

Ethnicity does not seem to interfere with the V/S dimension. In fact, in a naturalistic case–control study, V/S severity did not differ in 30 migrant HUD patients heading for Italy, compared with 30 Italian counterparts matched for age and gender [980]. Conversely, V/S severity was higher in Slovenian HUD patients than in Italian ones. Sixty-six Slovenians and 66 Italian HUD patients matched according to age and gender, at univariate analysis, showed a more severe V/S dimension, whereas multivariate discriminant analysis revealed a less significant difference between the two groups ($p < 0.026$) [981]. In the same study, V/S typology did not differ either in migrant vs. Italian HUD patients or in Slovenian vs. Italian ones.

The 5-factor SCL90 psychopathological dimensions are strongly correlated with HUD trait-conditions [343]. The presence and severity of addictive behaviours were recorded by utilizing CRAV-HERO, an inventory for assessing the behavioural covariates of craving in HUD patients. Thirteen behaviours were selected. We clustered the 13 behaviours in 6 operating models.

1. Exchange-related addictive behaviours (EXC-BX) that aimed to reveal the hierarchical approach applied by a subject to his/her values
2. Time-related addictive behaviours (TIME-BX) that test the subject's ability to wait and manage the substance and how much time is taken up by thinking about the substance
3. Risk-related addictive behaviours (RISK-BX) that are linked to the theme of risk in which the choice of whether to engage in substance use raises the question of endangering health, even life itself
4. Cue-induced/environment-related addictive behaviours (CUE/ENV-BX)

Based on the highest z scores obtained on the CRAV-HERO clusters, subjects can be assigned to one of these six mutually exclusive groups. For details see [982].

V/S dimension was closely correlated with heroin addictive behaviour (exchange and time items). The results of the canonical correlation analysis between five psychopathological dimensions and five different types of addictive behaviours showed that only one canonical variate was significant. Canonical variate set-one (SCL90), which accounts for 20.11% of the total variance, was saturated negatively by V/S, SS, and PA dimensions and positively (but at a superficial level) by the S/P dimension. Set-two (CRAV-HERO), which accounts for 83.68% of the total variance, was saturated negatively by TIME-BX, EXC-BX, RISK-BX, and CUE/ENV-BX. The addictive behaviour set was saturated positively (but at a superficial level) by CUE/ENV-BX. These sets were significantly correlated. V/S severity is, therefore, closely related to the severity of SS (withdrawal syndrome) and linked to the hierarchical approach applied by a subject to his/her values and to that subject's ability to wait and manage the substance and to how much time is taken up by thinking about the substance (Fig. 5.4).

The 5-factor SCL90 psychopathological dimensions can differentiate HUD patients from other psychopathological patients, but V/S was more severe and more frequent in MD patients [42]. We compared 972 HUD patients with 504 MD patients to estimate the magnitude of the differences, in terms of psychopathological symptoms. Prominent psychopathological domains were more frequent in HUD patients, in particular, W/BT, SS, and S/P. The V/S dimension was more frequent in MD patients, while the PA dimension failed to differentiate between the two groups. The prominent psychopathological groups are the most crucial factor in significantly differentiating between the two groups when drawing

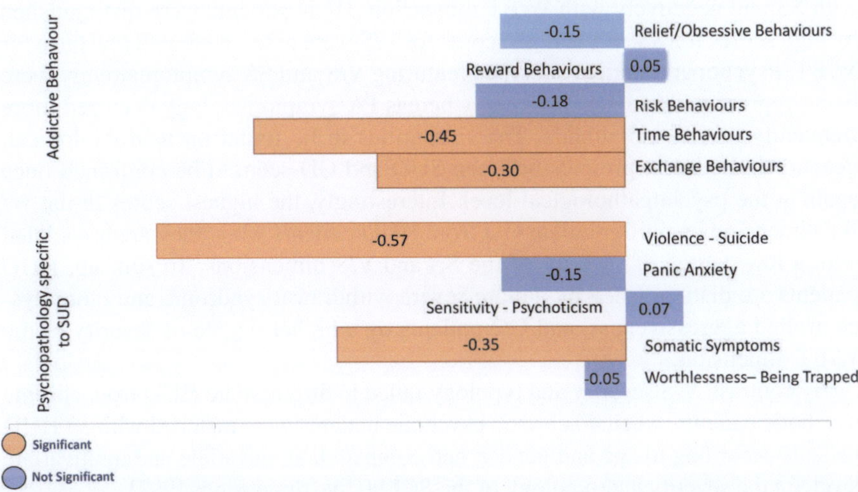

Fig. 5.4 Correlations between psychopathology specific to HUD and addictive behaviour in HUD patients

comparisons based on age, male gender, and the severity of psychopathological symptoms. The frequency of the association between addiction and mood disorders may be explained on both the neurobiological [983] and clinical levels [49, 984]. This study suggests that, in HUD patients, depressive symptomatology remains the most critical and frequent psychopathological aspect of HUD. Moreover, this symptomatology is less closely related to suicidal ideation than in depressed patients.

V/S severity and typology were shown to be more marked in non-psychiatric obese patients by comparing 972 HUD patients with 106 obese subjects; the severity of all psychopathological dimensions was, in fact, significantly higher in obese individuals. Discriminant analysis showed that PA and V/S severities were intense in obese patients, to a degree sufficient to allow differentiation between HUD (lower severity) and obese individuals (greater severity). At the reclassification level, 70.8% of obese individuals in the sample were reclassified as HUD patients. Psychopathological subtypes distinguished by PA and V/S typology were more frequent in obese patients, to a degree allowing discrimination between groups. Psychopathological subtypes characterized by W/BT, SS, and S/P symptomatology were more frequent among HUD patients, whereas PA and V/S symptomatologies were more frequent among obese individuals [985].

V/S severity and typology was more clear-cut in HUD than in gambling disorder (GD) patients [986]. We compared the severity and frequency of each of the five aspects found by us, in 972 HUD and 110 GD patients at univariate and multivariate levels. HUD patients showed higher general psychopathology indexes than GD patients. The severity of all five psychopathological dimensions was significantly greater in HUD patients. Discriminant analysis revealed that SS and V/S severities were able to discriminate between HUD (higher severity) and GD patients (lower severity), whereas PA and S/P were not. V/S correlated positively with SS and negatively with W/BT dimension. HUD patients were distinguished by high scores for SS, while high scores for V/S were associated with low ones for W/BT. Psychopathological subtypes featuring V/S and SS symptomatology were better represented in HUD patients, whereas PA symptomatology occurred more frequently in GD individuals. The similarities to be found on neurobiological, genetic, and clinical grounds between SUD and GD seem to be confirmed once again at the psychopathological level. Interestingly, the highest scores in the W/BT dimension can differentiate GD from HUD patients when they are associated with a low degree of severity of the SS and V/S dimensions. To sum up, HUD patients are distinguished by a more severe withdrawal syndrome and more dyscontrolled aggressiveness, and GD patients by a higher degree of severity of the W/BT dimension.

By contrast, V/S severity and typology failed to differentiate HUD from chronic psychotic patients, when 40 chronic psychotic patients were matched with 33 HUD patients according to age and gender, and compared, at univariate and multivariate level, on the severity and typology of the SCL90 five dimensions [987].

5.5 Therapeutic Aspects

5.5.1 Effect of Opioid Medications on Aggression

The presence of SCL90 hostility predicts an inadequate clinical response in NTX-treated HUD patients. NTX has been shown to have poor results on unselected populations of HUD patients. Its use is mostly confined to detoxification-related procedures, whereas its long-term effects and properties have been largely neglected. In one of our studies, we investigated the predictors of a successful outcome in a population of 149 patients diagnosed as HUD patients based on *DSM-IV* criteria and undergoing long-term NTX treatment (NTX maintenance). Favourable outcomes were related to on-going treatment, whereas negative outcomes were due to treatment discontinuation through addictive relapse. Retained individuals are more likely to have no problems at work and to be psychosocially adjusted. Earlier substance users are those most likely to drop out. Global psychopathological impairment, with reference to mood, aggressiveness, and delusions, is negatively related to treatment retention. NTX maintenance appears to be suitable for a subgroup of heroin users whose clinical pictures combine a low level of addictive disease with the absence of significant dysphoria, aggressive behaviour, and psychosis [44].

SCL90 Hostility severity predicts an inadequate clinical response in GPs' Office-Based MMTP. In one of our studies, we evaluated the effectiveness of methadone treatment carried out by GPs in Trieste, Italy, and we identified response treatment factors. Thirty-three subjects with heroin addiction according to the *DSM-IV-R* criteria were placed in an observational protocol with an average duration of 429 ± 273 days. The retention rate was used as a measure of outcome. Patients with greater severity of illness, problematic relationships with spouse/partner, difficulty with socialization and organization of leisure, with an altered mental state at the beginning of treatment; subjects with dual disorder (especially bipolar disorder), greater severity of obsessive-compulsive symptoms, interpersonal sensitivity, depression, violence, with greater severity of psychopathological symptoms, with the most significant number of problematic areas as regards the quality of life; and patients with a low dose of methadone given for treatment were those considered to be at highest risk of abandoning treatment [988].

Higher dosages of methadone are needed to stabilize violent patients. Using the SCL90's Hostility factor and the BDHI, in one of our studies we verified that methadone dosages depend on the grade of psychopathology and aggressiveness at treatment entrance. A sample of 20 subjects was divided into two clusters according to the baseline SCL90 score (high psychopathology vs. low psychopathology). All these subjects had been abstinent from various substances for a long time and had achieved a satisfactory level of psychosocial adaptation after a treatment period of variable length (1–96 months). Stabilization dosages ranged from 7 to 80, averaging 39 ± 23 mg/day. A higher degree of psychopathology corresponded to higher stabilization dosages (60 vs. 30 mg/day on average, the latter corresponding to a lower degree of psychopathology); similarly, higher aggressiveness accounted for higher stabilization dosages (50 vs. 30 mg/day for mildly aggressive subjects). Neither psychopathology nor aggressiveness appeared to vary with treatment duration. Methadone-sensitive psychopathology appeared to comprise depression, phobic anxiety, paranoia, physical features, and psychotic symptoms, with the latter two showing the strongest correlations. As regards BDHI-recorded aggressiveness, methadone dosage seemed to be related to unexpressed aggression, irritability, and violence, the most active associations emerging for the latter two. In conclusion, the higher the level of psychopathology and aggressiveness at treatment entrance, the higher the methadone dosage required for stabilization [50].

The question to be asked at this point is whether these psychopathological typologies, which can typify subjects with SUD, are affected by different medications used in the treatment of addiction. In the case of heroin addiction, for example, are methadone and buprenorphine equally effective on these psychopathological types, and what happens if the subject is not treated with medications, but, for instance, in a therapeutic community? In previous studies, we were able to demonstrate that, when the nine standard dimensions of the SCL90 were used, the effect was not specific, since almost all the nine psychopathological factors improved [703, 708].

In a sample of 213 HUD patients treated with opioid agonists (methadone or buprenorphine), at the end of the 12 months of observation, no significant outcome differences could be found in subjects who showed prominent symptoms of W/BT, SS, and PA—a result that could depend on the use of one of these two medications [703].

Patients who showed the presence of S/P symptomatology also showed higher retention in treatment if treated with methadone, regardless of gender, educational level, marital status, the presence of somatic and psychiatric comorbidity, social adjustment, legal problems, and polysubstance use at treatment entry. Achievement of a positive outcome was also independent of patients' age, age at the outset of heroin use, age at the onset of continuous use, how long dependence lasted, and age at first treatment. During follow-up, no differences in the use of opioids or cocaine were observed. It should be borne in mind that, at the start of treatment, working conditions in methadone-treated patients were worse than in those treated with buprenorphine. By contrast, patients showing V/S symptoms achieved significantly higher retention in treatment if they were treated with buprenorphine. This result was independent of patients' employment status, their educational level, civil status, social adjustment, the presence of somatic and psychiatric comorbidity, or legal problems, even polysubstance use. For these patients too, no differences were found in drug history or the efficacy of the two medications on substance use during treatment. In the sample group treated with buprenorphine, males were preponderant, showing more severe maladjustment in the social/leisure area. In the sample examined by us, therefore, methadone and buprenorphine showed the same impact on addiction pathology, as demonstrated by urinary tests, but different types of impact on the psychopathological subtypes we consider specific to SUD [43].

Gerra et al. investigated aggressive behaviour in a sample of 20 heroin-addicted patients in methadone or buprenorphine maintenance treatment, using a laboratory task, the Point Subtraction Aggression Paradigm. The aggressive response was found to be higher in the HUD patient group than in the control group, independently of agonist treatment [989]. Gerra and colleagues found a possible role of olanzapine in improving aggressiveness in HUD patients. A sample of 67 HUD patients in AOT with methadone or buprenorphine was co-administered with olanzapine (OLA group) or SSRIs (fluoxetine or paroxetine) and clonazepam (SSRI + BDZ group) for 12 weeks. Among those who completed the observational period ($n = 33$, 49.2%), a significant decrease in BDHI total scores and direct, indirect, verbal aggressiveness, irritability, and resentment subscale scores were found in the OLA group, whereas no differences were reported in the SSRI + BDZ group [990]. On the same wavelength, according to a 12-week Iranian trial, augmentation therapy with olanzapine or valproate can reduce aggressive behaviour in HUD patients in MMT. Notably, 201 HUD patients in MMT were randomized in two groups, the first receiving olanzapine (2.5–15 mg/day) plus placebo valproate ($n = 101$, OLA group), while the second took valproate (600–1000 mg/day) plus olanzapine placebo ($n = 100$). Patients were evaluated on the Overt Aggression Scale-Modified (OSA-M) at baseline and weekly. Among those who completed the trial ($n = 53$), OSA-M total score and aggression, irritability, and suicidality subscales decreased significantly, with olanzapine being more productive than valproate [991]. Evren et al. studied aggressiveness and impulsivity in a sample of 52 MM (methadone-maintained) HUD patients followed up for 12 months. Of them, 44.23% ($n = 23$) relapsed during the follow-up. Patients were assessed using the Barratt Impulsiveness Scale, version 11 (BIS-11), and the Buss–Perry Aggression Questionnaire at baseline (T0) and 12 months (T1). Compared with MM patients, relapsed patients showed higher mean verbal aggression (T0) and physical aggression and impulsivity scores (T1). On the whole, at T1, aggression and impulsivity were lower in MM patients (hostility, motor, and non-planning impulsivity), whereas they were higher in the relapsed group factors (motor and verbal aggression, attentional, and non-planning impulsivity). Interestingly, low verbal aggression and high motor impulsiveness at T0 and anger and motor impulsiveness at T1 may predict a relapse [992].

Thus, a series of studies indicates that opioid agonists are likely to be effective in controlling aggressive behaviour in opioid-addicted patients, as confirmed by the fall in levels of aggressiveness that followed adequate methadone treatment [453, 993]. Moreover, aggressive symptoms are among the features that may be found in the frequent situation of applying a self-medication theory [994]. In our study, buprenorphine showed better results than methadone in patients with prominently aggressive characteristics (in the V/S dominant group).

The observations reported in the literature and the results of our studies suggest that opioid agonists should be reconsidered, as they not only possess an anti-craving activity but are also able to act as psychotropic instruments in treating mental illness, with particular reference to mood, anxiety, and psychotic syndromes. In particular, methadone seems to be more effective in treating S/P aspects, whereas buprenorphine appears to be more effective in acting against aggressive behaviour (V/S). As a result, some DD patients may benefit from a treatment (methadone or buprenorphine) that not only targets their addictive problem but is also active in attenuating their mental disorder.

Is the psychopathological SUD typology proposed by us able to show its involvement in the results of residential treatment? To answer this question, 2016 subjects treated in various therapeutic communities were typified psychopathologically and monitored for up to 16 months [41]. Abandonment of the treatment was considered the focal event; it determined the level of retention in treating these subjects. The sample consisted of 2016 SUD patients diagnosed according to a clinical judgement; it comprised 1693 males and 323 females. At the end of the study, the cumulative retention rate was 0.39. The W/BT dimension was prominent in 298 patients, SS in 456, S/P in 406, PA in 518, and V/S in 338. Retention rates differed statistically between the five subgroups. In particular, V/S patients showed a lower retention rate than those for the W/BT, SS, S/P, and PA dimensions. Not having been detoxified at residential treatment entry and the presence of psychopathological symptoms were two factors that had a negative influence on the outcome. Prominent SS and V/S symptomatology at treatment entry correlated positively with dropout from the therapeutic community (Fig. 5.5).

In conclusion, TC programmes show a considerable variety of results, depending on the psychopathological typology of patients. Length of retention in treatment of

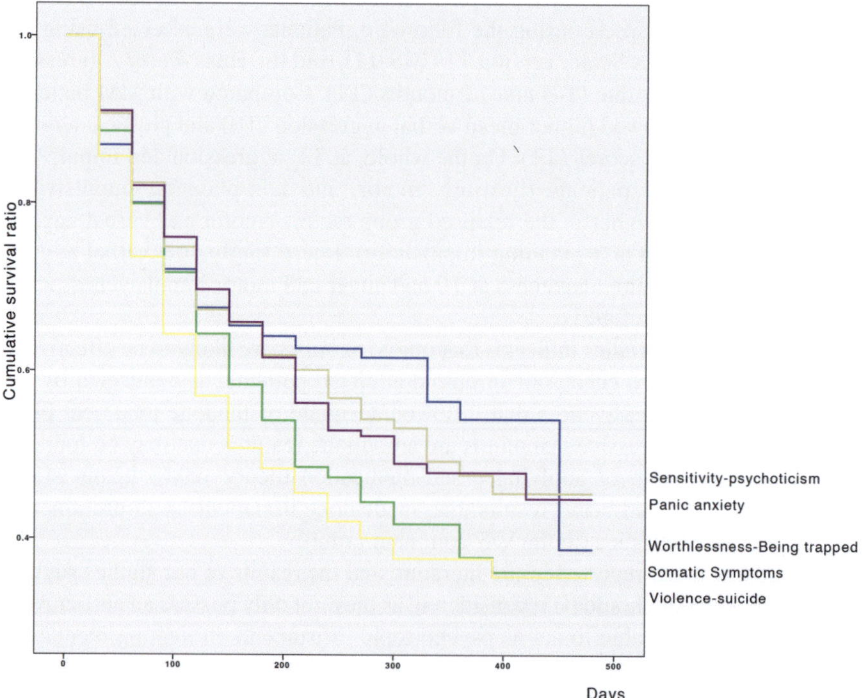

Fig. 5.5 Retention rate according to the prominent psychopathology of 2016 SUD patients treated in therapeutic community

patients entering TC treatment is significantly lower for those who have a more severe psychopathology. Moreover, V/S and SS patients may leave the treatment earlier than those allocated to the other three psychopathological dimensions resulting from the application of factor analysis to the SCL90 responses (i.e., W/BT, S/P, and PA). The SCL90 five-factorial structure of the psychopathology of substance dependence could turn out to be a useful tool when applied as a prognostic factor, together with age, detoxification status, and kind of substance of use, all of which have been shown to influence retention in treatment.

In summary, our studies show that 8 out of every 10 patients entering treatment show highly aggressive behaviour; in 2.5 out of every 10 this happens without physical contact; in 7.5 out of every 10 with physical contact; and 4.5 out of every 10 patients have an ego-syntonic perception of their aggressive behaviour. At treatment entry, BDHI Negativism and Assault clearly discriminate HUD patients from their NSU peers; violence and self-harm are found to be correlated in DD/HUD patients; in DD/BIP1-HUD suicidality increases; predominantly V/S patients are more frequent in younger HUD age brackets; the V/S dimension only minimally affects HUD state-conditions (choice of treatment, active substance use, psychiatric comorbidity, primary and secondary used substance, mono-substance use, and ethnicity); V/S dimension is strictly correlated with HUD trait-conditions (addictive behaviour and PTSD spectrum); and the V/S dimension can differentiate HUD from other psychiatric patients (depressed and psychotics) and non-psychiatric ones (obese), but is not able to differentiate patients affected by behavioural addictions (GD). On the therapeutic level, the presence of aggressive behaviour negatively influences GPs' office-based AOT and NTX maintenance. A higher methadone dosage is needed to stabilize AOT aggressive patients; predominantly V/S patients are well stabilized when in buprenorphine treatment.

We admit that our conclusions are based on clinical considerations. On the other hand, innovative strategies such as those presented here are often indispensable in clinical practice.

However, our studies suggest an in-depth psychopathological evaluation of the HUD patients, with particular attention to aggressive symptoms, before their entry into long-term opioid agonist treatment. Moreover, our data are compatible with Khantzian's self-medication theory, which looks at heroin addiction as a way of controlling violent manifestations. For this reason, the use of an adequate amount of opioid agonist seems to be crucial in the management of violent opioid addicts.

Alcohol Use Disorder and Polytoxicomania in Heroin Use Disorder Patients

6

6.1 Clinical Aspects

Several data from the literature define the relationship between depressive states and alcohol use, although controversy continues about the dynamics that link different kinds of depressive syndromes and alcohol-related problems. Most authors agree in considering heavy drinking as an equivalent, or a masked form, of depression. Patients who continue to drink, despite severe or advanced somatic consequences, display a peculiar form of depression [995]. Alcoholism stems from depressive states, which are mostly of minor severity and a disguised kind [996]. Other studies have described a significant association between bipolar disorders and alcohol use. According to Kraepelin, as many as 25% of bipolar patients used alcoholic drinks [204]. Several authors conclude that alcohol use mostly characterizes depressive states and is resorted to as a way to elate mood and soothe pain, whereas alcohol use during states of mood elation is a sign of excitement and impulsiveness [194]. DSM has suggested a close link between cyclothymia and alcohol use. Chronic depression too has been associated with alcohol use. It is not surprising, therefore, that alcohol use, which can stand as an addictive disease itself in some cases, is often found combined with substance non-medical use in general.

Studies in the literature have increasingly reported an association between heroin and alcohol use [157, 223, 402, 454, 997–1003]. Alcohol use seems to be related to polydrug use, and mainly affects young addicts; among these, lifetime rates for alcoholism range between 10% and 75%. The National Drug Alcohol Collaborative Project (NDACP) reported a rate of 43% for combined alcohol-heroin use in a sample of over 1500 HUD patients [1000]. Heroin was the first substance to be used in 99% of cases. Rounsaville reported a lifetime and index prevalence of alcohol dependence of 13% and 34%, respectively [1004]. Californian addicts have been reported to use alcohol at a rate of 53–75%, and 11% have been admitted to hospitals for alcohol-related somatic matters. Alcohol use occurs as often as 10–20% among street addicts, and up to 27% among methadone-maintained subjects [402,

© The Author(s), under exclusive license to Springer Nature Switzerland AG 2023

I. Maremmani et al., *Dual Disorder Heroin Addicts*,
https://doi.org/10.1007/978-3-031-30093-6_6

1001]. Some authors have tried to explain the increase in alcohol use during methadone treatment programmes, concluding that methadone-maintained addicts may use alcohol in order to counter the opioid-normalizing effect of methadone, and to go beyond the methadone-heightened opioid threshold [402, 1001, 1005]. When the correlation between alcohol use and heroin use among methadone-maintained addicts was examined in a large sample of HUD patients, it was pointed out that alcohol use during methadone treatment seems to be the result of an automatic behavioural pattern, according to which alcohol use tends to rise as street-opioid use falls, and the reverse [402]. Furthermore, Rounsaville, who supports this theory, also reports that alcohol use is mostly found in addicts who had once used alcohol, so displaying a relapse into a previous alcohol-related disorder [157].

On the basis of their clinical experience, Maremmani and Shinderman suggest that the use of alcohol, BDZs, and other types of drugs in HUD patients may be correlated with a condition of opioid dependence improperly compensated by street heroin or by substitution treatment dosages. Thus, the search for an appropriate methadone dosage during MMT is crucial not only because it raises the retention rate for patients within the treatment group, so allowing an improvement in social rehabilitation, but also because it lowers the risk of polydrug use [75].

6.2   Treatment of Alcohol Use Disorder in Heroin Use Disorder Patients

6.2.1   Heroin Use Disorder, Alcohol Use Disorder and Self-Help Groups

Anonymous or self-help groups are known to be a valid instrument in the treatment of alcohol dependence. The most active self-help groups are alcoholics anonymous (AA) and club for alcoholics in treatment (CAT). As regard AA, which is best represented in the USA, but is also active in Italy, American authors note that despite official guidelines laid down by the national committee (General Service Office for AA), stating the full compatibility of methadone treatment with AA activities, methadone treatment is often quickly eliminated, if not completely neglected. Progress has certainly been made in the field of self-help with the formation of institutional groups, which follow a well-defined, constant method and are directed by operators skilled in their specific task. Particularly interesting results have been achieved by the CAT organizations, started in Zagreb in 1964, by applying Hudolin's thought [1006]. They aim to provide members with a structured programme for the treatment of alcohol dependence. However, cultural bias should be neutralized, if the aim is to combine a self-help approach with methadone treatment; second, some changes should be made. For instance, CAT operators often reject the concept that alcohol dependence is a disease, preferring to speak of behavioural disorder. The concept of metabolic disease must, in any case, be accepted in order to get patients into a successful treatment and avoid any discrimination taking place. In fact, any refusal of this approach can be interpreted in terms of social and historical trends and has no clear correspondence with the theoretical system of self-help interventions. Hudolin himself stated that the first crucial step is to approach subjects as patients, a status they should be acknowledged as possessing if they are to receive appropriate treatment rather than blame. Nevertheless, self-help groups continue to judge it necessary to look beyond that concept, so as to avoid use less in-patient treatment and overtreatment by medical means; integrated approaches, they insist, should be preferred, to provide the best fit with each individual lifestyle. Scientifically speaking, these views appear to be meaningless, and they can be used as a basis for the proliferation of gratuitous belief and unskilled intervention due to the neglect of scientific principles. Another point made by most CAT operators is that by defining AUD patients as suffering from an illness, an excuse for controlled drinking may be introduced; this, they suspect, may result in contacts between people and alcohol being favoured, which is the origin of the whole problem. This statement cannot be wholly agreed upon, especially from an alcoholic's point of view. The true problem is a different one—the widespread lack of medical approaches to alcohol dependence, which leads to the view that any chemical compound, except for hepatoprotective preparations, is inappropriate. The conceptualization of alcoholism as a pathological state does not mean systematically referring AUD patients to in-patient treatments, to the detriment of integrated approaches. As long as the specific dynamic of this type of disorder is well understood, both kinds of approach can be applied, since both are supposed to contribute to a satisfactory outcome. The principle that a drug-free condition is to be achieved before any treatment approach is initiated should be looked at again. It has been widely accepted that disulfiram-treated patients are expected to meet no difficulty when enrolled in self-help programmes. Misunderstandings are, however, common when dealing with methadone-treated patients who continue to use alcohol or apply for self-help programmes while taking psychotropics for anxiety or mood disorders. Although CAT operators receive a thorough training in how to deal with relapsing behaviour as a crucial aspect of addictive diseases, they often regard a drug-free state as the only satisfactory outcome. If sodium oxybate (SMO) meets raised expectations, this view will turn out to be a misconception. A drug-free condition was originally conceived by Hudolin himself, within his hypothesis of an environmental approach, not as the ideal outcome, but as a way to achieve the true objective—the reversal of a dysfunctional lifestyle. That objective implies that a drug-free condition is perfectly compatible with pharmacotherapy, whether aversion therapy or some other form. It will be enough to know which drug to choose for a given phase of the disease: BDZs or SMO for withdrawal, serotoninergic agents to favour enduring abstinence, SMO to control craving, whether alone or associated with SSRIs, and acamprosate as an anti-craving agent in detoxified patients.

6.2.2 Agonist Opioid Treatment and Disulfiram Combination

Alcohol undoubtedly has a negative influence on the outcome of a methadone maintenance. It implies a more severe cognitive and behavioural disturbance, a higher prevalence of psychiatric disorders, and a lower degree of compliance, which often conditions an operator towards a quicker, premature tapering of methadone [148]. Moreover, alcohol dependence has more serious somatic consequences (e.g., chronic hepatic failure), which can lead to premature death or may favour overdosing accidents, due to interference with the methadone metabolism [1007]. Since both addictions need to be treated at the same time, disulfiram was tried first on methadone-maintained patients, but, although the complete safety of the combination was ascertained [1008–1010], its efficacy is still controversial, as disulfiram is mostly equivalent to placebo [1009]. The decrease in alcohol consumption appears to depend on a subject's compliance with the combined treatment; this depends in its turn on the level of the subject's awareness of the severity of the problem [1009]. It is awkward to get addicted patients to take disulfiram daily: as an alternative, subcutaneous implantations can be resorted to, as long as patients' consent; or else, methadone administration may be allowed, but only as long as compliance with disulfiram treatment is shown. Another strategy is not to provide patients with methadone if there is a positive result to the screening test for alcohol on the breath (revealing alcohol use during the previous 12 h) or abnormally high alcohol blood levels. This procedure does not guarantee that patients will abstain from alcohol after their methadone has been administered. Table 6.1 reports the feasible combinations of psychotropics with methadone, as observed by our research group.

The combined use of methadone and disulfiram should be limited to the most severe cases, or at least to cases in which non-compliance has hampered the feasibility of other treatments. Apart from such cases, different pharmacotherapies, supportive approaches, or psychosocial treatment should be used.

NTX, although useful in pure AUD patients, is unsuitable for AUD HUD patients. During NTX treatment, in fact, substance non-medical use (like BDZs and stimulants) has been reported to increase [406]. One possible explanation is the following: heroin is capable of inducing a strong craving, which reinforces heroin taking. NTX blocks the heroin-induced reward, so leading craving to extinction, but at the same time, it ends up by intensifying the hypophoria caused by lack of opioid stimulation. NTX-treated subjects may therefore resort to alcohol or BDZ to soothe late withdrawal symptoms and NTX-enhanced hypophoria.

Table 6.1 Drug interactions and methadone dosages in the experience of the PISA-V.P. Dole Research Group

	Dosage (mg/daily)		
	Mode	Min	Max
Methadone (stabilization dosage)	250	240	380
Sodium oxybate (cc/die)	30	10	60
Clonazepam	6	2	12
Trimipramine	50	25	100

6.2.3   SMO-Treatment for Heroin Use Disorder Patients with Concomitant Alcohol Use Disorder

6.2.3.1 Use of SMO in Alcohol Use Disorder Patients

In this book, the term SMO is used for referring to gammahydrossybutiric acid (GHB). SMO) is a natural compound which can be found as a metabolite in human nervous tissues; it binds to specific receptor sites in the brain. It exerts its action by modulating other systems too, or by affecting multiple-ligand receptor sites [1011–1013]. At different dose levels, SMO's effects may be primarily anaesthetic or euphoric. At lower dosages, it increases dopamine release, which is consistent with its documented anticraving properties, and its valuable impact on non-medical use liability and on the psychotic symptoms produced by overdosing [1014–1016]. The onset of its effects is rapid; its half-life is so short as to require dose-refraction at least into thirds during the course of the day in therapeutic regimens, or using greater refraction (with fractions at intervals as short as 3 h, corresponding to 8 fractions a day)—a procedure which results in more stable effects [1017–1020].

After failing to show antipsychotic properties in schizophrenic patients in two preliminary evaluations [1021, 1022], SMO proved effective against alcohol withdrawal and alcohol addiction [1023]. In these therapeutic settings, SMO was safe and well tolerated [1017]. As for the treatment of alcohol withdrawal, it is preferable to other agents because of its shorter half-life, which allows repeated administration free of the risks of late overdosing by accumulation. Its binding rate to plasma proteins is negligible, it is eliminated almost completely without producing metabolites, and it does not affect the liver's metabolic system [1017, 1020].

In the meantime, reports about its use, its use as a date rape drug, and its recreational use outside therapeutic settings have raised major concerns about the spread of SMO treatment. Hence, most of its therapeutic potential has been neglected in the attempt to avoid misuse. The outcome is that SMO, despite being one of the few effective drugs for the treatment of alcoholism, is rarely resorted to, and then mainly through inclusion in short-term schedules [1024].

SMO has proved to be superior to placebo, BDZs and clomethiazole in the management of alcohol withdrawal [1025, 1026]. When compared with flunitrazepam, SMO showed that it was more effective against autonomic symptoms (lower rate of adjunct clonidine administration), although less effective against psychotic symptoms related to the transient increase of dopaminergic transmission (higher rate of administered adjunct haloperidol). SMO is as effective as diazepam over the whole range of alcohol withdrawal, and it allows a quicker resolution of psychic symptoms [1027–1029].

Research has proved that SMO is effective in reducing alcohol use by addicted subjects during periods of variable length (3–12 months). On methodological grounds, the effectiveness of SMO may be questioned, because of the absence of randomized controlled trials. However, due to the lack of widely available, mainly effective medications for the average alcoholic, the behavioural effects of SMO must necessarily be compared with the spontaneous course of alcoholism when left untreated. Moreover, participants in SMO studies were selected either on the basis of documented resistance to other available treatments or on the grounds of a severe grade of alcoholism. In a multicentre study on 179 patients, complete response (sobriety) was achieved in 78% of the sample, the relapse rate being as high as 69.3% within a 6 month follow-up, and 78.6% in a 12 month follow-up after treatment discontinuation [1030]. In a 12-month study on treatment-resistant AUD patients, the retention rate was as high as 60%, with a 10% rate of complete response and a further 15% rate of partial response (comprising a reduction in drinking amounts and/or frequency). Interestingly, partial response was not associated with a worse outcome with respect to complete response. The possibility of achieving a complete response seems to be related to lower baseline consumption amounts.

Responsiveness to SMO seems to vary through time: in two separate studies, Addolorato and colleagues [1030, 1031] reported a momentous response rate of 78.1% at 6 months and of 67.8% among 2-month survivors. In the 12-month study by Maremmani and colleagues, complete response was less frequent, and less likely in the long term, although it must be noted that the subjects enrolled in this inquiry were all resistant to other treatments. Moreover, these authors regard retention in treatment (60%) as a parameter of effectiveness on addictive behaviour, although clearly not on consumption levels. Lastly, these authors have proved that equivalent results can be achieved with more severely ill subjects, regardless of sobriety, in terms of psychosocial adjustment and improvement [1032]. The short-term retention rate with SMO is higher: in the study by Maremmani and colleagues, no patients had dropped out by the end of the first month [1032], while Addolorato and colleagues report a survival rate above two-thirds at 2 months and of about two-thirds at 3 months, in two separate samples [1030]. The reduction recorded in the retention rate in moving from the shorter to the longer term should not be interpreted as a tendency for SMO to lose its apparent effectiveness; in reality, the long-term values simply yield a more realistic picture in reflecting SMO's therapeutic impact on a chronic relapsing disease such as alcoholism. As is true of the general stereotype of addiction, in alcoholism too, withdrawal and short-term compliance are quite likely to be accomplished for a variety of reasons; they represent non-specific behavioural features which can be observed during the early phase of treatment without possessing any therapeutic meaning. The longer the length of observation, the easier it becomes to recognize a behavioural change, or a gradually changing trend induced by ongoing treatment, so allowing discrimination from a transient phase of apparent remission.

Given its short half-life, SMO should be administered in refracted or repeated doses. Repeated dosing is needed in the management of withdrawal, to maintain the suppression of symptoms through time by the replacement of eliminated SMO with further oral amounts. In maintenance regimens, dosages are refracted: in this case, repeated dosing is meant to provide the brain with a tonic, stable, stimulation. The difference is that higher single doses produce stronger but quickly fading effects, which are phasic in nature, while lower doses that are administered more frequently, but with equal cumulative daily amounts, have a weaker but steadier effect, with a narrow concentration gap and a lower liability to use. On clinical grounds, a six-fraction schedule turned out to allow a higher retention rate than the less frequent administering of equal cumulative amounts [1019]. In another study [1031], the transition from a three- to a five-fraction schedule (with equal daily doses of 50 mg/day) appeared to permit a major improvement in treatment response; of 37 patients retained at 2 months with partial response, over two-thirds achieved and maintained sobriety during the following 2 months, after being shifted to the five-fraction schedule. Despite the large size of the sample ($n = 154$), no definitive statement can be made as to whether that improvement can be attributed to the change in schedule or to an increase in the short-term response to SMO through time for partial responders. In conclusion, on the one hand, it is advisable to increase the refraction ratio rather than increasing single dosages. On the other hand, it is not yet possible to achieve stable high levels of SMO in the blood by using high rates of refraction, that is, high levels of SMO tonic stimulation. A slow-release form of SMO would overcome this problem by allowing the use of SMO to produce slow-acting, long-lasting effects along a dose–response curve, as happens in the case of methadone. In this case, it would be possible to increase dosages up to the level required to neutralize severe alcohol craving.

SMO gives a better result than NTX and disulfiram in maintaining abstinence, and it has a better effect on craving than placebo or disulfiram. The problem is that about 30–40% of AUD patients are non-responders to SMO therapy. In our clinical practice, we speculate that by combining disulfiram with SMO treatment, we may be able to achieve a kind of antagonist effect by using the 'psychological threat' of disulfiram (adversative effect) while taking advantage of the anticraving effect of SMO, despite the limitation of its 'non-blockade' effect on alcohol. In this context, to improve the outcome in SMO long-term-treated AUD patients, we added disulfiram to SMO in the management of SMO treatment-resistant AUD patients. In this study, we compared retention in treatment of 52 patients who were treated with the SMO-disulfiram combination for up to 6 months with retention for the same subjects considering their most recent unsuccessful outpatient long-term treatment with SMO only. An additional comparison was carried out on the days of complete abstention from alcohol. Thirty-four patients (65.4%) successfully completed the protocol and were considered to be responders; 18 (34.6%) left the programme and were considered to be non-responders. Considering the days of complete abstinence from alcohol, 36 patients stayed in treatment longer with the SMO-disulfiram combination, 12 stayed for a shorter time and four for the same time. The results of this study seem to indicate a higher efficacy of the SMO-disulfiram association compared with SMO alone. Randomized controlled trials are now needed to verify this hypothesis [1033].

In a recent study, we described the cumulative post-marketing and clinical safety experience with SMO in AUD. We reported: safety data for SMO at approved posology in AUD were identified from:

- the clinical trial registries of the US-NIH (United States-National Institutes of Health) and the European Medicines Agency (EMA),
- reports from the biomedical literature, and

- available pharmacovigilance safety information from the EMA. We reported safety data from 3 recent large randomized clinical studies (520 participants) and 43 earlier clinical studies (2547 participants) showing that SMO has a good safety profile in AUD patients. The safety profile was confirmed by pharmacovigilance data resulting from 299,013 patients exposed to SMO in Austria and Italy. Main adverse events were transitory dizziness and vertigo. Serious adverse events were rare. No deaths attributable to SMO have been reported. Risks of use or dependence have proved to be low in patients without psychiatric comorbidities or polydrug use. The adverse events of SMO are transitory and do not require the discontinuation of treatment. SMO use or dependence are extremely rare in patients without psychiatric comorbidities or polydrug use [1034].

In conclusion, we therefore conclude that SMO is an effective, well-tolerated and safe treatment for withdrawal and relapse prevention treatment, especially in AUD patients with very high drinking risk level (VHDRL). The efficacy and safety of SMO in AUD patients with a VHDRL have been demonstrated [1035].

6.2.3.2 Withdrawal and Non-medical Use Liability

We can expect that administering SMO over the long term leads to the development of tolerance and heightens susceptibility to abrupt discontinuation in the form of rebound symptoms of variable severity conversely, in the short term, for instance, it is quite unlikely that patients will develop withdrawal from SMO, even after taking it as a substitution treatment for alcohol withdrawal [1036]; as far as the medium to long term is concerned, no cases of SMO withdrawal were reported in a group of narcoleptic patients to whom it had been administered at doses of 3 to 9 g/day [1037]. It therefore seems that SMO withdrawal is more typical of subjects taking high SMO dosages outside any therapeutic setting, as a recreational drug, or when patients misuse prescribed SMO [1038–1042]. Moreover, it may be that withdrawal develops accidentally in subjects who abruptly discontinue prescribed SMO without seeking medical advice: it is, however, improbable that AUD patients who take SMO for therapeutic purposes, when dropping out of programmes or showing unresponsiveness to SMO, will fail to react by increasing alcohol consumption, so avoiding any rebound. Apart from this, subjects compliant with therapeutic protocols will have their SMO gradually tapered, so no withdrawal can be expected. SMO withdrawal does stick to the general model of depressant withdrawal [1038, 1039]. It is characterized by a very quick onset (1 to 3 h after latest dose), an escalation to a delirium state which develops more rapidly than with other depressants, and a gradual extinction in times similar to those encountered with alcohol or short-acting withdrawal from BDZ. Psychic symptoms are more prominent than somatic ones [1043]. Diazepam treatment is quite effective [1030, 1044].

SMO is traded illegally as a recreational drug with pleasurable narcotic and euphoric effects. In particular, it is employed as a sex-enhancing drug, and, in some cases, it is administered to unsuspecting victims in order to make them prone to sexual intercourse and induce retrograde amnesia (a feature of date rape drugs), as happens with other substances, such as flunitrazepam. In a laboratory setting, SMO has euphoric effects at dosages of 30 mg/kg but not at 15 mg/kg [1045]. In a clinical sample of AUD patients receiving 50 mg/kg/die 3 times a day, non-medical use occurred in 10% of patients over a 6-month exposure period [1030]. A trend towards non-medical use may develop in the long term and be forerun by a period of balance. It is advisable to keep single doses low, so that the subject does not become conscious of the effects of SMO, because if he or she does, this usually acts as a predictor of subsequent non-medical use due to positive reinforcement. SMO non-medical use should be defined with reference to how subjects handle their SMO; some subjects, for instance, report taking SMO in order to avoid resorting to alcohol and may ask for increasing dosages in order to achieve better control of their alcohol craving. Such patients are neither SMO non-medical users nor those who keep on drinking alcohol although they are taking SMO. SMO non-medical users are those who run out of prescribed SMO due to a self-determined increase in dosages, and usually take larger dosages less often than prescribed (e.g., taking their whole daily dose in one single administration), because this reveals a specific craving for SMO. An overdose of SMO, below the coma level, may induce sedation, simple confusion or psychotic confusion (delirium) [1046, 1047]. Chronic non-medical users are expected to develop intoxication symptoms similar to those induced by alcohol or BDZs [1048].

Caputo et al. showed that the SMO/NTX (NTX) combination was more effective in maintaining abstinence from alcohol than either SMO and NTX used alone; in addition, the combined therapy could likely prevent relapses into heavy drinking and craving for SMO. It can be hypothesized that the synergic effect we found by employing the SMO/NTX combination derives from the combination of the reinforcing and the anti-reward effects which are typical of these drugs. Namely, the anti-reward effect induced by NTX could interfere with SMO-induced dopamine release, which is responsible for its rewarding activity, and this would lead to a modulation of the positive reinforcing effect of the drug. This could explain why patients receiving the combined therapy presented a significantly reduced number of relapses into heavy drinking and craving for SMO, and more successfully maintained a sustained abstinence from alcohol [1049].

SMO has proved to be effective in blocking opioid withdrawal in subjects tolerant to heroin or methadone [1036, 1050]: the onset of action is rapid, and the effects of SMO can be maintained by administering it repeatedly. During the period of observation, subjects stopped using opioids, as proved by negative urinalyses and negative naloxone challenges at the end of treatment [1036, 1050]. The mechanism of interaction between SMO and the opioid system is unclear, but it does not seem to be directly mediated by opioidergic receptors [1045, 1051]. In a small sample of HUD patients rendered tolerant to stable methadone doses, single doses of SMO caused no toxic effects [1045]. On these grounds, SMO has been used, in short-term or even rapid detoxification programmes, in subjects tolerant to heroin, for whom methadone or buprenorphine would have been more reasonable therapeutic options. Episodes of malpractice have happened too; SMO being employed to favour the accomplishment of medically supervised detoxification from therapeutic methadone. The liability of SMO to non-medical use, when it is administered as an anticraving agent to populations of methadone-maintained HUD patients, has not yet been measured. If slow-release SMO became available, research in this field would be more viable and the use of SMO would become safer.

6.2.3.3 SMO in the Treatment of Alcoholic HUD Patients

SMO may be effective in treating alcoholic HUD patients because of its opioid agonist action, and there are no scientific foundations for regarding alcohol-abusing HUD patients as unfit for this kind of treatment. The concurrent use of SMO and methadone is feasible and safe [168, 1052]. However, unlike methadone, SMO induces craving in certain patients; moreover, addicts in general are a population at risk, with a high incidence of impulsive and reckless subjects, so that it might be imprudent to expose addicted patients to a potential drug of non-medical use such as SMO. In any case, it should be remembered that, on behavioural grounds, HUD patients successfully maintained on methadone can be viewed as radically different from untreated HUD patients. Treatment responders do, in fact, display normalized behaviour, not only as far as opioid use is concerned but also in terms of impulsiveness associated with ongoing non-medical use of other substances: the behavioural stereotype of methadone-maintained subjects does not include proneness to substance non-medical use. In AUD patients with high levels of impulsiveness, habitual binge-drinking is incompatible with SMO prescription, due to the risk of toxic synergy. By contrast, in heroin-using HUD patients or alcohol-abusing methadone-maintained subjects, binge drinking is less likely; methadone treatment, even when ineffective in preventing or treating alcohol use, may modify the drinking pattern, and bring binge drinking to extinction. Paradoxically, some precautions, which are needed for pure AUD patients, may be inappropriate for heroin-addicted AUD patients.

It must, however, be added that SMO use is conceivable in an alcoholic heroin addict, once satisfactory behavioural stability has been achieved by means of agonist treatment.

In subjects who are given stable dosages of an opioid agonist, the addition of SMO does not produce unfavourable reactions [1045]. In our PISA-MMTP, a group of stabilized patients on an average methadone dose of 150 mg/day (range 60–380 mg/day) reduced alcohol consumption after being started on SMO at an average dosage of 4.725 g/day (range 1.75–5.25 g/day) [168, 1052].

In HUD patients, alcohol dependence can develop before heroin addiction or together with it [75, 1053–1055]; alternatively, it may mark a later-stage transition from a more expensive, illegal drug to a cheaper, legal one, across a common opioidergic bridge. Some HUD patients, incorrectly treated in short-term or agonist-free programmes, may resort to alcohol in order to stay detached from a heroin environment. Lastly, treatment with ineffective methadone dosages (known as 'undermedication') favours alcohol consumption and misuse during the programme [406, 1056]. Eventually, some HUD patients belonging to the previous categories will end up becoming actual AUD patients through a secondary form of alcohol misuse. Others may stay detached from alcohol, avoiding addiction at all stages, simply through the (re)introduction or dose-adjustment of agonist treatment [75, 1055,

1057, 1058]. In other words, SMO may be administered to HUD patients whose alcohol use fails to respond to effective dosages of methadone during a maintenance programme.

SMO may be administered to HUD patients, regardless of whether alcoholism is primary or secondary to heroin addiction in a chronological sense, after ascertaining that alcohol use is not an indirect expression of an unbalanced craving for opioids (masked heroinism). It would be useful to compare a maintenance regime at blocking dosages (100 mg/day) with a combined regimen of methadone and SMO, in order to clarify the interconnection between cravings for heroin and alcohol in this particular population of alcohol users. Moreover, SMO may be used to treat recently detoxified HUD patients who have recently experienced an intensifying craving for alcohol, so as to prevent its evolution towards secondary alcohol use. Lastly, SMO may be resorted to in the case of abstinent HUD patients who do not clearly need agonist treatment to be restored but show an increasing trend towards drinking.

6.2.3.4 SMO Use in Heroin Use Disorder Poly-User Patients

SMO may be employed as maintenance therapy and does allow the achievement of satisfactory levels of social adjustment in formerly impaired AUD patients, even when sobriety is not attained. Its mechanism of action seems to comprise pro-dopaminergic and GABAergic properties [1011–1013]. Due to its pro-dopaminergic action, SMO may turn out to be helpful both to polydrug users and poly-addicts, who are becoming increasingly frequent in the population of treatment-seeking AUD patients. On the other hand, polydrug users, due to their high level of impulsiveness, are not sufficiently reliable to be admitted to a structured treatment programme, both on decisional and behavioural grounds. Despite this limitation, one reasonable strategy is to target cravings one by one, starting with the most destabilizing substance and/or the most effective treatment regimen, and setting up a 'Chinese box' sequence. After putting up shutters against the first source of destabilization, a second treatment regimen may be added so that the second treatment may count on a greater level of baseline compliance. The effectiveness of some agents, even when hampered by a low level of compliance, may still be a usable resource. In the literature, it is still controversial whether SMO can be used for subjects who have used or are abusing other substances apart from alcohol, with special reference to narcotics. On the other hand, alcohol is seldom the only used substance in young drinkers, and polysubstance dependence is far from rare. Polydrug users may resort to alcohol secondarily, without being addicted to it, in order to handle intoxication from their substance of choice by enhancing its pleasurable effects or producing a pleasurable mixture. However, secondary use may turn into actual addiction, regardless of which substance was used first; some alcohol polydrug users may thus end up as AUD patients or poly-addicts. The selection of poly-using subjects for SMO treatment should account for differential diagnosis between alcohol use and addiction, rather than the chronological sequence of use. Also, the criteria for exclusion should include some behavioural trends or mental states which imply poor compliance and impulsiveness.

As long as cocaine consumption is out of control, and unless craving has been kept under control for some time, cocaine users should be regarded as unsuitable for SMO prescription. In fact, polydrug use pictures often feature cocaine as the main cause of global impulsiveness and unreliability, and no treatment option has proved of major efficacy against cocaine use in terms of compliance and the suppression of craving. Concurrent alcohol and BDZ use may develop in two ways: BDZs may either act as a replacement for alcohol episodically or cyclically, or be combined with it after specific craving drives, which signify an autonomously developed BDZ addiction. Independent BDZ addiction should be challenged with induction and stabilization with clonazepam at blocking dosages. As to the possible synergic effect of BDZs and SMO, the induction of GABA-A tolerance by higher clonazepam dosages allows patients a higher level of safety since it provides protection against intermittent GABA-A stimulation with used depressants. Cases reports have been described by Maremmani and Pacini [1056] and by Lamanna and Maremmani [1059].

6.2.3.5 Principles for the Safe and Effective Use of SMO

SMO's metabolic profile is the main limitation to the feasibility of maintenance treatment. In fact, its short half-life requires a certain level of compliance for effective dosages to be reached and maintained by self-administering on a regular basis. Addicts usually show poor compliance; in the specific case of HUD patients, this problem can be partly overcome by tying the patient to the treatment setting through his or her acquired tolerance to agonist medications. On the other hand, a long-acting formulation of SMO would be unsafe in the early phase of treatment, due to potentially unfavourable interactions with alcohol, just as in the case of long-acting disulfiram. On the one hand, the short latency of action of SMO is useful in the rapid buffering of alcohol withdrawal; on the other hand, it functions as the basis for SMO's non-medical use liability, together with its pro-dopaminergic action.

In order to minimize the risk of non-medical use, one must choose subjects for whom SMO treatment looms as feasible, and, second, select those at low risk of non-medical use behaviours. Whenever possible, SMO should be handed over to a third person (a significant one), whose duty is supervising its administration at prescribed doses and at regular intervals. Subjects should not handle large amounts of SMO, especially when self-administering it; limited supplies should be made available at regular intervals. It is advisable to divide daily dosages, right from the start, into four to six small fractions [1017–1020], so as to assess a patient's compliance and avoid the narcotic effects that would be elicited by large single doses. Apart from justified concerns about side-effects and possible interactions with other used substances, the aim of this strategy is to avoid SMO being discriminated by the brain as a source of euphoria. In particular, subjects who have already experienced opioid-induced euphoria are likely to discriminate SMO when it is administered at higher single doses, even when the cumulative daily amounts of exposure are equal [1045].

Once treatment has started, the persistence of drinking behaviours—though these will probably occur at lower levels—is not a reason for terminating treatment.

In fact, this kind of benefit constitutes a partial response to SMO (reduction in drinking frequency and/or amounts) and it resembles the outcome that constitutes a complete response (sobriety) [1032].

Alcohol use during SMO treatment cannot be regarded as SMO misuse, just as heroin use during methadone treatment cannot be classified as methadone misuse. Subjects taking lower SMO doses may try to achieve greater control over their craving by increasing their SMO doses autonomously. These behaviours should not be mistaken for SMO non-medical use, either; SMO non-medical use consists of the consumption of higher SMO doses in order to elicit euphoric effects.

SMO may be combined with other effective treatments for alcohol misuse. After some time, disulfiram can be added to a SMO regime, in order to proceed step by step towards complete sobriety after partial control over drinking has been achieved. In psychotic subjects, who are sensitive to SMO's dopaminergic effects, this combination is potentially harmful. A SMO-NTX combination is theoretically feasible, since doses of SMO do not seem to act directly via opioid receptors [1045, 1051].

In summary, SMO may be resorted to as means of alcohol use control even in polydrug users. Precautions must, however, be taken to counteract the higher level of impulsiveness in such populations, because the substance polydrug use tends to raise SMO's potential for non-medical use. SMO may be used in HUD patients who have already been stabilized on methadone treatment, due to the anti-impulsive effect of MMT and the minimization of secondary alcohol and depressant non-medical use with adequate methadone dosages. Cocaine users should not be given prescriptions of SMO in an outpatient setting; cocaine craving should, in fact, be targeted first, to increase compliance up to the minimum required to allow compliance with a maintenance, fractioned-dose SMO programme. The availability of a slow-acting, longer half-life SMO would change its pharmacokinetic profile into one more suitable for the healing of craving-related brain pathways. Its non-medical use potential would be minimized as a result, and its use could then be extended to impulsive individuals, as happens with methadone or buprenorphine.

6.2.3.6 Proposal

It should be borne in mind that the following precautions should be taken when exposing methadone-maintained HUD patients to SMO:

- The supervision of self-administered doses should be assigned to a significant one.
- Controlled availability of the drug, to prevent overdosing.
- The use of lower single doses, given that HUD patients are able to discriminate SMO when it is administered at higher single doses [1045].
- Assessment of subjective effects, in line with the rule according to which a stable, peak-less effect is associated with a low likelihood of non-medical use.
- SMO to be started separately from methadone, only after tolerance to opioids has become high or stable, and the patient has recently been abstinent from heroin.
- Methadone treatment is preliminary to SMO treatment; only subjects who have stopped using heroin should be started on SMO.

References

1. Tagliamonte A, Maremmani I. The problem of drug dependence. Heroin Addict Relat Clin Probl. 2001;3(2):7–20.
2. Tagliamonte A. Heroin addiction as normal illness. Heroin Addict Relat Clin Probl. 1999;1(1):9–12.
3. Maremmani I, Pacini M. Understanding the pathogenesis of drug addiction in order to implement a correct pharmacological intervention. Heroin Addict Relat Clin Probl. 2003;5(3):5–12.
4. Scholten W, Simon O, Maremmani I, Wells C, Kelly JF, Hammig R, Radbruch L. Access to treatment with controlled medicines rationale and recommendations for neutral, precise, and respectful language. Public Health. 2017;153:147–53.
5. Goldstein A. Dalla neurobiologia della dipendenza alla terapia dell'eroinismo. Italian J Addict. 1997;4(17):5–20.
6. Dole VP. Narcotic addiction, physical dependence and relapse. N Engl J Med. 1972;286(18):988–92.
7. Dole VP. Addictive behaviour. Sci Am. 1980;243:138–54.
8. Dole VP, Nyswander ME. Behavioral pharmacology and treatment of human drug abuse: methadone maintenance of narcotic addicts. In: Smith JE, Lane JD, editors. The neurobiology of opiate reward processes. Amsterdam: Elsevier Biomedical Press; 1983. p. 211–33.
9. Kreek MJ, Zhon Y, Schussman S. Craving in opiate, cocaine and alcohol addiction. Heroin Addict Relat Clin Probl. 2004;6(2–3):5–52.
10. Dole VP, Nyswander ME. Heroin addiction: a metabolic disease. Arch Intern Med. 1967;120:19–24.
11. Newman RG. Discontinuation symptoms are not addiction/dependence [letter]. Heroin Addict Relat Clin Probl. 2000;2(1):47–8.
12. Gessa GL. Ricadere in Tentazione. Medicina Delle Tossicodipendenze. Italian J Addict. 1997;5(14–15):20–7.
13. Quilici C, Pacini M, Maremmani I. The need for patient education. Opinions and attitudes on heroin addiction: changes in Italy over ten year (1995–2005). Heroin Addict Relat Clin Probl. 2007;9(4):35–54.
14. Goldstein RZ, Craig AD, Bechara A, Garavan H, Childress AR, Paulus MP, Volkow ND. The neurocircuitry of impaired insight in drug addiction. Trends Cogn Sci. 2009;13(9):372–80.
15. Verdejo-Garcia A, Perez-Garcia M. Substance abusers' self-awareness of the neurobehavioral consequences of addiction. Psychiatry Res. 2008;158(2):172–80.
16. Naqvi NH, Bechara A. The insula and drug addiction: an interoceptive view of pleasure, urges, and decision-making. Brain Struct Funct. 2010;214(5–6):435–50.
17. Jung JG, Kim JS, Kim GJ, Oh MK, Kim SS. Brief insight-enhancement intervention among patients with alcohol dependence. J Korean Med Sci. 2011;26(1):11–6.
18. Kim KM, Kim JS, Kim GJ, Kim SS, Jung JG, Kim SM, Pack HJ, Lee DH. The readiness to change and insight in alcohol dependent patients. J Korean Med Sci. 2007;22(3):453–8.

© The Editor(s) (if applicable) and The Author(s), under exclusive license to
Springer Nature Switzerland AG 2023
I. Maremmani et al., *Dual Disorder Heroin Addicts*,
https://doi.org/10.1007/978-3-031-30093-6

19. Yen CF, Hsiao RC, Chen CC, Lin HC, Yen CN, Ko CH, Yen JY, Chen CS. The role of insight to alcohol use disorders in insight to schizophrenia. Compr Psychiatry. 2009;50(1):58–62.
20. Moeller SJ, Maloney T, Parvaz MA, Alia-Klein N, Woicik PA, Telang F, Wang GJ, Volkow ND, Goldstein RZ. Impaired insight in cocaine addiction: laboratory evidence and effects on cocaine-seeking behaviour. Brain. 2010;133(Pt 5):1484–93.
21. Hester R, Simoes-Franklin C, Garavan H. Post-error behavior in active cocaine users: poor awareness of errors in the presence of intact performance adjustments. Neuropsychopharmacology. 2007;32(9):1974–84.
22. Sevy S, Robinson DG, Napolitano B, Patel RC, Gunduz-Bruce H, Miller R, McCormack J, Lorell BS, Kane J. Are cannabis use disorders associated with an earlier age at onset of psychosis? A study in first episode schizophrenia. Schizophr Res. 2010;120(1–3):101–7.
23. Hall W, Degenhardt L. Cannabis and the increased incidence and persistence of psychosis. BMJ. 2011;342:d719.
24. Kuepper R, van Os J, Lieb R, Wittchen HU, Hofler M, Henquet C. Continued cannabis use and risk of incidence and persistence of psychotic symptoms: 10 year follow-up cohort study. BMJ. 2011;342:d738.
25. Large M, Sharma S, Compton MT, Slade T, Nielssen O. Cannabis use and earlier onset of psychosis: a systematic meta-analysis. Arch Gen Psychiatry. 2011;68(6):555–61.
26. Miller R, Caponi JM, Sevy S, Robinson D. The insight-adherence-abstinence triad: an integrated treatment focus for cannabis-using first-episode schizophrenia patients. Bull Menn Clin. 2005;69(3):220–36.
27. Breitling LP, Rothenbacher D, Stegmaier C, Raum E, Brenner H. Older smokers' motivation and attempts to quit smoking: epidemiological insight into the question of lifestyle versus addiction. Dtsch Arztebl Int. 2009;106(27):451–5.
28. Falloon I. Comprehensive management of mental disorders. Buckingham: Buckingham Mental Health Service; 1988.
29. Falloon IRH, Fadden G. Integrated mental health care: a comprehensive, community-based approach. Cambridge: Cambridge University Press; 1995.
30. Falloon I. Chiama (community help to increase appropriate mental health services access). Paper presented at University of L'aquila, December 15. 1995.
31. Anderson CM, Reiss DJ, Hogarty GE. Schizophrenia and the family: a practitioner's guide to psychoeducation and management. New York: Guilford Press; 1986.
32. Bellack AS, Mueser KT. Psychosocial treatment for schizophrenia. Schizophr Bull. 1993;19(2):317–36.
33. Maremmani AGI, Rovai L, Rugani F, Pacini M, Lamanna F, Bacciardi S, Perugi G, Deltito J, Dell'Osso L, Maremmani I. Correlations between awareness of illness (insight) and history of addiction in heroin-addicted patients. Front Psych. 2012;3(61):1–11.
34. Szerman N, Martinez-Raga J, Baler R, Roncero C, Vega P, Basurte I, Grau-Lopez L, Torrens M, Casas M, Franco C, Spinnato G, Maremmani AGI, Maremmani I, Daulouede JP, Aguerretxe-Colina A, Ruiz P. Joint statement on dual disorders: addictions and other mental disorders. Addiction is a mental disorder, not a voluntary, self-indulgent act. Madrid: WADD, SEPD, WPA Section on DD, NIDA; 2017.
35. Pani PP, Trogu E, Vigna-Taglianti F, Mathis F, Diecidue R, Kirchmayer U, Amato L, Ghibaudi J, Camposeragna A, Saponaro A, Davoli M, Faggiano F, Maremmani AGI, Maremmani I. Psychopathological symptoms of heroin-addicted patients entering opioid agonist or therapeutic community treatment. Ann General Psychiatry. 2014;13:35.
36. Pani PP, Maremmani I, Trogu E, Gessa GL, Ruiz P, Akiskal HS. Delineating the psychic structure of substance abuse and addictions: should anxiety, mood and impulse-control dysregulation be included? J Affect Disord. 2010;122(3):185–97.
37. Pani PP, Maremmani AGI, Trogu E, Vigna-Taglianti F, Mathis F, Diecidue R, Kirchmayer U, Amato L, Ghibaudi J, Camposeragna A, Saponaro A, Davoli M, Faggiano F, Maremmani I. Psychopathology of addiction: may a SCL-90 based five dimensions structure be applied irrespectively of the involved drug? Ann General Psychiatry. 2016;15:13.

38. Pani PP, Maremmani AGI, Trogu E, Vigna-Taglianti F, Mathis F, Diecidue R, Kirchmayer U, Amato L, Davoli M, Ghibaudi J, Composeragna A, Saponaro A, Faggiano F, Maremmani I. Psychopathological symptoms in detoxified and non-detoxified heroin-dependent patients entering residential treatment. Heroin Addict Relat Clin Probl. 2015;17(2–3):17–24.
39. Pani PP, Maremmani AGI, Trogu E, Vigna-Taglianti F, Mathis F, Diecidue R, Kirchmayer U, Amato L, Davoli M, Ghibaudi J, Camposeragna A, Saponaro A, Faggiano F, Maremmani I. Psychic structure of opioid addiction: impact of lifetime psychiatric problems on SCL-90-based psychopathologic dimensions in heroin-dependent patients. Addict Disord Their Treat. 2016;15(1):6–16.
40. Maremmani I, Pani PP, Pacini M, Bizzarri JV, Trogu E, Maremmani AGI, Perugi G, Gerra G, Dell'Osso L. Subtyping patients with heroin addiction at treatment entry: factors derived Fron the SCL-90. Ann General Psychiatry. 2010;9(1):15.
41. Maremmani AGI, Pani PP, Trogu E, Vigna-Taglianti F, Mathis F, Diecidue R, Kirchmayer U, Amato L, Ghibaudi J, Camposeragna A, Saponaro A, Davoli M, Faggiano F, Maremmani I. The impact of psychopathological subtypes on retention rate of patients with substance use disorder entering residential therapeutic community treatment. Ann General Psychiatry. 2016;15:29.
42. Maremmani AGI, Cerniglia L, Cimino S, Bacciardi S, Rovai L, Rugani F, Massimetti E, Gazzarrini D, Pallucchini A, Pani PP, Akiskal HH, Maremmani I. Towards a specific psychopathology of heroin addiction. Comparison between heroin use disorder and major depression patients. Heroin Addict Relat Clin Probl. 2015;17(6):9–16.
43. Maremmani AGI, Rovai L, Pani PP, Pacini M, Lamanna F, Rugani F, Schiavi E, Dell'Osso L, Maremmani I. Do methadone and buprenorphine have the same impact on psychopathological symptoms of heroin addicts? Ann General Psychiatry. 2011;10:17.
44. Maremmani I, Pacini M, Giuntoli G, Lovrecic M, Perugi G. Naltrexone as maintenance therapy for heroin addiction: predictors of response. Heroin Addict Relat Clin Probl. 2004;6(1):43–52.
45. Maremmani I, Maremmani AGI, Pacini M. The psychic structure of the substance use disorder. Pisa: AU-CNS Press & Pacini Editore Medicina; 2019.
46. Lovrecic M, Lovrecic B, Dernovsek MZ, Tavcar R, Maremmani I. Unreported double frequency of heroin addicts visiting psychiatric services and addiction treatment services. Heroin Addict Relat Clin Probl. 2004;6(3):27–32.
47. Pacini M, Maremmani I. Malleus maleficarum . . . the superstition of psychosocially centred intervention in addictive diseases. Heroin addiction as case study. Heroin Addict Relat Clin Probl. 2013;15(3):9–18.
48. Uchtenhagen A. The role and function of heroin-assisted treatment at the treatment system level. Heroin Addict Relat Clin Probl. 2017;19(2):17–24.
49. Maremmani I, Perugi G, Pacini M, Akiskal HS. Toward a unitary perspective on the bipolar spectrum and substance abuse: opiate addiction as a paradigm. J Affect Disord. 2006;93(1–3):1–12.
50. Maremmani I, Zolesi O, Agueci T, Castrogiovanni P. Methadone doses and psychopathological symptoms during methadone maintenance. J Psychoactive Drugs. 1993;25(3):253–6.
51. Maremmani AGI, Rovai L, Rugani F, Bacciardi S, Dell'Osso L, Maremmani I. Substance abuse and psychosis. The strange case of opioids. Eur Rev Med Pharmacol Sci. 2014;18(3):287–302.
52. Maremmani AGI, Rovai L, Bacciardi S, Rugani F, Pacini M, Pani PP, Dell'Osso L, Akiskal HS, Maremmani I. The long-term outcomes of heroin dependent-treatment-resistant patients with bipolar 1 comorbidity after admission to enhanced methadone maintenance. J Affect Disord. 2013;151(2):582–9.
53. Bizzarri JV, Conca A, Maremmani I. Does a buprenorphine augmentation control manic symptoms in bipolar disorder with a past history of heroin addiction? A case report. Heroin Addict Relat Clin Probl. 2014;16(1):49–54.
54. Maremmani I, Canoniero S, Pacini M. Methadone dose and retention in treatment of heroin addicts with bipolar I disorder comorbidity. Preliminary results. Heroin Addict Relat Clin Probl. 2000;2(1):39–46.

55. Maremmani I, Zolesi O, Aglietti M, Marini G, Tagliamonte A, Shinderman M, Maxwell S. Methadone dose and retention during treatment of heroin addicts with axis I psychiatric comorbidity. J Addict Dis. 2000;19(2):29–41.

56. Maremmani I, Pacini M, Lubrano S, Perugi G, Tagliamonte A, Pani PP, Gerra G, Shinderman M. Long-term outcomes of treatment-resistant heroin addicts with and without DSM-IV axis I psychiatric comorbidity (dual diagnosis). Eur Addict Res. 2008;14(3):134–42.

57. Drake RE, Osher FC, Wallach MA. Alcohol use and abuse in schizophrenia. A prospective community study. J Nerv Ment Dis. 1989;177:408–14.

58. Osher FC, Drake RE, Noordsy DL, Teague GB, Hurlbut SC, Biesanz JC, Beaudett MS. Correlates and outcomes of alcohol use disorder among rural outpatients with schizophrenia. J Clin Psychiatry. 1994;55(3):109–13.

59. Swofford CD, Kasckow JW, Scheller-Gilkey G, Inderbitzin LB. Substance use: a powerful predictor of relapse in schizophrenia. Schizophr Res. 1996;20(1–2):145–51.

60. Kokkevi A, Stefanis N, Anastasopoulou E, Kostogianni C. Personality disorders in drug abusers: prevalence and their association with axis I disorders as predictors of treatment retention. Addict Behav. 1998;23(6):841–53.

61. Linszen DH, Dingemans PM, Lenior ME. Cannabis abuse and the course of recent-onset schizophrenia disorders. Arch Gen Psychiatry. 1994;51:273–9.

62. Brewer DD, Catalano RF, Haggerty K, Gainey RR, Fleming CB. A meta-analysis of predictors of continued drug use during and after treatment for opiate addiction. Addiction. 1998;93(1):73–92.

63. Maremmani AGI, Bacciardi S, Rovai L, Rugani F, Massimetti E, Gazzarrini D, Dell'Osso L, Maremmani I. Six-month outcome in bipolar Spectrum alcoholics treated with acamprosate after detoxification: a retrospective study. Int J Environ Res Public Health. 2014;11(12):12983–96.

64. Pacini M, Maremmani AGI, Rovai L, Rugani F, Bacciardi S, Maremmani I. Self-presentation and health issues of anonymous heroin addicts asking for a free internet medical consultation. Heroin Addict Relat Clin Probl. 2013;15(4):33–8.

65. Henriksen K, Waal H, Krajci P. Will non-compliant "hard-to-treat" opioid dependent patients profit from low threshold methadone treatment? A prospective 15-month evaluation of patients on low dosage methadone treatment at Oslo University Hospital. Heroin Addict Relat Clin Probl. 2016;18(3):23–8.

66. Pacini M, Maremmani AGI, Rovai L, Rugani F, Maremmani I. Treating heroin addicts. Blocking dosages and stimulation-stabilization of opioidergic system. Heroin Addict Relat Clin Probl. 2010;12(4):41–8.

67. Maremmani I, Pacini M, Canoniero S, Maremmani AGI, Tagliamonte A. Dose determination in dual diagnosed heroin addicts during methadone treatment. Heroin Addict Relat Clin Probl. 2010;12(1):17–24.

68. Maremmani AGI, Rovai L, Bacciardi S, Massimetti E, Gazzarrini D, Pallucchini A, Pani PP, Maremmani I. Relationships between addictive behaviours and dual disorders, as found in heroin use disorder patients at treatment entry. Heroin Addict Relat Clin Probl. 2016;18(2):5–12.

69. Prodromou M, Kyritsi E, Samartzis L. Dual disorders affects prognosis in patients with drug dependence in integrative care setting. Health Sci J. 2014;8(2):226–8.

70. Maremmani I, Pacini M, Perugi G, Deltito J, Akiskal H. Cocaine abuse and the bipolar spectrum in 1090 heroin addicts: clinical observations and a proposed pathophysiologic model. J Affect Disord. 2008;106(1–2):55–61.

71. Pacini M, Maremmani I, Vitali M, Romeo M, Santini P, Vermeil V, Ceccanti M. Cocaine abuse in 448 alcoholics: evidence for a bipolar connection. Addict Disord Their Treat. 2010;9(4):164–71.

72. Vitali M, Pacini M, Maremmani I, Romeo M, Ceccanti M. Pattern of cocaine consumption in a sample of Italian alcoholics. Int Clin Psychopharmacol. 2011;26:e98.

73. Maremmani AGI, Pacini M, Bacciardi S, Ceccanti M, Maremmani I. Current use of cannabis and past use of heroin as predictors of alcohol and concomitant cocaine use disorder. Alcologia. 2015;22(1):36–40.

74. Maremmani AGI, Pacini M, Pani PP, Ceccanti M, Bacciardi S, Akiskal HS, Maremmani I. Possible trajectories of addictions: the role of bipolar spectrum. Heroin Addict Relat Clin Probl. 2016;18(4):23–32.

75. Maremmani I, Shinderman MS. Alcohol, benzodiazepines and other drugs use in heroin addicts treated with methadone. Polyabuse or undermedication? Heroin Addict Relat Clin Probl. 1999;1(2):7–13.

76. Pacini M, Maremmani AGI, Ceccanti M, Maremmani I. Former heroin-dependent alcohol use disorder patients. Prevalence, addiction history and clinical features. Alcohol Alcohol. 2015;50(4):451–7.

77. Pacini M, Maremmani I, Vitali M, Santini P, Romeo M, Ceccanti M. Affective temperaments in alcoholic patients. Alcohol. 2009;43(5):397–404.

78. Maremmani I, Pacini M, Popovic D, Romano A, Maremmani AGI, Perugi G, Deltito J, Akiskal K, Akiskal H. Affective temperaments in heroin addiction. J Affect Disord. 2009;117(3):186–92.

79. Camacho A, Akiskal HS. Proposal for a bipolar-stimulant Spectrum: temperament, diagnostic validation and therapeutic outcomes with mood stabilizers. J Affect Disord. 2005;85:217–30.

80. Martin WR, Jasinski DR. Physiological parameters of morphine dependence in man, early abstinence, protracted abstinence. J Psychiatr Res. 1969;7:9–17.

81. Maremmani I, Pani PP, Mellini A, Pacini M, Marini G, Lovrecic M, Perugi G, Shinderman M. Alcohol and cocaine use and abuse among opioid addicts engaged in a methadone maintenance treatment program. J Addict Dis. 2007;26(1):61–70.

82. Pacini M, Maremmani I. Methadone reduces the need for antipsychotic and Antimanic agents in heroin addicts hospitalized for manic and/or acute psychotic episodes. Heroin Addict Relat Clin Probl. 2005;7(4):43–8.

83. Maremmani I, Pacini M, Pani PP, Perugi G, Deltito J, Akiskal H. The mental status of 1090 heroin addicts at entry into treatment: should depression be considered a 'dual diagnosis'? Ann General Psychiatry. 2007;6:31.

84. Akiskal HS, Pinto O. The evolving bipolar spectrum. Prototypes I, II, III, and IV. Psychiatr Clin North Am. 1999;22(3):517–34.

85. Maremmani I, Pacini M, Pani PP, Popovic D, Romano A, Maremmani AGI, Deltito J, Perugi G. Use of street methadone in Italian heroin addicts presenting for opioid agonist treatment. J Addict Dis. 2009;28(4):382–8.

86. Schifano F, Bargagli AM, Belleudi V, Amato L, Davoli M, Diecidue R, Versino E, Vigna-Taglianti F, Faggiano F, Perucci CA. Methadone treatment in clinical practice in Italy: need for improvement. Eur Addict Res. 2006;12(3):121–7.

87. Dole VP, Nyswander ME, Warner A. Successful treatment of 750 criminal addicts. JAMA. 1968;206:2708–11.

88. Dole VP, Nyswander ME, Kreek MJ. Narcotic blockade. Arch Intern Med. 1966;118:304–9.

89. Dole VP. What have we learned from three decades of methadone maintenance treatment. Drug Alcohol Rev. 1994;13(3):330–8.

90. Dole VP. Research on methadone maintenance treatment. Int J Addict. 1970;5:360–3.

91. Isbell H, Vogel VH. The addiction liability of methadon (Amidone, Dolophine, 10820) and its use in the treatment of the morphine abstinence syndrome. Am J Psychiatry. 1949;105:909–14.

92. Weppner RS, Stephens RC, Conrad HT. Methadone: some aspects of its legal and illegal use. Am J Psychiatry. 1972;129(4):451–5.

93. Berger H. Prevention of the diversion of clinic methadone to the street market. Proc Natl Conf Methadone Treat. 1973;2:1264–6.

94. Bourne PG. Methadone diversion. Proc Natl Conf Methadone Treat. 1973;2:839–41.

95. Resnick RB. Problems of methadone diversion and implications for control. Int J Addict. 1977;12(7):803–6.

96. Goldman FR, Thistel CI. Diversion of methadone: illicit methadone use among applicants to two metropolitan drug abuse programs. Int J Addict. 1978;13(6):855–62.

97. Hough G, Washton AM, Resnick RB. Addressing the diversion of take-home methadone: laam as the sole treatment choice for patients seeking maintenance therapy. NIDA Res Monogr. 1983;43:302–9.

98. Ritter A, Di Natale R. The relationship between take-away methadone policies and methadone diversion. Drug Alcohol Rev. 2005;24(4):347–52.

99. Verebey KE. Opioids in mental illness: theories, clinical observations and treatment possibilities. Ann N Y Acad Sci. 1982;398:1–512.

100. Kreek MJ. Pharmacological treatment of addiction: normalization of physiology and aids risk reduction. In: Tagliamonte A, Maremmani I, editors. Drug addiction and related clinical problems. Wien: Springer-Verlag; 1995. p. 165–74.

101. Maremmani AGI, Pallucchini A, Rovai L, Bacciardi S, Spera V, Maiello M, Perugi G, Maremmani I. The long-term outcome of patients with heroin use disorder/dual disorder (chronic psychosis) after admission to enhanced methadone maintenance. Ann General Psychiatry. 2018;17:14.

102. Ochoa Mangado E, Lopez-Ibor Alino JJ, Perez de los Cobos Peris JC, Cebollada Gracia A. Detoxification treatment with naltrexone in opiate dependence. Actas Luso Esp Neurol Psiquiatr Cienc Afines. 1992;20(5):215–29.

103. Lopez-Ibor Alino JJ, Perez de los Cobos JC, Ochoa E, Hernandez Herreros M. Maintenance treatment for opiate dependence at a naltrexone clinic. Actas Luso Esp Neurol Psiquiatr Cienc Afines. 1990;18(5):296–305.

104. Resnick RB, Schuyten-Resnick E, Washton A. Narchotic antagonists in the treatment of opioid dependence: review and commentary. Compr Psychiatry. 1979;20:116–25.

105. Hollister L. Clinical evaluation of naltrexone treatment of opiate-dependent individuals: report of the National Research Council Committee on clinical evaluation of narcotic antagonists. Arch Gen Psychiatry. 1978;35:335–41.

106. Comer SD, Sullivan MA, Yu E, Rothenberg JL, Kleber HD, Kampman K, Dackis C, O'Brien CP. Injectable, sustained-release naltrexone for the treatment of opioid dependence: a randomized, placebo-controlled trial. Arch Gen Psychiatry. 2006;63(2):210–8.

107. Krupitskii EM, Nunes EV, Ling U, Gastfrend DR, Memisoglu A, Blokhina EA, Silverman BL. Injectable extended-release naltrexone for opioid dependence: an open label study of long-term safety and efficacy. Zh Nevrol Psikhiatr Im S S Korsakova. 2014;114(11):49–56.

108. Mogali S, Khan NA, Drill ES, Pavlicova M, Sullivan MA, Nunes E, Bisaga A. Baseline characteristics of patients predicting suitability for rapid naltrexone induction. Am J Addict. 2015;24(3):258–64.

109. Sideroff SN, Charauwasta VC, Farvik ME. Craving in heroin addicts maintained on the opiate antagonist naltrexone. Am J Drug Alcohol Abuse. 1978;5:415–23.

110. Ritter AJ. Naltrexone in the treatment of heroin dependence: relationship with depression and risk of overdose. Aust N Z J Psychiatry. 2002;36(2):224–8.

111. Rothman RB, Gorelick DA, Heishman SJ, Eichmiller PR, Hill BH, Norbeck J, Liberto JG. An open-label study of a functional opioid kappa antagonist in the treatment of opioid dependence. J Subst Abus Treat. 2000;18(3):277–81.

112. Waldron VD, Klimt CR, Seibel JE. Methadone overdose treated with naloxone infusion. JAMA. 1973;225(1):53.

113. Bradberry JC, Raebel MA. Continuous infusion of naloxone in the treatment of narcotic overdose. Drug Intell Clin Pharm. 1981;15(12):945–50.

114. Tandberg D, Abercrombie D. Treatment of heroin overdose with endotracheal naloxone. Ann Emerg Med. 1982;11(8):443–5.

115. Wermeling DP. A response to the opioid overdose epidemic: naloxone nasal spray. Drug Deliv Transl Res. 2013;3(1):63–74.

116. Hansen A. Norway tries naloxone in spray form to prevent deaths from drug overdose. BMJ. 2014;348:g1686.

117. Loimer N, Hofmann P, Chaudhry HR. Nasal administration of naloxone is as effective as the intravenous route in opiate addicts. Int J Addict. 1994;29(6):819–27.

118. Behar E, Santos GM, Wheeler E, Rowe C, Coffin PO. Brief overdose education is sufficient for naloxone distribution to opioid users. Drug Alcohol Depend. 2015;148:209–12.
119. Bagley SM, Peterson J, Cheng DM, Jose C, Quinn E, O'Connor PG, Walley AY. Overdose education and naloxone rescue kits for family members of opioid users: characteristics, motivations and naloxone use. Subst Abus. 2015;36(2):149–54. https://doi.org/10.1080/0889707 7.2014.989352.
120. Walley AY, Xuan Z, Hackman HH, Quinn E, Doe-Simkins M, Sorensen-Alawad A, Ruiz S, Ozonoff A. Opioid overdose rates and implementation of overdose education and nasal naloxone distribution in Massachusetts: interrupted time series analysis. BMJ. 2013;346:f174.
121. Dorus W, Senay EC. Depression demographic dimensions, and drug abuse. Am J Psychiatry. 1980;137:669–704.
122. Rounsaville BJ, Weissman MM, Rosenberger PH, Wilbur CH, Kleber HD. Detecting depressive disorders in drug abusers: a comparison of screening instruments. J Affect Disord. 1979;1:255–67.
123. Robins PR. Depression and drug addiction. Psychoanal Q. 1974;48:375–86.
124. Lehman WX, De Angelis GC. Adolescents, methadone, and psychoterapeutic agents. In: Proceedings of the national conference on methadone treatment. New York: National Association for the Prevention of the Addiction to Narcotics; 1972. p. 95–104.
125. Weissman MM, Slobetz F, Prusoff BA, Mesritz M, Howard PAT. Clinical depression among narcotic addicts maintained on methadone in the community. Am J Psychiatry. 1976;133:1434–8.
126. Steer RA, Kotzer E. Affective changes in Male and female methadone patients. Drug Alcohol Depend. 1980;5:115–22.
127. McLellan AT, O'Brien CP, Kron R. Matching substance abuse patients to appropriate treatment: a conceptual and methodological approach. Drug Alcohol Depend. 1980;5:189–95.
128. Jainchill N, De Leon G, Pinkham L. Psychiatric diagnosis among substance abusers in therapeutic community treatment. J Psychoactive Drugs. 1986;18(3):209–13.
129. Khantzian EJ, Treece CD. Heroin addiction: the diagnostic dilemma for psychiatry. In: Pickens RW, Heston LL, editors. Psychiatric factors in drug abuse. New York: Grune and Stratton; 1979. p. 21–45.
130. Brienza RS, Stein MD, Chen M, Gogineni A, Sobota M, Maksad J, Hu P, Clarke J. Depression among needle exchange program and methadone maintenance clients. J Subst Abus Treat. 2000;18(4):331–7.
131. Hendriks WJ. Use of multifamily counseling groups in treatment of male narcotics addicts. Int J Group Psychother. 1971;21:34–90.
132. De Jong AJ, Van Den Brink W, Hartveld FM. Personality disorders in alcoholics and drug addicts. Compr Psychiatry. 1993;34(2):87–94.
133. Inman DJ, Bascue LO, Scoloda T. Identifications of borderline personality disorders among substance abuse in-patients. J Subst Abuse Treat. 1985;2(4):229–32.
134. Khantzian EJ, Treece C. DSM-III psychiatric diagnosis of narcotic addicts: recent findings. Arch Gen Psychiatry. 1985;42:1067–77.
135. O'Doherty F, Davies JB. Life events and addiction: a critical review. Br J Addict. 1987;82(2):127–37.
136. Pope HG. Drug abuse and psychopatology. N Engl J Med. 1979;301(24):1341–2.
137. Rounsaville BJ, Weissman MM, Crits-Christoph K, Wilber C, Kleber H. Diagnosis and symptoms of depression in opiate addicts. Course and relationship to treatment outcome. Arch Gen Psychiatry. 1982;39(2):151–6.
138. Woody GE, McLellan AT, Luborsky L, O'Brien CP. Psychiatric severity as a predictor of benefits from psychotherapy: the Penn-VA study. Am J Psychiatry. 1984;141:1172–7.
139. Abbott PJ, Weller SB, Walker SR. Psychiatric disorders of opioid addicts entering treatment: preliminary data. J Addict Dis. 1994;13(3):1–11.
140. Bela GLA, Folke J, Von Knorring L, Terenius L, Wahlstrom A. Endorphins in chronic pain. Differences in CSF endorphin levels between organic and psychogenic pain syndromes. Pain. 1978;5:153–62.

141. Chen CC, Tsai SY, Su LW, Yang TW, Tsai CJ, Hwu HG. Psychiatric co-morbidity among male heroin addicts: differences between hospital and incarcerated subjects in Taiwan. Addiction. 1999;94(6):825–32.

142. Darke S, Swift W, Hall W. Prevalence, severity and correlates of psychological morbidity among methadone maintenance clients. Addiction. 1994;89(2):211–7.

143. Khantzian EJ. The self-medication hypothesis of addictive disorders: focus on heroin and cocaine dependence. Am J Psychiatry. 1985;142:1259–64.

144. Mason BJ, Kocsis JH, Melia D, Khuri ET, Sweeney J, Wells A, Borg L, Millman RB, Kreek MJ. Psychiatric comorbidity in methadone maintained patients. J Addict Dis. 1998;17(3):75–89.

145. Mintz J, O'Brien CP, Woody GE, Beck AT. Depression in treated narcotic addicts, ex addicts, non addicts, and suicide attempters: validation of a very brief depression scale. Am J Drug Alcohol Abuse. 1979;6:385–96.

146. Mirin SR, Meyer RE, McNamee B. Psychopatology and mood duration in heroin use: acute and chronic effects. Arch Gen Psychiatry. 1976;33:1503–8.

147. Pilowsky I, Katsikitis M. Depressive illness and dependency. Acta Psychiatr Scand. 1983;68:11–4.

148. Ross HE, Glaser FB, Germanson T. The prevalence of psychiatric disorders in patients with alcohol and other drug problems. Arch Gen Psychiatry. 1988;45(11):1023–31.

149. Shaw BF, Steer RA, Beck AT, Schut J. Structure of depression in heroin addicts. Br J Addict. 1979;74:295–303.

150. von Limbeek J, Wouters L, Kaplan CD, Geerlings PJ, von Alem V. Prevalence of psychopathology in drug-addicted Dutch. J Subst Abus Treat. 1992;9(1):43–52.

151. Krausz M, Verthein U, Degkewitz P, Haasen C, Raschke P. Maintenance treatment of opiate addicts in Germany with medications containing codeine: results of follow-up study. Addiction. 1998;93:1161–7.

152. Clerici M, Capitanio C, Garini R, Carta I. Tossicodipendenza Ed Interventi Psicoterapeutici: Il Profilo Psicopatologico Del Tossicodipendente Da Eroina. Arch Psicol Neurol Psichiatr. 1987;48:546–59.

153. Dackis CA, Gold MS. Opiate addiction and depression: cause or effect. Drug Alcohol Depend. 1983;11:105–9.

154. Rounsaville BJ. Epidemiology of drug use and abuse in adults. In: Cavenar JO, editor. Psychiatry. New York: Basic Books; 1985. p. 137–43.

155. Rounsaville BJ, Rosenberger PH, Wilber CH, Weissman MM, Kleber HB. A comparison of the SAD/RDC and the DSM-III, diagnosing drug abusers. J Nerv Ment Dis. 1980;168:90–7.

156. Rounsaville BJ, Weissman MM, Kleber HD. An evaluation of depression in opiate addicts. Res Commun Ment Health. 1983;3:257–89.

157. Rounsaville BJ, Weissman MM, Kleber H, Wilber C. Heterogeneity of psychiatric diagnosis in treated opiate addicts. Arch Gen Psychiatry. 1982;39:161–6.

158. Gold MS, Pottash ALC, Sweeney DR, Martin D, Extein I. Antimanic, antidepressant, and antipanic effects of opiate: clinical, neuro-anatomical, and biochemical evidence. Ann N Y Acad Sci. 1982;398:140–50.

159. Mirin SM, Weiss R, Michael J, Griffin M. Psychopathology in substance abusers: diagnosis and treatment. Am J Drug Alcohol Abuse. 1988;14(2):139–57.

160. Mirin SM, Weiss RD. Psychiatric comorbidity in drug/alcohol addiction. In: Miller NS, editor. Comprehensive handbook of drug and alcohol addiction. White Plains, NY: Mercel Dekker; 1991. p. 65–77.

161. Maremmani I, Capone MR, Aglietti M, Castrogiovanni P. Heroin dependence and bipolar disorders. New Trends Exp Clin Psychiat. 1994;10:179–82.

162. Maremmani I, Canoniero S, Pacini M, Lazzeri A, Placidi GF. Opioids and cannabinoids abuse among bipolar patients. Heroin Addict Relat Clin Probl. 2000;2(2):35–42.

163. Maremmani AGI, Bacciardi S, Gehring ND, Cambioli L, Schutz C, Jang K, Krausz M. Substance use among homeless individuals with schizophrenia and bipolar disorder. J Nerv Ment Dis. 2017;205(3):173–7.

164. Maremmani AGI, Bacciardi S, Gehring ND, Cambioli L, Schutz C, Akiskal HS, Jang K, Krausz M. The impact of mood symptomatology on pattern of substance use among homeless. J Affect Disord. 2015;176:164–70.
165. Volovka SJ, Anderson B, Koz G. Naloxone and naltrexone in mental illness and tardive dyskinesia. Ann N Y Acad Sci. 1982;398:143–52.
166. O'Brien CP. Research advances in the understanding and treatment of addiction. Am J Addict. 2003;12(Suppl 2):S36–47.
167. Judd LL, Akiskal HS. The prevalence and disability of bipolar spectrum disorders in the us population: re-analysis of the ECA database taking into account subthreshold cases. J Affect Disord. 2003;73(1–2):123–31.
168. Maremmani I, Pacini M, Lubrano S, Lovrecic M, Perugi G. Dual diagnosis heroin addicts. The clinical and therapeutic aspects. Heroin Addict Relat Clin Probl. 2003;5(2):7–98.
169. Akiskal HS. The prevalent clinical spectrum of bipolar disorders: beyond DSM IV. J Clin Psychopharmacol. 1996;17(Suppl 3):117–22.
170. Perugi G, Akiskal HS. The soft bipolar spectrum redefined: focus on the cyclothymic anxious-sensitive, impulse discontrol, and binge-eating connection in bipolar II and related condition. Psychiatr Clin North Am. 2002;25(4):713–37.
171. American Psychiatric Association. Diagnostic and statistical manual of mental disorders, DSM-5. Washington, DC: American Psychiatric Association; 2013.
172. Akiskal HS, Djenderedjian AM, Rosenthal RH. Cyclothymic disorder: validating criteria for inclusion in the bipolar affective group. Am J Psychiatry. 1977;134:1227–33.
173. Akiskal HS, Khani MK, Scott-Strauss A. Cyclothymic temperamental disorders. Psychiatr Clin North Am. 1979;2:527–54.
174. Angst J. The etiology and nosology of endogenous depressive psychoses. Monogr Gesamtgeb Neurol Psychiatr. 1966;112:1–118.
175. Fieve RR, Dunner DL. Unipolar and bipolar affective states. In: Flach FF, Draghi SS, editors. The nature and treatment of depression. New York: Wiley; 1975. p. 145–60.
176. Akiskal HS. The bipolar spectrum: new concepts in classification and diagnosis. In: Grinspoon L, editor. Psychiatry update: the American Psychiatric Association annual review, vol. 11. Washington, DC: American Psychiatric Press; 1983. p. 271–92.
177. Akiskal HS, Mallya G. Criteria for the 'soft' bipolar spectrum: treatment implications. Psychopharmacol Bull. 1987;23:68–73.
178. Akiskal HS, Bourgeois ML, Angst J, Post R, Moller H, Hirschfeld R. Re-evaluating the prevalence of and diagnostic composition within the broad clinical spectrum of bipolar disorders. J Affect Disord. 2000;59(Suppl 1):S5–S30.
179. World Health Organization. The ICD-10 classification of mental and behavioural disorders. Clinical descriptions and diagnostic guidelines. Geneva: WHO; 1992.
180. Bowden CL. Lithium-responsive depression. Compr Psychiatry. 1978;19(3):227–31.
181. Strober M, Carlson G. Bipolar illness in adolescents with major depression: clinical, genetic, and psychopharmacologic predictors in a three- to four-year prospective follow-up investigation. Arch Gen Psychiatry. 1982;39:549–55.
182. Akiskal HS, Hantouche EG, Allilaire J-F, Sechter D, Bourgeois M, Azorin JM, Chatenêt-Duchêne L, Lancrenon S. Validating antidepressant-associated hypomania (bipolar III): a systematic comparison with spontaneous hypomania (bipolar II). J Affect Disord. 2003;73:65–74.
183. Rosenthal TL, Akiskal HS, Scott-Strauss A, Rosenthal RH, David M. Familial and developmental factors in characterological depressions. J Affect Disord. 1981;3:183–92.
184. Akiskal HS, Choen SE, Davis GC, Punzantian VR, Kashgarian M, Bolinger JM. Borderline: an adjective in search of a noun. J Clin Psychiatry. 1985;46:41–8.
185. Perugi G, Akiskal HS, Ramacciotti S, Nassini S, Toni C, Milanfranchi A, Musetti L. Depressive comorbidity of panic, social phobic, and obsessive-compulsive disorders re-examined: is there a bipolar II connection? J Psychiatr Res. 1999;33:53–61.

186. Akiskal HS, Maser JD, Zeller PJ, Endicott J, Coryell W, Keller M, Warshaw M, Clayton P, Goodwin F. Switching from unipolar to bipolar II. An 11-year prospective study of clinical and temperamental predictors in 559 patients. Arch Gen Psychiatry. 1995;52:114–23.

187. Henry C, Bellivier F, Sorbara F, Tangwongchai S, Lacoste J, Faure-Chaigneau M, Leboyer M. Bipolar sensation seeking is associated with a propensity to abuse rather than to temperamental characteristics. Eur Psychiatry. 2001;16(5):289–92.

188. Signoretta S, Maremmani I, Liguori A, Perugi G, Akiskal HS. Affective temperament traits measured by temps-I and emotional-behavioral problems in clinically-well children, adolescents, and young adults. J Affect Disord. 2005;85(1–2):169–80.

189. Akiskal HS. Subaffective disorders: dysthymic, cyclothymic and bipolar II disorders in the 'borderline' realm. Psychiatr Clin North Am. 1981;4:25–46.

190. Alneas R, Torgensen S. Personality and personality disorders among patients with major depression in combination with dysthymic or cyclothymic disorders. Acta Psychiatr Scand. 1989;79:363–9.

191. Perugi G, Akiskal HS, Lattanzi L, Cecconi D, Mastrocinque C, Patronelli A, Vignoli S, Bemi E. The high prevalence of 'soft' bipolar (II) features in atypical depression. Compr Psychiatry. 1998;39(2):63–71.

192. Rozin P, Stoess C. Is there a general tendency to become addicted? Addict Behav. 1993;18:81–7.

193. Brady KT, Lydiard RB. Bipolar affective disorder and substance abuse. J Clin Pharmacol. 1992;12(1):17S–22S.

194. Brady KT, Sonne SC. The relationship between substance abuse and bipolar disorder. J Clin Psichiatry. 1995;56(3):19–24.

195. Himmelhoch JM, Mulla D, Neil JF, Detre TP, Kupfer DJ. Incidence and significance of mixed affective states in a bipolar population. Arch Gen Psychiatry. 1976;33:1062–7.

196. Sherwood Brown E, Suppes T, Adinoff B, Ryan Thomas N. Drug abuse and bipolar disorder: comorbidity or misdiagnosis? J Affect Disord. 2001;65(2):105–15.

197. Strakowski SM, Del Bello MP, Fleck DE, Arndt S. The impact of substance abuse on the course of bipolar disorder. Biol Psychiatry. 2000;48(6):477–85.

198. Winokur G, Coryell W, Akiskal HS, Maser J, Keller MB, Endicott J, Mueller T. Alcoholism in manic-depressive (bipolar) illness: familial illness, course of illness and the primary-secondary distinction. Am J Psychiatry. 1995;152:365–72.

199. Estroff TW, Dackis CA, Gold MS, Pottash ALC. Drug abuse and bipolar disorders. Int J Psychiatry Med. 1985;15:37–40.

200. Miller FT, Busch F, Tanenbaum JH. Drug abuse in schizophrenia and bipolar disorders. Am J Drug Alcohol Abuse. 1989;15(3):291–5.

201. Ackerknecht EH. A short history of psychiatry. New York: Hafner; 1959.

202. Zilboorg G. A history of medical psychology. New York: W. W. Norton; 1941.

203. Whitwell JR. Historical notes on psychiatry (early times-end of 16th century). London: HK Lewis; 1936.

204. Kraepelin E. Manic-depressive insanity and paranoia. Translated by Rm Barclay. New York: Arno Press; 1976.

205. Rottanburg D, Robins AH, Oved B, Ben-Arie O, Teggin A, Elk R. Cannabis-associated psychosis with hypomanic features. Lancet. 1982;18(2):1364–6.

206. Lacoursiere RB, Swatek R. Adverse interaction between disulfiram and marijuana: a case report. Am J Psychiatry. 1983;140(2):243–4.

207. Stoll AL, Cole JO, Lukas SE. A case of mania as result of fluoxetine-marijuana interaction. J Clin Psychiatry. 1991;52(6):280–1.

208. Cocores JA, Petel MD, Gold MS, Pottash AC. Cocaine abuse, attention deficit disorder, and bipolar patients. J Nerv Ment Dis. 1987;175(7):431–2.

209. Wilens TE, Biederman J, Mick E, Faraone SV, Spencer T. Adhd is associated with early onset substance use disorders. J Nerv Ment Dis. 1997;185(8):475–82.

210. Lemere F. Lithium treatment of cocaine addiction. Am J Psychiatry. 1991;148(2):276–7.

211. Goldberg JF, Garno JL, Portera L, Leon AC, Kocsis JH, Whiteside JE. Correlates of suicidal ideation in dysphoric mania. J Affect Disord. 1999;56(1):75–81.
212. Weiss RD, Mirin SM, Michael JL, Sollogub AC. Psychopathology in chronic cocaine abusers. Am J Drug Alcohol Abuse. 1986;12(1–2):17–29.
213. Kalivas PW, Volkow ND. The neural basis of addiction: a pathology of motivation and choice. Am J Psychiatry. 2005;162:1403–13.
214. Grove WM, Eckert ED, Heston L, Bouchard TJJ, Segal N, Lykken DT. Heritability of substance abuse and antisocial behavior: a study of monozygotic twins reared apart. Biol Psychiatry. 1990;27(12):1293–304.
215. Kendler KS, Gardner COJ. Twin studies of adult psychiatric and substance dependence disorders: are they biased by differences in the environmental experiences of monozygotic and dizygotic twins in childhood and adolescence? Psychol Med. 1998;28(3):625–33.
216. Pickens RW, Svikis DS, McGue M, et al. Heterogeneity in the inheritance of alcoholism: a study of male and female twins. Arch Gen Psychiatry. 1991;48:19–28.
217. Woody GE, Blaine JD. Depression in narcotic addicts: quite possibly more than a chance association. In: Dupont RL, Goldstein A, O'Donnell J, editors. Handbook on drug abuse, National Institute on Drug Abuse Pub. No. 277–286. Washington, DC: U.S. Government Printing Office; 1979.
218. Mirin SM, Meyer RE, McNamee B. Psychopathology and mood during heroin use: acute vs. chronic effects. Arch Gen Psychiatry. 1976;33:1503–8.
219. Rounsaville BJ, Kosten TR, Weissman MM, Kleber HD. Evaluating and treating depressive disorders in opiate addicts. Rockville, MD: National Institute on Drug Abuse; 1985.
220. Martin WR, Hewett BB, Baken AJ, Heartzen CA. Aspects of the psychopathology and pathophysiology of addiction. Drug Alcohol Depend. 1977;2:185–202.
221. Linnoila MI. Anxiety and alcoholism. J Clin Psychiatry. 1989;50:26–9.
222. Mirin SM, Weiss RD. Substance abuse and mental illness. In: Frances RJ, Miller SI, editors. Clinical textbook of addictive disorders. New York: Guilford Press; 1991. p. 271–98.
223. Mirin SN, Weiss RD, Griffin ML, Michael JL. Psychopathology in drug abusers and their families. Compr Psychiatry. 1991;32:36–51.
224. Nunes EV, McGrath PJ, Quitkin FM, Stewart JP, Harrison W, Tricamo E, Ocepek-Welikson K. Imipramine treatment of alcoholism with comorbid depression. Am J Psychiatry. 1993;150:963–5.
225. Nunes EV, Quitkin FM, Brady R, Stewart JW. Imipramine treatment of methadone maintenance patients with affective disorders and illicit drug use. Am J Psychiatry. 1991;148:667–9.
226. Lovrecic M, Lovrecic B, Rovai L, Rugani F, Maremmani AGI, Maremmani I. Further evidence of no relationship between anxiety-depressive mental status and dual diagnosis in heroin addicts entering treatment. Heroin Addict Relat Clin Probl. 2011;13(4):27–34.
227. Deglon JJ. Le Traitement À long Terme des Héroînomanes par La Mèthadone. Genève: Editions Mèdicine et Hygiène; 1982.
228. Kleber HD, Weissman MM, Rounsaville BJ, Prusoff BA, Wilbur CH. Imipramine as treatment for depression in opiate addicts. Arch Gen Psychiatry. 1983;40:649–53.
229. Varga E, Sugerman AA, Apter J. The effect of codeine on involutional and senile depression. Ann N Y Acad Sci. 1982;398:103–5.
230. Inturrisi CE, Alexopoulos GS, Lipman RS, Foley K, Rossier J. Beta-endorphin Immunoreactivity in the plasma of psychiatric patients receiving electroconvulsive treatment. In: Verebey K, editor. Opioids in mental illness: theories, clinical observations and treatment possibilities, Annals of the New York Academy of Sciences, vol. 398. New York: New York Academy of Sciences; 1982.
231. Dilsaver S. The pathophysiologies of substance abuse and affective disorders: an integrative model? J Clin Pharmacol. 1987;7:1–10.
232. Madden JD, Chappel JM, Zuspan F, Gumpel J, Mejia A, Davis R. Observation and treatment of neonatal narcotic withdrawal. Am J Obstet Gynecol. 1977;127:190–9.

233. Maremmani AGI, Rovai L, Rugani F, Bacciardi S, Massimetti E, Gazzarrini D, Dell'Osso L, Fengyi T, Akiskal HS, Maremmani I. Chronology of illness in dual diagnosis heroin addicts. The role of mood disorders. J Affect Disord. 2015;179:156–60.

234. Kessler RC. The epidemiology of dual diagnosis. Biol Psychiatry. 2004;56(10):730–7.

235. Merikangas K, Stevens DE. Substance abuse among women: familial factors and comorbidity. In: Wetherington CL, Roman AB, editors. Drug addiction research and the health of women. NIDA: Bethesda, MD; 1998. p. 245–69.

236. Sareen J, Chartier M, Kjernisted KD, Stein MB. Comorbidity of phobic disorders with alcoholism in a Canadian community sample. Can J Psychiatr. 2001;46(8):733–40.

237. Swendsen JD, Merikangas KR. The comorbidity of depression and substance use disorders. Clin Psychol Rev. 2000;20(2):173–89.

238. Hagnell O, Grasbeck A. Comorbidity of anxiety and depression in the Lundby 25-year prospective study: the pattern of subsequent episodes. In: Maser JD, Cloninger CR, editors. Comorbidity of mood and anxiety disorders. Washington, DC: American Psychiatric Press; 1990. p. 139–52.

239. Murphy JM. Diagnostic comorbidity and symptom co-occurrence: the Stirling County study. In: Maser JD, Cloninger CR, editors. Comorbidity of mood and anxiety disorders. Washington, DC: American Psychiatric Press; 1990. p. 139–52.

240. Weiss RD, Mirin SM. Substance abuse as an attempt at self-medication. Psychiatr Med. 1985;3(4):357–67.

241. Clouet DH. A biochemical and neurophysiological comparison of opioids and antipsychotics. Ann N Y Acad Sci. 1982;398:130–9.

242. Kosten TR, Rounsaville BJ, Kleber HD. Relationship of depression to psychosocial stressors in heroin addicts. J Nerv Ment Dis. 1983;171:97–104.

243. Prusoff BA, Thompson DW, Sholomskas D, Riordan CE. Psychosocial stressors and depression among former heroin dependent patients maintained on methadone. J Nerv Ment Dis. 1977;165:57–63.

244. De Leon D. The therapeutic community: study of effectiveness. Treatment research monograph series. Washington, DC: National Istitute on Drug Abuse; 1984.

245. De Leon D, Jainchill N. Male and female drug abusers: social and psychological status 2 years after treatment in a therapeutic community. Am J Drug Alcohol Abuse. 1981;8(4):380–2.

246. Higgins ST, Silverman K. Motivating behavior change among illicit-drug abusers. Washington, DC: American Psychological Association; 1998.

247. Maremmani AGI, Bacciardi S, Rovai L, Rugani F, Akiskal HS, Maremmani I. Do bipolar patients use street opioids to stabilize mood? Heroin Addict Relat Clin Probl. 2013;15(4):25–32.

248. Maremmani AGI, Rugani F, Bacciardi S, Rovai L, Pacini M, Dell'Osso L, Maremmani I. Does dual diagnosis affect violence and moderate/superficial self-harm in heroin addiction at treatment entry? J Addict Med. 2014;8(2):116–22.

249. Maremmani AGI, Rugani F, Bacciardi S, Rovai L, Massimetti E, Gazzarrini D, Dell'Osso L, Maremmani I. Differentiating between the course of illness in bipolar 1 and chronic-psychotic heroin-dependent patients at their first agonist opioid treatment. J Addict Dis. 2015;34(1):43–54.

250. Bandettini Di Poggio A, Fornai F, Paparelli A, Pacini M, Perugi G, Maremmani I. Comparison between heroin and heroin-cocaine Polyabusers: a psychopathological study. Ann N Y Acad Sci. 2006;1074:438–45.

251. Mitchell JD, Brown ES, Rush AJ. Comorbid disorders in patients with bipolar disorder and concomitant substance dependence. J Affect Disord. 2007;102(1–3):281–7.

252. Leweke FM, Koethe D. Cannabis and psychiatric disorders:it is not only addiction. Addict Biol. 2008;13:264–75.

253. Keup W. Psychotic symptoms due to cannabis abuse. Dis Nerv Syst. 1970;31:119–26.

254. Chopra GS, Smith JW. Psychotic reactions following cannabis use in east Indians. Arch Gen Psychiatry. 1974;30:24–7.

255. Mathers DC, Ghodse AH. Cannabis and psychotic illness. Br J Psychiatry. 1992;161:648–53.

256. Gruber AJ, Pope HG. Cannabis psychotic disorder: does it exist? Am J Addict. 1994;3(1):72–83.
257. Sembhi S, Lee JW. Cannabis use in psychotic patients. Aust N Z J Psychiatry. 1999;33(4):529–32.
258. Hall W, Degenhardt L, Teesson M. Cannabis use and psychotic disorders: an update. Drug Alcohol Rev. 2004;23:433–43.
259. Guaiana G. Past or current drug or alcohol use disorders increase the likelihood of a switch from depressive to manic, mixed or hypomanic states in patients with bipolar disorder. Evid Based Ment Health. 2010;13(3):78.
260. Swendsen JD, Tennen H, Carney MA, Affleck G, Willard A, Hromi A. Mood and alcohol consumption: an experience sampling test of the self-medication hypothesis. J Abnorm Psychol. 2000;109(2):198–204.
261. Bolton JM, Robinson J, Sareen J. Self-medication of mood disorders with alcohol and drugs in the National Epidemiologic Survey on alcohol and related conditions. J Affect Disord. 2009;115(3):367–75.
262. Weiss RD, Greenfield SF, Najavits LM, Soto JA, Wyner D, Tohen M, Griffin M. Medication compliance among patients with bipolar disorder and substance use disorder. J Clin Psychiatry. 1998;59(4):172–4.
263. Khalkho IP, Khess CR. Drug non-compliance in mania: the Indian experience. Indian J Psychiatry. 1999;41(2):108–10.
264. Hong J, Reed C, Novick D, Haro JM, Aguado J. Clinical and economic consequences of medication non-adherence in the treatment of patients with a manic/mixed episode of bipolar disorder: results from the European mania in bipolar longitudinal evaluation of medication (EMBLEM) study. Psychiatry Res. 2011;190(1):110–4.
265. Husted JR. Insight in severe mental illness: implications for treatment decisions. J Am Acad Psychiatry Law. 1999;27(1):33–49.
266. Francis JL, Penn DL. The relationship between insight and social skill in persons with severe mental illness. J Nerv Ment Dis. 2001;189(12):822–9.
267. Vender S, Poloni N. Is the insight a Favourable prognostic factor in the treatment of mental disorders? Recenti Prog Med. 2006;97(10):565–70.
268. Murphy JM, Waller MB, Gatto G. Effects of fluoxetina on the intragastric self-administration of ethanol in the alcohol preferring P line of rats. Alcohol. 1988;5:283–6.
269. Rich CL, Fowler RC, Young D. Substance abuse and suicide: the San Diego study. Ann Clin Psychiatry. 1989;1:70–9.
270. Hasin D, Grant B, Endicott J. Treated and untreated suicide attempts in substance abuse patients. J Nerv Ment Dis. 1988;176:289–93.
271. Barraclough B, Bunch J, Nelson B. A hundred cases of suicide: clinical aspects. Br J Psychiatry. 1974;25:350–5.
272. Dorpat T, Woodhall K. A study of suicide in the Seattle area. Compr Psychiatry. 1960;1:340–9.
273. Rich CL, Young D, Fowler RC. The San Diego suicide study: young vs old subjects. Arch Gen Psychiatry. 1986;43:570–7.
274. Rich CL, Fowler RC, Fogarthy LA. The San Diego suicide study: III relationship between diagnosis and stressors. Arch Gen Psychiatry. 1988;45:580–9.
275. Volkow ND, Fowler JS, Wolf AP, Hitzemann R, Dewey S, Bendriem B, Alpert R, Hoff A. Changes in brain glucose metabolism in cocaine dependence and withdrawal. Am J Psychiatry. 1991;148:621–6.
276. Galanter M, Castaneda R. Self-destructive behaviour in the substance abuser. Psychiatr Clin North Am. 1985;8:250–1.
277. Humeniuk R, Ali R, White J, Hall W, Farrel M. Proceedings of the expert workshop on induction and stabilisation of patients onto methadone. Adelaide: NIDA; 2000.
278. Miles CP. Conditions predisposing to suicide: a review. J Nerv Ment Dis. 1977;164:230–1.
279. Stimmel B, Goldberg J, Murphy R. Fetal outcome in narcotic dependent women: the importance of the type of maternal narcotic used. Am J Drug Alcohol Abuse. 1983;9:373–95.

280. Ward NG, Schuckit M. Factors associated with suicidal behavior in polydrug abusers. J Clin Psychiatry. 1980;41:370–9.

281. Vaillant GE. A twelve-year follow-up of New York narcotic addicts, IV: some characteristics and determinants of abstinence. Am J Psychiatry. 1966;123:575–85.

282. Bewley TH, Ben-Arie O, James JP. Morbidity and mortality from heroin dependence. Br Med J. 1968;1:720–5.

283. Marzuk PM, Mann JJ. Suicide and substance abuse. Psychiatr Ann. 1988;18:630–9.

284. Renaud J, Brent DA, Birmaher B, Chiappetta L, Bridge J. Suicide in adolescents with disruptive disorders. J Am Acad Child Adolesc Psychiatry. 1999;38(7):846–51.

285. Flower RC, Rich CL, Young D. San Diego suicide study: II substance abuse in young cases. Arch Gen Psychiatry. 1986;43:960–2.

286. Mino A, Bousquet A, Broers B. Substance abuse and drug related death, suicidal ideation and suicide: a review. Crisis. 1999;20(1):28–35.

287. Cornelius JR, Thase ME, Salloum IM, Cornelius MD, Black A, Mann JJ. Cocaine use associated with increased suicidal behaviour in depressed alcoholics. Addict Behav. 1998;23(1):119–21.

288. Tondo L, Baldessarini RJ, Hennen J, Minnai GP, Salis P, Scamonatti L, Masia M, Ghiani C, Mannu P. Suicide attempts in major affective disorder patients with comorbid substance use disorders. J Clin Psychiatry. 1999;60(Suppl 2):63–9.

289. Pirkola SP, Isometsa ET, Heikkinen ME, Henriksson MM, Marttunen MJ, Lonnqvist JK. Female psychoactive substance dependent suicide victims differ from male-results FRM a nationwide psychological autopsy study. Compr Psychiatry. 1999;40(2):101–7.

290. Grant BF, Hasin DS. Suicidal ideation among the United States drinking population: results from National Longitudinal Alcohol Epidemiologic Survey. J Stud Alcohol. 1999;60(3):422–9.

291. Miotto K, McCann MJ, Rawson RA, Frosch D, Ling W. Overdose, suicide attemps and death among a cohort of naltrexone treated opioid addicts. Drug Alcohol Depend. 1997;45(1–2):131–4.

292. Nordström P, Asberg M, Aberg-Wistedt A, Nordin C. Attempted suicide predicts suicide risk in mood disorders. Acta Psychiatr Scand. 1995;92:345–50.

293. Appleby L, Cooper J, Amos T, Faragher B. Psychological autopsy study of suicides by people aged under 35. Br J Psychiatry. 1999;175:168–74.

294. Suokas J, Suominen K, Isometsä E, Ostamo A, Lönnqvist J. Long-term risk factors for suicide mortality after attempted suicide—findings of a 14-year follow-up study. Acta Psychiatr Scand. 2001;104:117–21.

295. Rihmer Z, Kiss K. Bipolar disorders and suicidal behaviour. Bipolar Disord. 2002;4(Suppl 1):21–5.

296. Rihmer Z, Bels N, Kiss K. Strategies for suicide preventon. Curr Opin Psychiatry. 2002;15:83–7.

297. Beautrais AL, Joyce PR, Mulder RT, Fergusson DM, Deavoli BJ, Nightingale SK. Prevalence and comorbidity of mental disorders in persons making serious suicide attempts: a case-control study. Am J Psychiatry. 1996;153(8):1009–14.

298. Beautrais AL, Joyce PR, Mulder RT. Risk factors for serious attempts among youths aged 13 through 24 years. J Am Acad Child Adolesc Psychiatry. 1996;35(9):1174–82.

299. Kessler RC, Borges C, Walters EE. Prevalence and risk factors for lifetime suicide attempts in the National Comorbidity Survey. Arch Gen Psychiatry. 1999;56:617–26.

300. Weissman MM, Bland RC, Canino GJ, Greenwald S, Hwu HG, Joyce PR, Karam EG, Lee CK, Lellouch J, Lepine JP, Newman SC, Rubio-Stipec M, Wells PJ, Wickramarante PJ, Wittcjhen HU, Yeh EK. Prevalence of suicide ideation and suicide attempts in nine countries. Psychol Med. 1999;29:9–17.

301. Beck AT, Brown GP, Berchick RJ, Stewart BL, Steer RA. Relationship between hopelessness and ultimate suicide: a replication with psychiatric outpatients. Am J Psychiatry. 1990;147:190–5.

302. Fawcett J, Schefiner WA, Fogg L, Clark DC, Young MA, Hedeker D, Gibbons R. Time-related prediction of suicide in major affective disorder. Am J Psychiatry. 1990;147:1189–94.
303. Maremmani I, Pani PP, Canoniero S, Pacini M, Perugi G, Rihmer Z, Akiskal HS. Is the bipolar spectrum the psychopathological substrate of suicidality in heroin addicts? Psychopathology. 2007;40(5):269–77.
304. Lynch TR, Johnson CS, Mendelson T, Robins CJ, Krishan KRR, Blazer DG. New onset and remission of suicidal ideation among a depressed adult sample. J Affect Disord. 1999;56:49–54.
305. Goldney RD, Dal Grande E, Fisher LJ, Wilson D. Population Attributale risk of major depression for suicidal ideation in a random and representative community sample. J Affect Disord. 2003;74:267–72.
306. Dalton EJ, Cate-Carter TD, Mundo E, Parikh SV, Kennedy JL. Suicide risk in bipolar patients: the role of co-morbid substance use disorders. Bipolar Disord. 2003;5:58–61.
307. Levy JC, Deykin EY. Suicidality, depression and substance abuse in adolescence. Am J Psychiatry. 1989;146(11):1462–7.
308. Martin WR. Opioid antagonists. Pharmacol Rev. 1967;19:463–521.
309. Martin WR, Jasinski DR, Mansky PA. Naltrexone, an antagonist for the treatment of heroin dependence. Arch Gen Psychiatry. 1973;28:784–91.
310. Pacini M, Maremmani I. Il Problema Della Personalità Tossicofilica Nella Patogenesi Del Disturbo Da Uso Di Sostanze Psicoattive. Revisione Della Letteratura E Recenti Acquisizioni. Italian J Psychopathol. 2001;7(2):185–99.
311. Maremmani AGI, Pani PP, Rovai L, Bacciardi S, Maremmani I. Towards the identification of a specific psychopathology of substance use disorders. Front Psych. 2017;8:68.
312. Carbone MG, Maiello M, Spera V, Manni C, Pallucchini A, Maremmani AGI, Maremmani I. The SCL90-based psychopathological structure may be applied in substance use disorder patients independently of the drug involved, even in heroin, alcohol and cocaine monodrug users. Heroin Addict Relat Clin Probl. 2018;20(5):29–34.
313. Maremmani AGI, Rovai L, Maremmani I. Heroin addicts' psychopathological subtypes. Correlations with the natural history of illness. Heroin Addict Relat Clin Probl. 2012;14(1):11–22.
314. Maremmani I, Iantomasi C, Pani PP, AGI M, Mathis F, for the VOECT Group. A prospective study of psychopathology stability and changes after 3 month drug-abstinence in Italian substance use disorder patients during a residential treatment. Heroin Addict Relat Clin Probl. 2020;22(2):35–43.
315. Brook DW, Brook JS, Zhang C, Cohen P, Whiteman M. Drug use and the risk of major depressive disorder, alcohol dependence, and substance use disorders. Arch Gen Psychiatry. 2002;59:1039–44.
316. Blum K, Braverman ER, Holder JM, Lubar JF, Monastra VJ, Miller D, Lubar JO, Chen TJ, Comings DE. Reward deficiency syndrome: a biogenetic model for the diagnosis and treatment of impulsive, addictive, and compulsive behaviors. J Psychoactive Drugs. 2000;32(Suppl I–IV):1–112.
317. Schuckit MA, Tipp JE, Bergman M, Reich W, Hesselbrock VM, Smith TL. Comparison of induced and independent major depressive disorders in 2,945 alcoholics. Am J Psychiatry. 1997;154(7):948–57.
318. Gerra G, Angioni L, Zaimovic A, Moi G, Bussandri M, Bertacca S, Santoro G, Gardini S, Caccavari R, Nicoli MA. Substance use among high-school students: relationships with temperament, personality traits, and parental care perception. Subst Use Misuse. 2004;39(2):345–67.
319. Conner BT, Noble EP, Berman SM, Ozkaragoz T, Ritchie T, Antolin T, Sheen C. DRD2 genotypes and substance use in adolescent children of alcoholics. Drug Alcohol Depend. 2005;79(3):379–87.
320. Volman SF, Lammel S, Margolis EB, Kim Y, Richard JM, Roitman MF, Lobo MK. New insights into the specificity and plasticity of reward and aversion encoding in the mesolimbic system. J Neurosci. 2013;33(45):17569–76.

321. Post RM, Kalivas P. Bipolar disorder and substance misuse: pathological and therapeutic implications of their comorbidity and cross-sensitisation. Br J Psychiatry. 2013;202(3):172–6.
322. Hunt GE, Malhi GS, Lai HMX, Cleary M. Prevalence of comorbid substance use in major depressive disorder in community and clinical settings, 1990–2019: systematic review and meta-analysis. J Affect Disord. 2020;266:288–304.
323. Boden JM, Fergusson DM. Alcohol and depression. Addiction. 2011;106(5):906–14.
324. Foulds JA, Adamson SJ, Boden JM, Williman JA, Mulder RT. Depression in patients with alcohol use disorders: systematic review and meta-analysis of outcomes for independent and substance-induced disorders. J Affect Disord. 2015;185:47–59.
325. Gomez-Coronado N, Sethi R, Bortolasci CC, Arancini L, Berk M, Dodd S. A review of the neurobiological underpinning of comorbid substance use and mood disorders. J Affect Disord. 2018;241:388–401.
326. Camardese G, Di Giuda D, Di Nicola M, Cocciolillo F, Giordano A, Janiri L, Guglielmo R. Imaging studies on dopamine transporter and depression: a review of literature and suggestions for future research. J Psychiatr Res. 2014;51:7–18.
327. Hagele C, Schlagenhauf F, Rapp M, Sterzer P, Beck A, Bermpohl F, Stoy M, Strohle A, Wittchen HU, Dolan RJ, Heinz A. Dimensional psychiatry: reward dysfunction and depressive mood across psychiatric disorders. Psychopharmacology. 2015;232(2):331–41.
328. Berk M, Post R, Ratheesh A, Gliddon E, Singh A, Vieta E, Carvalho AF, Ashton MM, Berk L, Cotton SM, McGorry PD, Fernandes BS, Yatham LN, Dodd S. Staging in bipolar disorder: from theoretical framework to clinical utility. World Psychiatry. 2017;16(3):236–44.
329. Belujon P, Grace AA. Dopamine system Dysregulation in major depressive disorders. Int J Neuropsychopharmacol. 2017;20(12):1036–46.
330. Butelman ER, Yuferov V, Kreek MJ. Kappa-opioid receptor/dynorphin system: genetic and pharmacotherapeutic implications for addiction. Trends Neurosci. 2012;35(10):587–96.
331. Carlezon WAJ, Konradi C. Understanding the neurobiological consequences of early exposure to psychotropic drugs: linking behavior with molecules. Neuropharmacology. 2004;47(Suppl 1):47–60.
332. George O, Le Moal M, Koob GF. Allostasis and addiction: role of the dopamine and Corticotropin-releasing factor systems. Physiol Behav. 2012;106(1):58–64.
333. George O, Koob GF, Vendruscolo LF. Negative reinforcement via motivational withdrawal is the driving force behind the transition to addiction. Psychopharmacology. 2014;231(19):3911–7.
334. Koob GF, Volkow ND. Neurocircuitry of addiction. Neuropsychopharmacology. 2010;35(1):217–38.
335. Koob GF, Volkow ND. Neurobiology of addiction: a neurocircuitry analysis. Lancet Psychiatry. 2016;3(8):760–73.
336. McEwen BS, Gianaros PJ. Stress- and allostasis-induced brain plasticity. Annu Rev Med. 2011;62:431–45.
337. Nemeroff CB. New vistas in neuropeptide research in neuropsychiatry: focus on corticotropin-releasing factor. Neuropsychopharmacology. 1992;6:69–75.
338. Stam R, Bruijnzeel AW, Wiegant VM. Long-lasting stress sensitisation. Eur J Pharmacol. 2000;405:217–24.
339. Sarnyai Z, Shaham Y, Heinrichs SC. The role of corticotropinreleasing factor in drug addiction. Pharmacol Rev. 2001;53:209–43.
340. Weiss F, Ciccocioppo R, Parsons LH, Katner S, Liu X, Zorrilla EP, Valdez GR, Ben Shahar O, Angeletti S, Richter RR. Compulsive drug-seeking behavior and relapse. Neuroadaptation, stress, and conditioning factors. Ann N Y Acad Sci. 2001;937:1–26.
341. Brady KT, Sinha R. Co-occurring mental and substance use disorders: the neurobiological effects of chronic stress. Am J Psychiatry. 2005;162(8):1483–93.
342. Maremmani AGI, Pani PP, Rovai L, Bacciardi S, Rugani F, Dell'Osso L, Pacini M, Maremmani I. The effects of agonist opioids on the psychopathology of opioid dependence. Heroin Addict Relat Clin Probl. 2013;15(2):47–56.

343. Della Rocca F, Maremmani AGI, Rovai L, Bacciardi S, Lamanna F, Maremmani I. Further evidence of a specific psychopathology of heroin use disorder. Relationships between psychopathological dimensions and addictive behaviors. Heroin Addict Relat Clin Probl. 2017;19(6):13–20.

344. Maremmani I, Maremmani AGI, Rugani F, Rovai L, Pacini M, Bacciardi S, Deltito J, Dell'Osso L, Akiskal HS. Clinical presentations of substance abuse in bipolar heroin addicts at time of treatment entry. Ann General Psychiatry. 2012;11(1):23.

345. Della Rocca F, Novi M, Maremmani AGI, Pani PP, Miccoli M, Maremmani I. Exploring the depressive syndrome of heroin use disorder patients. Relationships between worthlessness/being trapped, deficit reward and post-withdrawal syndromes. Heroin Addict Relat Clin Probl. 2021;23(3):61–74.

346. Baharudin A, Mislan N, Ibrahim N, Sidi H, Nik Jaafar NR. Depression in male patients on methadone maintenance therapy. Asia Pac Psychiatry. 2013;5(Suppl 1):67–73.

347. Seidman SN, Roose SP. The relationship between depression and erectile dysfunction. Curr Psychiatry Rep. 2000;2(3):201–5.

348. Quaglio G, Lugoboni F, Pattaro C, Melara B, Mezzelani P, Des Jarlais DC. Erectile dysfunction in Male heroin users, receiving methadone and buprenorphine maintenance treatment. Drug Alcohol Depend. 2008;94(1–3):12–8.

349. Spring WDJ, Willenbring ML, Maddux TL. Sexual dysfunction and psychological distress in methadone maintenance. Int J Addict. 1992;27(11):1325–34.

350. Blum K, Sheridan PJ, Wood RC, Braverman ER, Chen TJ, Cull JG, Comings DE. The D2 dopamine receptor gene as a determinant of reward deficiency syndrome. J R Soc Med. 1996;89(7):396–400.

351. Gold MS, Blum K, Febo M, Baron D, Modestino EJ, Elman I, Badgaiyan RD. Molecular role of dopamine in anhedonia linked to reward deficiency syndrome (RDS) and anti- reward systems. Front Biosci (Schol Ed). 2018;10(2):309–25.

352. Comings DE, Blum K. Reward deficiency syndrome: genetic aspects of behavioral disorders. Prog Brain Res. 2000;126:325–41.

353. Surguladze S, Keedwell P, Phillips M. Neural system underlying affective disorders. Adv Psychiat Treat. 2003;9:446–55.

354. Blum K, Werner T, Carnes S, Carnes P, Bowirrat A, Giordano J, Oscar-Berman M, Gold M. Sex, drugs, and rock 'N' roll: hypothesizing common mesolimbic activation as a function of reward gene polymorphisms. J Psychoactive Drugs. 2012;44(1):38–55.

355. Martin WR. Pathophysiology of narcotic addiction: possible role of protracted abstinence in relapse. In: Zarafonetis CJD, editor. Drug abuse. Philadelphia: Lea and Febiger; 1972. p. 153–9.

356. Martin J, Ingles J. Pain tolerance and narcotic addiction. Br J Soc Psychol. 1965;4:224–9.

357. Rovai L, Maremmani AGI, Pacini M, Pani PP, Rugani F, Lamanna F, Schiavi E, Mautone S, Dell'Osso L, Maremmani I. Negative dimensions in psychiatry. amotivation syndrome as a paradigme of negative symptoms in substance abuse. Riv Psichiatr. 2013;48(1):1–9.

358. Kreek MJ, Koob GF. Drug dependence: stress and dysregulation of brain reward pathways. Drug Alcohol Depend. 1998;51(1–2):23–47.

359. Maremmani I, Castrogiovanni P, Daini L, Zolesi O. Use of fluoxetine in heroin addiction. Br J Psychiatry. 1992;160:570–1.

360. Bacciardi S, Maremmani AGI, Rovai L, Rugani F, Pani PP, Pacini M, Dell'Osso L, Akiskal HS, Maremmani I. Drug (heroin) addiction, bipolar spectrum and impulse control disorders. Heroin Addict Relat Clin Probl. 2013;15(2):29–36.

361. Akiskal HS, Judd LL, Gillin JC, Lemmi H. Subthreshold depressions: clinical and Polysomnographic validation of dysthymic, residual and masked forms. J Affect Disord. 1997;45(1–2):53–63.

362. Koob GF. Drugs of abuse: anatomy, pharmacology and function of reward patways. Trends Pharmacol Sci. 1992;13:177–84.

363. Lesch KP, Laux G, Schulte HM, Pfulle RH, Beckmann H. Corticotropin and cortisol response to human CRH as a probe for HPA system integrity in major depressive disorder. Psychiatry Res. 1988;24(1):25–34.

364. Nunes EV, Sullivan MA, Levin FR. Treatment of depression in patients with opiate dependence. Biol Psychiatry. 2004;56(10):793–802.

365. Maremmani I, Spera V, Maremmani AGI, Carli M, Scarselli M. Is trazodone contramid® useful in inducing patients to refrain from using cocaine after detoxification, so avoiding early relapse? A case Series. Addict Disord Their Treat. 2019;18(2):105–12.

366. Zijlstra F, Booij J, van den Brink W, Franken IH. Striatal dopamine D2 receptor binding and dopamine release during cue-elicited craving in recently abstinent opiate-dependent males. Eur Neuropsychopharmacol. 2008;18(4):262–70.

367. Land BB, Bruchas MR, Lemos JC, Xu M, Melief EJ, Chavkin C. The dysphoric component of stress is encoded by activation of the dynorphin kappa-opioid system. J Neurosci. 2008;28(2):407–14.

368. Shirayama Y, Ishida H, Iwata M, Hazama GI, Kawahara R, Duman RS. Stress increases dynorphin immunoreactivity in limbic brain regions and dynorphin antagonism produces antidepressant-like effects. J Neurochem. 2004;90(5):1258–68.

369. Pani PP, Maremmani M, Icro AG, Pacini M, Trogu E, Gessa GL, Ruiz P, Maremmani I. Delineating the psychic structure of substance abuse and addictions: from neurobiology to clinical implications: ten years later. J Clin Med. 2020;9:1913.

370. Maremmani I, Zolesi O, Daini L, Castrogiovanni P, Tagliamonte A. Fluoxetine improves outcome in addicted patients treated with opioid antagonists. Am J Addict. 1995;4(3):267–71.

371. Zaaijer ER, van Dijk L, de Bruin K, Goudriaan AE, Lammers LA, Koeter MW, van den Brink W, Booij J. Effect of extended-release naltrexone on striatal dopamine transporter availability, depression and anhedonia in heroin-dependent patients. Psychopharmacology. 2015;232(14):2597–607.

372. Galynker II, Eisenberg D, Matochik JA, Gertmenian-King E, Cohen L, Kimes AS, Contoreggi C, Kurian V, Ernst M, Rosenthal RN, Prosser J, London ED. Cerebral metabolism and mood in remitted opiate dependence. Drug Alcohol Depend. 2007;90(2–3):166–74.

373. Emrich HM. Endorphins in psychiatry. Psychiatr Dev. 1984;2(2):97–114.

374. Kline NS, Li CH, Lehmann E, Lajtha A, Laski E, Cooper T. Beta-endorphin-induced changes in schizophrenic and depressed patients. Arch Gen Psychiatry. 1977;34:111–3.

375. Diana M, Young SJ, Groves PM. Modulation of dopaminergic terminal excitability by D1 selective agents: further characterization. Neuroscience. 1991;42:441–9.

376. Iribarne C, Picart D, Dreano Y, Berthou F. In vitro interactions between fluoxetine or fluvoxamine and methadone or buprenorphine. Fundam Clin Pharmacol. 1998;12(2):194–9.

377. Bertschy G, Baumann P, Eap CB, Baetting D. Probable metabolic interaction between methadone and fluvoxamine in addict patients. Ther Drug Monit. 1994;16(1):42–5.

378. Kreek MJ, Levran O, Reed B, Schlussman SD, Zhou Y, Butelman ER. Opiate addiction and cocaine addiction: underlying molecular neurobiology and genetics. J Clin Invest. 2012;122(10):3387–93.

379. Kreek MJ, Nielsen DA, Butelman ER, La Forge KS. Genetic influences on impulsivity, risk taking, stress responsivity and vulnerability to drug abuse and addiction. Nat Neurosci. 2005;8(11):1450–7.

380. Lopez-Quintero C, Anthony JC. Drug use disorders in the polydrug context: new epidemiological evidence from a foodborne outbreak approach. Ann N Y Acad Sci. 2015;1349:119–26.

381. Brecht ML, Huang D, Evans E, Hser YI. Polydrug use and implications for longitudinal research: ten-year trajectories for heroin, cocaine, and methamphetamine users. Drug Alcohol Depend. 2008;96(3):193–201.

382. Godley SH, Dennis ML, Godley MD, Funk RR. Thirty-month relapse trajectory cluster groups among adolescents discharged from out-patient treatment. Addiction. 2004;99(Suppl 2):129–39.

383. Nosyk B, Li L, Evans E, Huang D, Min J, Kerr T, Brecht ML, Hser YI. Characterizing longitudinal health state transitions among heroin, cocaine, and methamphetamine users. Drug Alcohol Depend. 2014;140:69–77.
384. Murphy DA, Hser YI, Huang D, Brecht ML, Herbeck DM. Self-report of longitudinal substance use: a comparison of the UCLA natural history interview and the addiction severity index. J Drug Issues. 2010;40(2):495–516.
385. Peters J, Pattij T, De Vries TJ. Targeting cocaine versus heroin memories: divergent roles within ventromedial prefrontal cortex. Trends Pharmacol Sci. 2013;34(12):689–95.
386. Badiani A, Belin D, Epstein D, Calu D, Shaham Y. Opiate versus psychostimulant addiction: the differences do matter. Nat Rev Neurosci. 2011;12(11):685–700.
387. Levran O, Peles E, Randesi M, Correa da Rosa J, Ott J, Rotrosen J, Adelson M, Kreek MJ. Synaptic plasticity and signal transduction gene polymorphisms and vulnerability to drug addictions in populations of European or African ancestry. CNS Neurosci Ther. 2015;21(11):898–904.
388. Levran O, Randesi M, Li Y, Rotrosen J, Ott J, Adelson M, Kreek MJ. Drug addiction and stress-response genetic variability: association study in African Americans. Ann Hum Genet. 2014;78(4):290–8.
389. Ceccanti M, Vitali M. Alcoholics with a history of heroin consumption: clinical features and chronology of substance abuse. Heroin Addict Relat Clin Probl. 2009;11(3):35–8.
390. Maremmani I, Pacini M, Pani PP, on behalf of the 'Basics on Addiction Group'. Basics on addiction: a training package for medical practitioners or psychiatrists who treat opioid dependence. Heroin Addict Relat Clin Probl. 2011;13(2):5–40.
391. Maremmani I, Pacini M, Perugi G. Addictive disorders, bipolar spectrum and the impulsive link: the psychopathology of a self-regenerating pathway. Heroin Addict Relat Clin Probl. 2005;7(3):33–46.
392. Pacini M, Mellini A, Attilia ML, Ceccanti M, Maremmani I. Alcohol abuse in heroin addicts: an unfolding metabolic destiny. Heroin Addict Relat Clin Probl. 2005;7(1):31–8.
393. Bendimerad P, Blecha L. Benefits in reducing alcohol consumption: how nalmefene can help. Encéphale. 2014;40(6):495–500.
394. Kleber GE. Treatment of drug dependence: what works. Int Rev Psychiatry. 1989;1:81–100.
395. Kleber HD. Concomitant use of methadone with other psychoactive drugs in the treatment of opiate addicts with other DSM-III diagnosis. In: Cooper JR, Altman F, Brown BS, Czechowicz D, editors. Research on the treatment of narcotic addiction: state of the art. Rockville, MD: NIDA; 1983. p. 119–58.
396. McLellan AT, Childress AR, Griffith J, Woody GE. The psychiatrically severe drug abuse patient: methadone maintenance or therapeutic community? Am J Drug Alcohol Abuse. 1984;10(1):77–95.
397. Griffiths RR, McLeod DR, Bigelow GE, Liebson IA, Roache JD. Relative abuse liability of diazepam and oxazepam: behavioral and subjective dose effects. Psychopharmacology. 1984;84(2):147–54.
398. Sellers EM, Ciraulo DA, DuPont RL, Griffiths RR, Kosten TR, Romach MK, Woody GE. Alprazolam and benzodiazepine dependence. J Clin Psychiatry. 1993;54(Suppl 10):64–75.
399. Maremmani AGI, Bacciardi S, Rugani F, Rovai L, Massimetti E, Gazzarrini D, Dell'Osso L, Pani PP, Pacini M, Maremmani I. Is it possible to treat heroin addicts with severe comorbid benzodiazepines addiction combining enhanced methadone maintenance and clonazepam maintenance treatments? Heroin Addict Relat Clin Probl. 2014;16(4):15–24.
400. Maremmani AGI, Bacciardi S, Rugani F, Rovai L, Massimetti E, Gazzarrini D, Dell'Osso L, Pani PP, Pacini M, Maremmani I. Outcomes of clonazepam maintained benzodiazepine-heroin addicted patients during methadone maintenance: a descriptive case series. Heroin Addict Relat Clin Probl. 2014;16(3):55–64.
401. Maremmani AGI, Rovai L, Rugani F, Bacciardi S, Pacini M, Dell'Osso L, Maremmani I. Clonazepam as agonist substitution treatment for benzodiazepine dependence: a case report. Case Rep Psychiatry. 2013;2013:367594. https://doi.org/10.1155/2013/367594.

402. Anglin MD, Almong IJ, Fisher DG, Peters KR. Alcohol use by heroin addicts: evidence for an inverse relationship: a study of methadone maintenance and drug-free treatment samples. Am J Drug Alcohol Abuse. 1989;15:191–207.

403. Ball JC, Ross A. Follow-up study of 105 patients who left treatment. In: Ball JC, Ross A, editors. The effectiveness of methadone maintenance treatment. New York: Springer-Verlag; 1991. p. 176–87.

404. Barglow P, Kotun J, Dunteman GH, Condelli WS, Fairbank JA. Methadone and cocaine [2]. Hosp Community Psychiatry. 1992;43:1245–6.

405. Stimmel B, Cohen M, Sturiano V, Hanbury R, Korts D, Jackson G. Is treatment for alcoholism effective in persons on methadone maintenance? Am J Psychiatry. 1983;140:862–6.

406. Maremmani I, Balestri C, Sbrana A, Tagliamonte A. Substance (ab)use during methadone and naltrexone treatment. Interest of adequate methadone dosage. J Mainten Addict. 2003;2(1–2):19–36.

407. Stine SM, Freeman M, Burns B, Charney DS, Kosten TR. Effects of methadone dose on cocaine abuse in a methadone program. Am J Addict. 1992;1:294–303.

408. Spensley J. Doxepin: a useful adjunct in the treatment of heroin addicts in a methadone program. Int J Addict. 1976;11:191–7.

409. Woody GE, O'Brien CP, Rickels K. Depression and anxiety in heroin addicts: a placebo controlled study of doxepin in combination with methadone. Am J Psychiatry. 1975;132:447–50.

410. Strain EC, Stitzer ML, Bigelow GE. Early treatment time course of depressive symptoms in opiate addicts. J Nerv Ment Dis. 1991;179:215–21.

411. Wieland WF, Sola S. Depression in opiate addicts measured by objective tests. In: Proceedings of the national conference on methadone treatment. New York: AMTA; 1970. p. 187–202.

412. Stimmel B, Cohen MJ, Hambury R. Alcoholism and polydrugs abuse in persons on methadone maintenance. Ann N Y Acad Sci. 1978;311:99–109.

413. Cohen MJ, Hanbury R, Simmel B. Abuse of amitriptiline. JAMA. 1978;240:1372–3.

414. Moreno Brea MR, Rojas Corrales O, G-R J, Mico JA. Drug interactions of methadone with CNS-active agents. Actas Espaniolas Psyquiatricas. 1999;27(2):103–10.

415. De Maria PAJ, Serota RD. A therapeutic use of the methadone fluvoxamine drug interaction. J Addict Dis. 1999;18(4):5–12.

416. Cronson AJ, Flemenbaum A. Antagonism of cocaine highs by lithium. Am J Psychiatry. 1978;135:856–7.

417. Nunes EW, McGrath PJ, Wager S, Quitkin FM. Lithium treatment for cocaine abusers with bipolar spectrum disorders. Am J Psychiatry. 1990;147(5):655–7.

418. Gawin F, Allen D, Humblestone B. Outpatient treatment of 'crack' cocaine smocking with flupenthixol decanoate. Arch Gen Psychiatry. 1989;46:322–5.

419. Jasinski DR, Nutti JG, Haertzen CA, Griffith JD. Lithium: effects on subjective functioning and morphine-induced euphoria. Science. 1977;195:582–4.

420. Jensen J. The effect of prolonged lithium ingestion on morphine actions in the rat. Acta Pharmacol Toxicol. 1974;35:395–402.

421. Angst J, Autenrieth F, Brem F, Koukkou M, Meyer H, Stassen HH, Storck U. Preliminary results of treatment with beta-endorphin in depression. In: Udsin E, Bunney WEJ, Kline NS, editors. Endorphins in mental health research. London: Macmillan; 1979. p. 518–28.

422. Gerner RH, Catlin DH, Gorelick DA, Hui KK, Li CH. Beta-endorphin. Intravenous infusion causes behavioral change in psychiatric inpatients. Arch Gen Psychiatry. 1980;37:642–7.

423. Exstein I, Pickard D, et al. Methadone and morphine in depression. Pharmacological Bulletin. 1981;17:29–33.

424. Extein I, Pottash ALC, Gold MS. A possible opioid receptor dysfunction in some depressive disorders. Ann N Y Acad Sci. 1982;398:113–9.

425. Mendelson JH, Ellingboe J, Keuhnle JC, Mello NK. Effects of naltrexone on mood and neuroendocrine function in normal adult males. Psychoneuroendocrinology. 1978;3(3–4):231–6.

426. Sullivan MA, Nunes EV. New-onset mania and psychosis following heroin detoxification and naltrexone maintenance. Am J Addict. 2005;14(5):486–7.

427. Levinson I, Galynker II, Rosenthal RN. Methadone withdrawal psychosis. J Clin Psychiatry. 1995;56(2):73–6.
428. Shariat SV, Hosseinifard Z, Taban M, Shabani A. Mania precipitated by opioid withdrawal: a retrospective study. Am J Addict. 2013;22(4):338–43.
429. Malcolm R, O'Neil PM, Von JM, Dickerson PC. Naltrexone and dysphoria: a double-blind placebo controlled trial. Biol Psychiatry. 1987;22(6):710–6.
430. Hatsukami DK, Mitchell JE, Morley JE, Morgan SF, Levine AS. Effect of naltrexone on mood and cognitive functioning among overweight men. Biol Psychiatry. 1986;21(3):293–300.
431. Miotto K, McCann M, Basch J, Rawson R, Ling W. Naltrexone and dysphoria: fact or myth? Am J Addict. 2002;11(2):151–60.
432. Crowley TJ, Wagner JE, Zerbe G, Macdonald M. Naltrexone-induced dysphoria in former opioid addicts. Am J Psychiatry. 1985;142(9):1081–4.
433. Emrich HM, Vogt P, Herz A. Possible antidepressive effects of opioids: action of buprenorphine. Ann N Y Acad Sci. 1982;398:108–12.
434. Carlezon WA Jr, Beguin C, Knoll AT, Cohen BM. Kappa-opioid ligands in the study and treatment of mood disorders. Pharmacol Ther. 2009;123(3):334–43.
435. Berrocoso E, Sanchez-Blazquez P, Garzon J, Mico JA. Opiates as antidepressants. Curr Pharm Des. 2009;15(14):1612–22.
436. Gold MS, Pottash AC, Sweeney DR, Kleber HD, Redmond E. Rapid opiate detoxification: clinical evidence of antidepressant and antpanic effects of opiates. Am J Psychiatry. 1979;136:982–3.
437. Maremmani I, Marini G, Fornai F. Naltrexone-induced panic attacks. Am J Psychiatry. 1998;155:447.
438. Salamina G, Diecidue R, Vigna-Taglianti F, Jarre P, Schifano P, Bargagli AM, Davoli M, Amato L, Perucci CA, Faggiano F. Effectiveness of therapies for heroin addiction in retaining patients in treatment: results from the Vedette study. Subst Use Misuse. 2010;45(12):2076–92.
439. D'Ippoliti D, Davoli M, Perucci CA, Pasqualini F, Bargagli AM. Retention in treatment of heroin users in Italy: the role of treatment type and of methadone maintenance dosage. Drug Alcohol Depend. 1998;52(2):167–71.
440. Faggiano F, Vigna-Taglianti F, Versino E, Lemma P. Methadone maintenance at different dosages for opioid dependence. Cochrane Database Syst Rev. 2003;3:CD002208.
441. Brady TM, Salvucci S, Sverdlov LS, Male A, Kyeyune H, Sikali E, DeSale S, Yu P. Methadone dosage and retention: an examination of the 60 mg/day threshold. J Addict Dis. 2005;24(3):23–47.
442. Pollack HA, D'Aunno T. Dosage patterns in methadone treatment: results from a National Survey, 1988–2005. Health Serv Res. 2008;43(6):2143–63.
443. Maremmani I, Pacini M, Lamanna F, Pani PP, Perugi G, Deltito J, Salloum IM, Akiskal HS. Mood stabilizers in the treatment of substance use disorders. CNS Spectr. 2010;15(2):95–109.
444. Rounsaville BJ, Cacciola J, Weissman MM, Kleber HD. Diagnostic concordance in a follow-up study of opiate addicts. J Psychiatr Res. 1981;16:191–201.
445. Farrell M, Howes S, Taylor C, Lewis G, Jenkins R, Bebbington P, Jarvis M, Brugha M, Gill B, Meltzer H. Substance misuse and psychiatric comorbidity: an overview of the OPCS National Psychiatric Morbidity Survey. Addict Behav. 1998;23(5):909–18.
446. De Leon G, Rosenthal M, Brodney K. Therapeutic community for drug addicts, long term measurement of emotional changes. Psychol Rep. 1971;29:595–600.
447. De Leon G, Skodon A, Rosenthal MS. Phoenix house. Changes in psychopatology signs of resident drug addicts. Arch Gen Psychiatry. 1973;28(1):131–5.
448. Haddox V, Jacobson M. Psychological adjustment, mood and personality fluctuations in long term methadone maintenance patients. Int J Addict. 1972;7:619–27.
449. Jacobs PE, Doft EB, Koger J. A study of SCL-90 scores of 264 methadone patients in treatment. Int J Addict. 1981;16:541–8.
450. Korin H. Comparison of psychometric measures in psychiatric patients using heroin and other drugs. J Abnorm Psychol. 1974;83:208–12.

451. Krausz M, Degkwitz P, Haasen C, Verthein U. Opioid addiction and Suicidality. Crisis. 1996;17(4):175–81.

452. Kessler RC, McGonagle KA, Zhao S, Nelson CB, Hughes M, Eshleman S, Wittchen HU, Kendler KS. Lifetime and 12-month prevalence of DSM-III-R psychiatric disorders in the United States. Results from the National Comorbidity Survey. Arch Gen Psychiatry. 1994;51(1):8–19.

453. Haney M, Miczek KA. Morphine effects on maternal aggression, pup care and analgesia in mice. Psychopharmacology (Berl). 1989;98(1):68–74.

454. Scrima L, Hartman PG, Johnson FH Jr, Hiller FC. Efficacy of gamma-hydroxibutyrrate vs placebo in treating narcolepsy cataplexy; double-blind subjective measures. Biol Psychiatry. 1989;26:331–43.

455. Wurmser L. The question of specific psychopathology in compulsive drug use. Ann N Y Acad Sci. 1982;398:33–43.

456. Ray R, Pal H, Kumar R, Maulick P, Mangla R. Post-marketing surveillance of buprenorphine. Pharmacoepidemiol Drug Saf. 2004;13(9):615–9.

457. Senay EC, Adams EH, Geller A, Inciardi JA, Munoz A, Schnoll SH, Woody GE, Cicero TJ. Physical dependence on ultram (tramadol hydrochloride): both opioid-like and atypical withdrawal symptoms occur. Drug Alcohol Depend. 2003;69(3):233–41.

458. Luby ED, Marrazzi MA, Kinzie J. Treatment of chronic anorexia nervosa with opiate blockade. J Clin Pharmacol. 1987;7(1):52–3.

459. Kane FJJ, Pokorny A. Mental and emotional disturbance with pentazocine (Talwin) use. South Med J. 1975;68(7):808–11.

460. Liebowitz MR, Gorman JM, Fyer AJ, Dillon DJ, Klein DF. Effects of naloxone on patients with panic attacks. Am J Psychiatry. 1984;141(8):995–7.

461. Ahmad B, Mufti KA, Farooq S. Psychiatric comorbidity in substance abuse (opioids). J Pak Med Assoc. 2001;51(5):183–6.

462. Rosen MI, Kosten T. Cocaine associated panic attacks in methadone maintained patients. Am J Drug Alcohol Abuse. 1992;18(1):57–62.

463. Sullivan MD, Edlund MJ, Steffick D, Unutzer J. Regular use of prescribed opioids: association with common psychiatric disorders. Pain. 2005;119(1–3):95–103.

464. Gold MS, Pottash AL, Sweeney DR, Davies RK, Kleber HD. Clonidine decreases opiate withdrawal-related anxiety: possible opiate noradrenergic interaction in anxiety and panic. Subst Alcohol Actions Misuse. 1980;1(2):239–46.

465. Gold MS, Pottash AC, Extein IL, Kleber HD. Neuroanatomical sites of action of clonidine in opiate withdrawal: the locus Coeruleus connection. Prog Clin Biol Res. 1981;71:285–98.

466. Stine SM, Southwick SM, Petrakis IL, Kosten TR, Charney DS, Krystal JH. Yohimbine-induced withdrawal and anxiety symptoms in opioid-dependent patients. Biol Psychiatry. 2002;51(8):642–51.

467. Kleber HD. Methadone maintenance treatment—a reply. Am J Drug Alcohol Abuse. 1977;4:267–72.

468. Woody GE, Mintz J, O'Hare K, O'Brien OF, Greenstein RA, Hargrove HE. Diazepam use by patients in a methadone program: how seriuos a problem? J Psychedelic Drugs. 1975;7:373–9.

469. Woody GE, O'Brien CP, Greenstein RA. Misuse and abuse of diazepam: an increasingly common medical problem. J Addict. 1975;10:843–8.

470. Shannon HE, Holtzman SG, Davis DC. Interactions between narcotic analgesics and benzodiazepine derivatives on behavior in the mouse. J Pharmacol Exp Ther. 1976;199:389–99.

471. Budd RD, Walkin E, Jain NC, Sneath TC. Frequency of use of diazepam in individuals on probation and in methadone maintenance programs. Am J Drug Alcohol Abuse. 1979;6:511–4.

472. Kryspin-Exner K, Demel I. The use of tranquilizer in the treatment of mixed drug abuse. Int J Clin Pharmacol. 1975;12:13–8.

473. Schimidt LG, Muller-Oerlinghausen B, Schlunder M. Benzodiazepines and barbiturates in chronic alcoholic and opiate addicts. An epidemiological study of hospitalized addicts. Deutsche Medizine. 1987;112(48):1849–54.

474. Hunt WA, Dalton TK. Regional brain acetylcholine levels in rats acutely treated with ethanol or rendered ethanol-dependence. Brain Res. 1976;109:628–31.
475. Hartog J, Tusen DJ. Valium use and abuse by methadone maintainance clients. Int J Addict. 1987;22:1147–0.
476. Winokur A, Rickels K, Greenblatt DJ, Snyder PJ, Schatz NJ. Withdrawal reaction from long-term, low dosage administration of diazepam. Arch Gen Psychiatry. 1980;37:101–5.
477. Gastfriend DR. Pharmacological treatments for psychiatric symptoms in addiction populations. In: Miller NS, editor. The principles and practice of addictions in psychiatry. Philadelphia: W.B. Saunders; 1997. p. 486–95.
478. Brands B, Blake J, Marsh DC, Sproule B, Jeyapalan R, Li S. The impact of benzodiazepine use on methadone maintenance treatment outcomes. J Addict Dis. 2008;27(3):37–48.
479. Somers CJ, O'Connor J. Retrospective study of outcomes, for patients admitted to a drug treatment centre board. Ir Med J. 2012;105(9):295–8.
480. Eiroa-Orosa FJ, Haasen C, Verthein U, Dilg C, Schafer I, Reimer J. Benzodiazepine use among patients in heroin-assisted vs. methadone maintenance treatment: findings of the German randomized controlled trial. Drug Alcohol Depend. 2010;112(3):226–33.
481. Ghitza UE, Epstein DH, Preston KL. Self-report of illicit benzodiazepine use on the addiction severity index predicts treatment outcome. Drug Alcohol Depend. 2008;97(1–2):150–7.
482. DeMaria PA Jr, Sterling R, Weinstein SP. The effect of stimulant and sedative use on treatment outcome of patients admitted to methadone maintenance treatment. Am J Addict. 2000;9(2):145–53.
483. Shaffer HJ, LaSalvia TA. Patterns of substance use among methadone maintenance patients. Indicators of outcome. J Subst Abus Treat. 1992;9(2):143–7.
484. McCowan C, Kidd B, Fahey T. Factors associated with mortality in Scottish patients receiving methadone in primary care: retrospective cohort study. BMJ. 2009;338:b2225.
485. Kamal F, Flavin S, Campbell F, Behan C, Fagan J, Smyth R. Factors affecting the outcome of methadone maintenance treatment in opiate dependence. Ir Med J. 2007;100(3):393–7.
486. Drake S, Swift W, Hall W, Ross M. Drug use, HIV risk-taking and psychosocial correlates of benzodiazepine use among methadone maintenance clients. Drug Alcohol Depend. 1993;34(1):67–70.
487. Peles E, Schreiber S, Adelson M. 15-year survival and retention of patients in a general hospital-affiliated methadone maintenance treatment (MMT) Center in Israel. Drug Alcohol Depend. 2010;107(2–3):141–8.
488. Lintzeris N, Mitchell TB, Bond A, Nestor L, Strang J. Interactions on mixing diazepam with methadone or buprenorphine in maintenance patients. J Clin Psychopharmacol. 2006;26(3):274–83.
489. Reed LJ, Glasper A, de Wet CJ, Bearn J, Gossop M. Comparison of buprenorphine and methadone in the treatment of opiate withdrawal: possible advantages of buprenorphine for the treatment of opiate-benzodiazepine codependent patients? J Clin Psychopharmacol. 2007;27(2):188–92.
490. Weizman T, Gelkopf M, Melamed Y, Adelson M, Bleich A. Treatment of benzodiazepine dependence in methadone maintenance treatment patients: a comparison of two therapeutic modalities and the role of psychiatric comorbidity. Aust N Z J Psychiatry. 2003;37(4):458–63.
491. Dole VP, Joseph H. Long term outcome of patients treated with methadone maintenance. Ann N Y Acad Sci. 1978;311:181–9.
492. Siassi I, Angle BP, Alston DC. Comparison of the effect of high and low doses of methadone on treatment outcome. Int J Addict. 1977;12(8):993–1005.
493. Strain EC, Stitzer ML, Liebson IA, Bigelow GE. Methadone dose and treatment outcome. Drug Alcohol Depend. 1993;33(2):105–17.
494. Blaney T, Craig RJ. Methadone maintenance. Does dose determine differences in outcome? J Subst Abus Treat. 1999;16(3):221–8.
495. Fareed A, Casarella J, Roberts M, Sleboda M, Amar R, Vayalapalli S, Drexler K. High dose versus moderate dose methadone maintenance: is there a better outcome? J Addict Dis. 2009;28(4):399–405.

496. Kritz S, Chu M, John-Hull C, Madray C, Louie B, Brown LS Jr. Opioid dependence as a chronic disease: the interrelationships between length of stay, methadone dose, and age on treatment outcome at an urban opioid treatment program. J Addict Dis. 2009;28(1):53–6.

497. Foster DJ, Somogyi AA, Bochner F. Methadone N-demethylation in human liver microsomes: lack of stereoselectivity and involvement of CYP3A4. Br J Clin Pharmacol. 1999;47:403–12.

498. Chen CH, Wang SC, Tsou HH, Ho IK, Tian JN, Yu CJ, Hsiao CF, Chou SY, Lin YF, Fang KC, Huang CL, Su LW, Fang YC, Liu ML, Lin KM, Hsu YT, Liu SC, Chen A, Liu YL. Genetic polymorphisms in CYP3A4 are associated with withdrawal symptoms and adverse reactions in methadone maintenance patients. Pharmacogenomics. 2011;12(10):1397–406.

499. Kharasch ED, Stubbert K. Role of cytochrome P4502B6 in methadone metabolism and clearance. J Clin Pharmacol. 2013;53(3):305–13.

500. Shinderman M, Maxwell S, Brawand-Amey M, Golay KP, Baumann P, Eap CB. Cytochrome P4503A4 metabolic activity, methadone blood concentrations, and methadone doses. Drug Alcohol Depend. 2003;69(2):205–11.

501. Wang JS, DeVane CL. Involvement of CYP3A4, CYP2C8 and CYP2D6 in the metabolism of (R)- and (S)- methadone in vitro. Drug Metab Dispos. 2003;31:742–7.

502. Anggard E. Disposition of methadone in methadone maintenance. Clin Pharmacol Ther. 1974;17(3):258–66.

503. Verebely K, Volavka J, Mule S, Resnick R. Methadone in man: pharmacokinetic and excretion studies in acute and chronic treatment. Clin Pharmacol Ther. 1975;18:180–90.

504. Wilkinson GR. Cytochrome P4503A (CYP3A) metabolism: prediction of in vivo activity in humans. J Pharmacokinet Biopharm. 1996;24:475–90.

505. Goodwin B, Redimbo MR, Kliewer SA. Regulation of CYP3A gene transcription by the Pregnane X receptor. Annu Rev Pharmacol Toxicol. 2002;42:1–23.

506. Oda Y, Kharasch ED. Metabolism of methadone and levo-alpha-acetylmethadol (laam) by human intestinal cytochrome P4503A4 (CYP3A4): potential contribution of intestinal metabolism to presystemic clearance and bioactivation. J Pharmacol Exp Ther. 2001;298(3):1021–32.

507. Baigent M. Managing patients with dual diagnosis in psychiatric practice. Curr Opin Psychiatry. 2012;25(3):201–5.

508. Gonzalez-Pinto A, Alberich S, Barbeito S, Alonso M, Vieta E, Martinez-Aran A, Saenz M, Lopez P. Different profile of substance abuse in relation to predominant polarity in bipolar disorder: the Vitoria long-term follow-up study. J Affect Disord. 2010;124(3):250–5.

509. Sajatovic M, Ignacio RV, West JA, Cassidy KA, Safavi R, Kilbourne AM, Blow FC. Predictors of nonadherence among individuals with bipolar disorder receiving treatment in a community mental health clinic. Compr Psychiatry. 2009;50(2):100–7.

510. Amato L, Minozzi S, Davoli M, Vecchi S. Psychosocial and pharmacological treatments versus pharmacological treatments for opioid detoxification. Cochrane Database Syst Rev. 2011;9:CD005031.

511. Liebrenz M, Boesch L, Stohler R, Caflisch C. Agonist substitution: a treatment alternative for high-dose benzodiazepine dependent patients? Addiction. 2010;105(11):1870–4.

512. Wu LT, Ling W, Burchett B, Blazer DG, Shostak J, Woody GE. Gender and racial/ethnic differences in addiction severity, HIV risk, and quality of life among adults in opioid detoxification: results from the National Drug Abuse Treatment Clinical Trials Network. Subst Abus Rehabil. 2010;2010(1):13–22.

513. Loga S, Loga-Zec S, Spremo M. Cannabis and psychiatric disorders. Psychiatr Danub. 2010;22(2):296–7.

514. Gonzalez-Pinto A, Vega P, Ibanez B, Mosquera F, Barbeito S, Gutierrez M, Ruiz de Azua S, Ruiz I, Vieta E. Impact of cannabis and other drugs on age at onset of psychosis. J Clin Psychiatry. 2008;69(8):1210–6.

515. Dragt S, Nieman DH, Becker HE, van de Fliert R, Dingemans PM, de Haan L, van Amelsvoort TA, Linszen DH. Age of onset of cannabis use is associated with age of onset of high-risk symptoms for psychosis. Can J Psychiatr. 2010;55(3):165–71.

516. Maremmani I, Lazzeri A, Pacini M, Lovrecic M, Placidi GF, Perugi G. Diagnostic and symptomatological features in chronic psychotic patients according to cannabis use status. J Psychoactive Drugs. 2004;36(2):235–41.
517. Srisurapanont M, Arunpongpaisal S, Wada K, Marsden J, Ali R, Kongsakon R. Comparisons of methamphetamine psychotic and schizophrenic symptoms: a differential item functioning analysis. Prog Neuro-Psychopharmacol Biol Psychiatry. 2011;35(4):959–64.
518. Karila L, Petit A, Cottencin O, Reynaud M. Methamphetamine dependence: consequences and complications. Presse Med. 2010;39(12):1246–53.
519. Schep LJ, Slaughter RJ, Beasley DM. The clinical toxicology of metamfetamine. Clin Toxicol (Phila). 2010;48(7):675–94.
520. Floyd AG, Boutros NN, Struve FA, Wolf E, Oliwa GM. Risk factors for experiencing psychosis during cocaine use: a preliminary report. J Psychiatr Res. 2006;40(2):178–82.
521. Marona-Lewicka D, Nichols CD, Nichols DE. An animal model of schizophrenia based on chronic LSD administration: old idea, new results. Neuropharmacology. 2011;61(3):503–12.
522. Carls KA, Ruehter VL. An evaluation of phencyclidine (PCP) psychosis: a retrospective analysis at a state facility. Am J Drug Alcohol Abuse. 2006;32(4):673–8.
523. Perala J, Kuoppasalmi K, Pirkola S, Harkanen T, Saarni S, Tuulio-Henriksson A, Viertio S, Latvala A, Koskinen S, Lonnqvist J, Suvisaari J. Alcohol-induced psychotic disorder and delirium in the general population. Br J Psychiatry. 2010;197(3):200–6.
524. Greenberg DM, Lee JW. Psychotic manifestations of alcoholism. Curr Psychiatry Rep. 2001;3(4):314–8.
525. Jordaan GP, Nel DG, Hewlett RH, Emsley R. Alcohol-induced psychotic disorder: a comparative study on the clinical characteristics of patients with alcohol dependence and schizophrenia. J Stud Alcohol Drugs. 2009;70(6):870–6.
526. Smith MJ, Thirthalli J, Abdallah AB, Murray RM, Cottler LB. Prevalence of psychotic symptoms in substance users: a comparison across substances. Compr Psychiatry. 2009;50(3):245–50.
527. McKenna GJ. Methadone and opiate drugs: psychotropic effect and self-medication. Ann N Y Acad Sci. 1982;398:44–55.
528. Maremmani I, Pacini M, Pani PP. Effectiveness of buprenorphine in double diagnosed patients. Buprenorphine as Psychothropic drug. Heroin Addict Relat Clin Probl. 2006;8(1):31–48.
529. Fein G, Di Sclafani V, Finn P, Scheiner DL. Sub-diagnostic psychiatric comorbidity in alcoholics. Drug Alcohol Depend. 2007;87:139–45.
530. Hulse GK, Saunders JB, Roydhouse RM, Stockwell TR, Basso MR. Screening for hazardous alcohol use and dependence in psychiatric in-patients using the audit questionnaire. Drug Alcohol Rev. 2000;19(3):291–8.
531. Rovai L, Maremmani AGI, Bacciardi S, Gazzarrini D, Pallucchini A, Spera V, Perugi G, Maremmani I. Opposed effect of Hyperthymic and cyclothymic temperament in substance use disorder (heroin or alcohol dependent patients). J Affect Disord. 2017;218:339–45.
532. Keverne EB. Gaba-Ergic neurons and the neurobiology of schizophrenia and other psychoses. Brain Res Bull. 1999;48(5):467–73.
533. Sakata S, Nakamura J. Delirium tremens. Ryoikibetsu Shokogun Shirizu. 2003;40:432–6.
534. Ros LT. Alcoholic withdrawal delirium. Wiad Lek. 1995;48(1–12):135–9.
535. Griffin RE, Gross GA, Teitelbaum HS. Delirium tremens: a review. J Am Osteopath Assoc. 1993;93(9):924, 929–932, 935.
536. Gleason OC. Delirium. Am Fam Physician. 2003;67(5):1027–34.
537. McKeon A, Frye MA, Delanty N. The alcohol withdrawal syndrome. J Neurol Neurosurg Psychiatry. 2008;79(8):854–62.
538. Yost DA. Alcohol withdrawal syndrome. Am Fam Physician. 1996;54(2):657–64. 669
539. Wustmann T, Gutmann P. Palinacousis in alcohol Hallucinosis. Psychiatr Prax. 2007;34(6):302–4.
540. Michael A, Mirza S, Mirza KA, Babu VS, Vithayathil E. Morbid jealousy in alcoholism. Br J Psychiatry. 1995;167(5):668–72.

541. Soyka M. Alcohol hallucinosis and jealous delusion. Fortschr Neurol Psychiatr. 2006;74(6):346–52; quiz 353–344.

542. Koster A, Lajer M, Lindhardt A, Rosenbaum B. Gender differences in first episode psychosis. Soc Psychiatry Psychiatr Epidemiol. 2008;43(12):940–6.

543. Barrigon ML, Gurpegui M, Ruiz-Veguilla M, Diaz FJ, Anguita M, Sarramea F, Cervilla J. Temporal relationship of first-episode non-affective psychosis with cannabis use: a clinical verification of an epidemiological hypothesis. J Psychiatr Res. 2010;44(7):413–20.

544. Arendt M, Rosenberg R, Foldager L, Perto G, Munk-Jorgensen P. Cannabis-induced psychosis and subsequent schizophrenia-spectrum disorders: follow-up study of 535 incident cases. Br J Psychiatry. 2005;187(6):510–5.

545. Mason O, Morgan CJ, Dhiman SK, Patel A, Parti N, Curran HV. Acute cannabis use causes increased psychotomimetic experiences in individuals prone to psychosis. Psychol Med. 2009;39(6):951–6.

546. Barkus E, Lewis S. Schizotypy and psychosis-like experiences from recreational cannabis in a non-clinical sample. Psychol Med. 2008;38(9):1267–76.

547. Anglin DM, Corcoran CM, Brown AS, Chen H, Lighty Q, Brook JS, Cohen PR. Early cannabis use and schizotypal personality disorder symptoms from adolescence to middle adulthood. Schizophr Res. 2012;137(1–3):45–9.

548. Pacini M, Maremmani I. Substance-related psychotic chronicity and schizoaffective pictures: is there a bipolar connection? In: Murray WH, editor. Schizoaffective disorder: new research. Hauppauge, NY: Nova Science Publishers; 2006. p. 221–8.

549. Semple DM, McIntosh AM, Lawrie SM. Cannabis as a risk factor for psychosis: systematic review. J Psychopharmacol (Oxf). 2005;19(2):187–94.

550. D'Souza DC, Sewell RA, Ranganathan M. Cannabis and psychosis/schizophrenia: human studies. Eur Arch Psychiatry Clin Neurosci. 2009;259(7):413–31.

551. Ornstein J, Stone J. Cannabis and psychosis. Br J Psychiatry. 2010;197(4):333.

552. Vernex N, Dagher G, Touzeau D. Cannabis and premonitory symptoms of schizophrenia: what is the time sequence? Heroin Addict Relat Clin Probl. 2009;11(3):29–34.

553. Malone DT, Hill MN, Rubino T. Adolescent cannabis use and psychosis: epidemiology and neurodevelopmental models. Br J Pharmacol. 2010;160(3):511–22.

554. Kuepper R, Morrison PD, van Os J, Murray RM, Kenis G, Henquet C. Does dopamine mediate the psychosis-inducing effects of cannabis? A review and integration of findings across disciplines. Schizophr Res. 2010;121(1–3):107–17.

555. Zuardi AW, Crippa JA, Hallak JE, Pinto JP, Chagas MH, Rodrigues GG, Dursun SM, Tumas V. Cannabidiol for the treatment of psychosis in Parkinson's disease. J Psychopharmacol. 2009;23(8):979–83.

556. Marco EM, Garcia-Gutierrez MS, Bermudez-Silva FJ, Moreira FA, Guimaraes F, Manzanares J, Viveros MP. Endocannabinoid system and psychiatry: in search of a neurobiological basis for detrimental and potential therapeutic effects. Front Behav Neurosci. 2011;5:63.

557. Schubart CD, Sommer IE, van Gastel WA, Goetgebuer RL, Kahn RS, Boks MP. Cannabis with high Cannabidiol content is associated with fewer psychotic experiences. Schizophr Res. 2011;130(1–3):216–21.

558. Kulhalli V, Isaac M, Murthy P. Cannabis-related psychosis: presentation and effect of abstinence. Indian J Psychiatry. 2007;49(4):256–61.

559. Schimmelmann BG, Conus P, Cotton SM, Kupferschmid S, Karow A, Schultze-Lutter F, McGorry PD, Lambert M. Cannabis use disorder and age at onset of psychosis—a study in first-episode patients. Schizophr Res. 2011;129(1):52–6.

560. Dragt S, Nieman DH, Schultze-Lutter F, van der Meer F, Becker H, de Haan L, Dingemans PM, Birchwood M, Patterson P, Salokangas RK, Heinimaa M, Heinz A, Juckel G, Graf von Reventlow H, French P, Stevens H, Ruhrmann S, Klosterkotter J, Linszen DH, EPOS Group. Cannabis use and age at onset of symptoms in subjects at clinical high risk for psychosis. Acta Psychiatr Scand. 2012;125(1):45–53.

561. Compton MT, Kelley ME, Ramsay CE, Pringle M, Goulding SM, Esterberg ML, Stewart T, Walker EF. Association of pre-onset cannabis, alcohol, and tobacco use with age at

onset of prodrome and age at onset of psychosis in first-episode patients. Am J Psychiatry. 2009;166(11):1251–7.

562. McGrath J, Welham J, Scott J, Varghese D, Degenhardt L, Hayatbakhsh MR, Alati R, Williams GM, Bor W, Najman JM. Association between cannabis use and psychosis-related outcomes using sibling pair analysis in a cohort of young adults. Arch Gen Psychiatry. 2010;67(5):440–7.

563. Mahoney JJ 3rd, Hawkins RY, De La Garza R 2nd, Kalechstein AD, Newton TF. Relationship between gender and psychotic symptoms in cocaine-dependent and methamphetamine-dependent participants. Gend Med. 2010;7(5):414–21.

564. Dluzen DE, Liu B. Gender differences in methamphetamine use and responses: a review. Gend Med. 2008;5(1):24–35.

565. McGuire PK, Cope H, Fahy TA. Diversity of psychopathology associated with use of 3,4-metylendioximethamphetamine (ecstasy). Br J Psychiatry. 1994;165:391–5.

566. McGuire P. Long term psychiatric and cognitive effects of MDMA use. Toxicol Lett. 2000;112–113:153–6.

567. Creighton FJ, Black DL, Hyde CE. Ecstasy psychosis and flashbacks. Br J Psychiatry. 1991;159:713–5.

568. Gouzoulis E, Borchardt D, Hermle L. A case of toxic psychosis induced by 'Eve' (3,4-methylene-dioxyethylam-phetamine). Arch Gen Psychiatry. 1993;50(1):75.

569. Ujike H, Katsu T, Okahisa Y, Takaki M, Kodama M, Inada T, Uchimura N, Yamada M, Iwata N, Sora I, Iyo M, Ozaki N, Kuroda S. Genetic variants of D2 but not D3 or D4 dopamine receptor gene are associated with rapid onset and poor prognosis of methamphetamine psychosis. Prog Neuro-Psychopharmacol Biol Psychiatry. 2009;33(4):625–9.

570. Dawe S, Davis P, Lapworth K, McKetin R. Mechanisms underlying aggressive and hostile behavior in amphetamine users. Curr Opin Psychiatry. 2009;22(3):269–73.

571. Gerra G, Zaimovic A, Giusti F, Delsignore R, Raggi MA, Laviola G, Macchia T, Brambilla F. Experimentally-induced aggressive behaviour in subjects with 3,4-methylenedioxy-methanfetamine (MDMA; "ecstasy") use hystory; psychobiological correlates. J Subst Abuse. 2001;13:471–91.

572. Milas M. Acute psychosis with aggressive behavior as a consequence of MDMA (ecstasy) consumption. Lijec Vjesn. 2000;122(1–2):27–30.

573. Wan L, Baldridge RM, Colby AM, Stanford MS. Enhanced intensity dependence and aggression history indicate previous regular ecstasy use in abstinent Polydrug users. Prog Neuro-Psychopharmacol Biol Psychiatry. 2009;33(8):1484–90.

574. Lapworth K, Dawe S, Davis P, Kavanagh D, Young R, Saunders J. Impulsivity and positive psychotic symptoms influence hostility in methamphetamine users. Addict Behav. 2009;34(4):380–5.

575. Rugani F, Bacciardi S, Rovai L, Pacini M, Maremmani AGI, Deltito J, Dell'Osso L, Maremmani I. Symptomatological features of patients with and without ecstasy use during their first psychotic episode. Int J Environ Res Public Health. 2012;9(7):2283–92.

576. Schifano F. Chronic atypical psychosis associated with Mdma (ecstasy) abuse (letter). Lancet. 1991;338:1335.

577. Landabaso MA, Iraurgi I, Jimenez-Lerma JM, Calle R, Sanz J, Gutierrez-Fraile M. Ecstasy-induced psychotic disorder: six-month follow-up study. Eur Addict Res. 2002;8(3):133–40.

578. Vecellio M, Schopper C, Modestin J. Neuropsychiatric consequences (atypical psychosis and complex-partial seizures) of ecstasy use: possible evidence for toxicity-vulnerability predictors and implications for preventative and clinical care. J Psychopharmacol. 2003;17(3):342–5.

579. Potash MN, Gordon KA, Conrad KL. Persistent psychosis and medical complications after a single ingestion of MDMA "ecstasy": a case report and review of the literature. Psychiatry. 2009;6(7):40–4.

580. Hartel-Petri R, Rodler R, Schmeisser U, Steinmann J, Wolfersdorf M. Increasing prevalence of amphetamine—and methamphetamine-induced psychosis. Psychiatr Prax. 2005;32(1):13–7.

581. Dore G, Sweeting M. Drug-induced psychosis associated with crystalline methamphetamine. Australas Psychiatry. 2006;14(1):86–9.
582. McKetin R, McLaren J, Lubman DI, Hides L. The prevalence of psychotic symptoms among methamphetamine users. Addiction. 2006;101(10):1473–8.
583. McGuire P, Fahy T. Chronic paranoid psychosis after misuse of MDMA ("ecstasy"). BMJ. 1991;302(6778):697.
584. Demirkiran M, Jankovic J, Dean JM. Ecstasy intoxication: an overlap between serotonin syndrome and neuroleptic malignant syndrome. Clin Neuropharmacol. 1996;19(2):157–64.
585. Yui K, Goto K, Ikemoto S, Nishijima K, Yoshino T, Ishiguro T. Susceptibility to subsequent episodes of spontaneous recurrence of methamphetamine psychosis. Drug Alcohol Depend. 2001;64(2):133–42.
586. Vaiva G, Bailly D, Boss V, Thomas P, Lestavel P, Goudemand M. A case of acute psychotic episode after a single dose of ecstasy. L'Encephale. 2001;27(2):198–202.
587. Marchesi C, Tonna M, Maggini C. Obsessive-compulsive disorder followed by psychotic episode in long-term ecstasy misuse. World J Biol Psychiatry. 2009;10(4 Pt 2):599–602.
588. Van Kampen J, Katz M. Persistent psychosis after a single ingestion of 'Ecstasy'. Psychosomatics. 2001;42(6):525–7.
589. Mooney M, Sofuoglu M, Dudish-Poulsen S, Hatsukami DK. Preliminary observations of paranoia in a human laboratory study of cocaine. Addict Behav. 2006;31(7):1245–51.
590. Satel SL, Edell WS. Cocaine-induced paranoia and psychosis proneness. Am J Psychiatry. 1991;148:1708–11.
591. Kuzenko N, Sareen J, Beesdo-Baum K, Perkonigg A, Hofler M, Simm J, Lieb R, Wittchen HU. Associations between use of cocaine, amphetamines, or psychedelics and psychotic symptoms in a community sample. Acta Psychiatr Scand. 2011;123(6):466–74.
592. Kalayasiri R, Kranzler HR, Weiss R, Brady K, Gueorguieva R, Panhuysen C, Yang BZ, Farrer L, Gelernter J, Malison RT. Risk factors for cocaine-induced paranoia in cocaine-dependent sibling pairs. Drug Alcohol Depend. 2006;84(1):77–84.
593. Kalayasiri R, Gelernter J, Farrer L, Weiss R, Brady K, Gueorguieva R, Kranzler HR, Malison RT. Adolescent cannabis use increases risk for cocaine-induced paranoia. Drug Alcohol Depend. 2010;107(2–3):196–201.
594. Roncero C, Daigre C, Gonzalvo B, Valero S, Castells X, Grau-Lopez L, Eiroa-Orosa FJ, Casas M. Risk factors for cocaine-induced psychosis in cocaine-dependent patients. Eur Psychiatry. 2013;28(3):141–6.
595. Brady KT, Lydiard RB, Malcolm R, Ballenger JC. Cocaine-induced psychosis. J Clin Psychiatry. 1991;52(12):509–12.
596. Reid MS, Ciplet D, O'Leary S, Branchey M, Buydens-Branchey L, Angrist B. Sensitization to the psychosis-inducing effects of cocaine compared with measures of cocaine craving and cue reactivity. Am J Addict. 2004;13(3):305–15.
597. Cubells JF, Feinn R, Pearson D, Burda J, Tang Y, Farrer LA, Gelernter J, Kranzler HR. Rating the severity and character of transient cocaine-induced delusions and hallucinations with a new instrument, the scale for assessment of positive symptoms for cocaine-induced psychosis (SAPS-CIP). Drug Alcohol Depend. 2005;80(1):23–33.
598. Mitchell J, Vierkant AD. Delusions and hallucinations of cocaine abusers and paranoid schizophrenics: a comparative study. J Psychol. 1991;125(3):301–10.
599. Roth ME, Cosgrove KP, Carroll ME. Sex differences in the vulnerability to drug abuse: a review of preclinical studies. Neurosci Biobehav Rev. 2004;28(6):533–46.
600. Zhang Y, Lu C, Zhang J, Hu L, Song H, Li J, Kang L. Gender differences in abusers of amphetamine-type stimulants and ketamine in southwestern China. Addict Behav. 2012;38(1):1424–30.
601. Honey GD, Corlett PR, Absalom AR, Lee M, Pomarol-Clotet E, Murray GK, McKenna PJ, Bullmore ET, Menon DK, Fletcher PC. Individual differences in psychotic effects of ketamine are predicted by brain function measured under placebo. J Neurosci. 2008;28(25):6295–303.
602. Johnson M, Richards W, Griffiths R. Human hallucinogen research: guidelines for safety. J Psychopharmacol. 2008;22(6):603–20.

603. Goff DC, Coyle JT. The emerging role of glutamate in the pathophysiology and treatment of schizophrenia. Am J Psychiatry. 2001;158(9):1367–77.
604. Corlett PR, Honey GD, Fletcher PC. From prediction error to psychosis: ketamine as a pharmacological model of delusions. J Psychopharmacol. 2007;21(3):238–52.
605. Iasevoli F, Polese D, Ambesi-Impiombato A, Muscettola G, de Bartolomeis A. Ketamine-related expression of Glutamatergic postsynaptic density genes: possible implications in psychosis. Neurosci Lett. 2007;416(1):1–5.
606. Lahti AC, Koffel B, LaPorte D, Tamminga CA. Subanesthetic doses of ketamine stimulate psychosis in schizophrenia. Neuropsychopharmacology. 1995;13(1):9–19.
607. Javitt DC, Zukin SR. Recent advances in the phencyclidine model of schizophrenia. Am J Psychiatry. 1991;148(10):1301–8.
608. Rosse RB, Collins JP Jr, Fay-McCarthy M, Alim TN, Wyatt RJ, Deutsch SI. Phenomenologic comparison of the idiopathic psychosis of schizophrenia and drug-induced cocaine and phencyclidine psychoses: a retrospective study. Clin Neuropharmacol. 1994;17(4):359–69.
609. Erard R, Luisada PV, Peele R. The PCP psychosis: prolonged intoxication or drug-precipitated functional illness? J Psychedelic Drugs. 1980;12:235–52.
610. Pomarol-Clotet E, Honey GD, Murray GK, Corlett PR, Absalom AR, Lee M, McKenna PJ, Bullmore ET, Fletcher PC. Psychological effects of ketamine in healthy volunteers. Phenomenological study. Br J Psychiatry. 2006;189:173–9.
611. Pearlson GD. Psychiatric and medical syndromes associated with phencyclidine (PCP) abuse. Johns Hopkins Med J. 1981;148(1):25–33.
612. Aniline O, Pitts FN. Phencyclidine: a review and perspectives. Crit Rev Toxicol. 1982;10:145–7.
613. Pal HR, Berry N, Kumar R, Ray R. Ketamine dependence. Anaesth Intensive Care. 2002;30(3):382–4.
614. Rainey JM, Crowder MK. Prolonged psychosis attributed to phencyclidine—report of 3 cases. Am J Psychiatry. 1975;132(10):1076–8.
615. Okudaira K, Yabana T, Takahashi H, Iizuka H, Nakajima K, Saito A. Inhalant abusers and psychiatric symptoms. Seishin Shinkeigaku Zasshi. 1996;98(4):203–12.
616. Bowen SE, Wiley JL, Jones HE, Balster RL. Phencyclidine- and diazepam-like discriminative stimulus effects of inhalants in mice. Exp Clin Psychopharmacol. 1999;7(1):28–37.
617. Shelton KL, Balster RL. Effects of abused inhalants and gaba-positive modulators in dizocilpine discriminating inbred mice. Pharmacol Biochem Behav. 2004;79(2):219–28.
618. Riegel AC, Zapata A, Shippenberg TS, French ED. The abused inhalant toluene increases dopamine release in the nucleus accumbens by directly stimulating ventral tegmental area neurons. Neuropsychopharmacology. 2007;32(7):1558–69.
619. Howard MO, Bowen SE, Garland EL, Perron BE, Vaughn MG. Inhalant use and inhalant use disorders in the United States. Addict Sci Clin Pract. 2011;6(1):18–31.
620. Rao NP, Gupta A, Sreejayan K, Chand PK, Benegal V, Murthy P. Toluene associated schizophrenia-like psychosis. Indian J Psychiatry. 2009;51(4):329–30.
621. Saito T, Sekito Y, Ikeda N, Taniguchi E, Kadowaki I, Ashizawa T. A case report of volatile solvent psychosis. Nihon Arukoru Yakubutsu Igakkai Zasshi. 1996;31(5):475–82.
622. Saito T, Ikeda N, Miyashita H, Yanbe K, Shirasaka T. Clinical manifestation of volatile solvent psychosis. Nihon Arukoru Yakubutsu Igakkai Zasshi. 1997;32(3):189–96.
623. Wada K, Nakayama K, Koishikawa H, Katayama M, Hirai S, Yabana T, Aoki T, Iwashita S. Symptomatological structure of volatile solvent-induced psychosis: is "solvent psychosis" a discernible syndrome? Nihon Arukoru Yakubutsu Igakkai Zasshi. 2005;40(5):471–84.
624. Lin BF, Ou MC, Chung SS, Pang CY, Chen HH. Adolescent toluene exposure produces enduring social and cognitive deficits in mice: an animal model of solvent-induced psychosis. World J Biol Psychiatry. 2010;11(6):792–802.
625. Perron BE, Howard MO. Adolescent inhalant use, abuse and dependence. Addiction. 2009;104(7):1185–92.
626. Shoval G, Zalsman G, Nahshoni E, Weizman A. The use of illicit substances in adolescent schizophrenia inpatients. Int J Adolesc Med Health. 2006;18(4):643–8.

627. Maremmani AGI, Dell'Osso L, Pacini M, Popovic D, Rovai L, Torrens M, Perugi G, Maremmani I. Dual diagnosis and chronology of illness in 1090 treatment seeking Italian heroin dependent patients. J Addict Dis. 2011;30(2):123–35.

628. Gold MS, Redmond DE, Donabedian RK, Goodwin FK, Extein I. Increase in serum prolactin by exogenous and endogenous opiates: evidence for antidopamine and antipsychotic effects. Am J Psychiatry. 1978;135:1415–6.

629. Bart G, Borg L, Schluger JH, Green M, Ho A, Kreek MJ. Suppressed prolactin response to dynorphin A1-13 in methadone-maintained versus control subjects. J Pharmacol Exp Ther. 2003;306(2):581–7.

630. Schmauss C, Yassouridis A, Emrich HM. Antipsychotic effect of buprenorphine in schizophrenia. Am J Psychiatry. 1987;144(10):1340–2.

631. Holtzman SG. Phencyclidine-like discriminative stimulus properties of psychotomimetic opioids. Ann NY Acad Sci. 1982;398:230–9.

632. Jaffee JH, Martin WR. Opioid analgesics and antagonists. In: Gilman AG, Rall WR, Nies AS, Taylor P, editors. Goodman and gilmans: the pharmacological basis of therapeutics. 8th ed. New York: Pergamon Press; 1990. p. 488–521.

633. Heikkila L, Rimon R, Terenius L. Dynorphin a and substance P in the cerebrospinal fluid of schizophrenic patients. Psychiatry Res. 1990;34(3):229–36.

634. Volavka J, Anderson B, Koz G. Naloxone and naltrexone in mentall illness and tardive diskynesia. Ann N Y Acad Sci. 1982;398:97–102.

635. Shreeram SS, McDonald T, Dennison S. Psychosis after ultrarapid opiate detoxification. Am J Psychiatry. 2001;158(6):970.

636. Weibel S, Mallaret M, Bennouna-Greene M, Bertschy G. A case of acute psychosis after buprenorphine withdrawal: abrupt versus progressive discontinuation could make a difference. J Clin Psychiatry. 2012;73(6):e756.

637. Bell M. Morphine and morphinomania. N Y State Med J. 1911;93:680–2.

638. Schwartz JM, Ksir C, Koob GF, Bloom FE. Changes in Locomotor response to beta-endorphin microinfusion during and after opiate abstinence syndrome—a proposal for a model of the onset of mania. Psychiatry Res. 1982;7(2):153–61.

639. Pfeffer AZ, Ruble DC. Chronic psychoses and addiction to morphine. Arch Neurol Psychiatr. 1946;56:655–72.

640. Gerard DL, Kornetsky C. Adolescent opiate addiction: a study of control and addict sujects. Psychoanal Q. 1955;19:457–86.

641. Cobo J, Ramos MM, Pelaez T, Garcia G, Marsal F. Psychosis related to methadone withdrawal. Acta Neuropsychiatrica. 2006;18(1):50–1.

642. Karila L, Berlin I, Benyamina A, Reynaud M. Psychotic symptoms following buprenorphine withdrawal. Am J Psychiatry. 2008;165(3):400–1.

643. American Psychiatric Association. Diagnostic and statistical manual of mental disorders, DSM-IV. Washington, DC: American Psychiatric Association; 1994.

644. Evans JD, Heaton RK, Paulsen JS, McAdams LA, Heaton SC, Jeste DV. Schizoaffective disorder: a form of schizophrenia or affective disorder? J Clin Psychiatry. 1999;60(12):874–82.

645. Akiskal HS, Puzantian VR. Psychotic forms of depression and mania. Psychiatr Clin North Am. 1979;2:419–39.

646. Dervaux A, Bayle FJ, Laqueille X, Bourdel MC, Le Borgne MH, Olie JP, Krebs MO. Is substance abuse in schizophrenia related to impulsivity, sensation seeking or anhedonia? Am J Psychiatry. 2001;158(3):492–4.

647. Mueser KT, Yarnold PR, Rosenberg SD, Swett CJ, Miles KM, Hill D. Substance use disorder in hospitalized severely mentally ill psychiatric patients: prevalence, correlates, and subgroupds. Schizophr Bull. 2000;26(1):179–92.

648. Kane JM, Carson WH, Saha AR, McQuade RD, Ingenito GG, Zimbroff DL, Ali MW. Efficacy and safety of aripiprazole and haloperidol versus placebo in patients with schizophrenia and schizoaffective disorder. J Clin Psychiatry. 2002;63(9):763–71.

649. Meltzer HY, Arvanitis L, Bauer D, Rein W. Meta-Trial Study Group. Placebo-controlled evaluation of four novel compounds for the treatment of schizophrenia and schizoaffective disorder. Am J Psychiatry. 2004;161(6):975–84.
650. Potkin SG, Saha AR, Kujawa MJ, Carson WH, Ali M, Stock E, Stringfellow J, Ingenito GG, Marder SR. Aripiprazole, an antipsychotic with a novel mechanism of action, and risperidone vs placebo in patients with schizophrenia and schizoaffective disorder. Arch Gen Psychiatry. 2003;60(7):681–90.
651. Sharma RP, Strakowski SM. A double-blind, randomized, prospective evaluation of the efficacy and safety of risperidone versus haloperidol in the treatment of schizoaffective disorder. J Clin Psychopharmacol. 2001;21(4):360–8.
652. Simpson GM, Glick ID, Weiden PJ, Romano SJ. Randomized, controlled, double-blind multicenter comparison of the efficacy and tolerability of ziprasidone and olanzapine in acutely ill inpatients with schizophrenia or schizoaffective disorder. Am J Psychiatry. 2004;161(10):1837–47.
653. Small JP, Klapper MH, Malloy FW, Steadman TM. Tolerability and efficacy of clozapine combined with lithium in schizophrenia and schizoaffective disorder. J Clin Psychopharmacol. 2003;23(3):223–8.
654. Volavka J, Czobor P, Sheitman B, Lindenmayer JP, Citrome L, McEvoy JP, Cooper TB, Chakos M, Lieberman JA. Clozapine, olanzapine, risperidone, and haloperidol in the treatment of patients with chronic schizophrenia and schizoaffective disorder. Am J Psychiatry. 2002;159(2):255–62.
655. Marneros A. Expanding the group of bipolar disorders. J Affect Disord. 2001;62(1–2):39–44.
656. Spitzer RL, Endicott J, Robins E. Research diagnostic criteria (RDC). New York: New York State Psychiatric Institute; 1975.
657. Andreasson S, Allebeck P, Engstrom A, Rydberg U. Cannabis and schizophrenia. Lancet. 1987;2:1483–5.
658. Andreasson S, Allebeck P, Ryberg U. Schizophrenia in users and nonusers of cannabis: a longitudinal study in Stockolm County. Acta Psychiatr Scand. 1989;79:505–10.
659. Bell DS. Comparison of amphetamine psychosis and schizophrenia. Br J Psychiatry. 1965;3:701–6.
660. Connell PH. Amphetamine psychosis. In: Maudsley monographs, N°5. New York: Oxford University Press; 1958. p. 15–36.
661. Kolansky H, Moore WT. Effects of marihuana on adolescents and young adults. JAMA. 1971;216:486–92.
662. Post R. Cocaine psychosis: a continuum model. Am J Psychiatry. 1975;132:225–30.
663. Rounsaville B, Anton S, Carroll K, Budde D, Prusoff BA, Gawin F. Psychiatric diagnosis of treatment seeking cocaine abusers. Arch Gen Psychiatry. 1991;48:43–51.
664. Sato M, Chen CC, Akiyama K, Otsuki S. Acute exacerbation of paranoid psychotic state after long-term abstinence in patients with previous methamphetamine psychosis. Biol Psychiatry. 1983;18:429–40.
665. Nakatani Y, Yoshizawa J, Yamada H, Iwanami A, Sakaguchi M, Katoh N. Methamphetamine psychosis in Japan: a survey. Br J Addict. 1989;84:1548–9.
666. Yukitaki EA. Amphetamine psychosis in Tokio: its clinical features and social problems. Enolia Psychiatrica and Neurologica Japonica. 1983;37:115–20.
667. Utena H. Behavioral aberrations in methamphetamine intoxicated animals and chemical correlates in the brain. In: Tokizanet T, Schade JP, editors. Brain res. Amsterdam: Elsevier; 1966. p. 192–207.
668. Series H, Boeles S, et al. Psychiatric complications of 'ecstasy' use. J Psychopharmacol (Oxf). 1994;8:60–1.
669. Davis BL. The PCP epidemic: a critical review. Int J Addict. 1982;17:1137–55.
670. Tomiyama G. Chronic schizophrenia-like states in methamphetamine psychosis. Jpn J Psychiatry Neurol. 1990;44:531–9.
671. Krausz M, Verthein U, Dekwitz P. Prevalence of psychiatric disorders in opiate dependent patients in contact with the drug treatment system. Nervenarzt. 1998;69(7):557–67.

672. McLellan AT, Woody GE, O'Brien CP. Development of psychiatric illness in drug abusers: possible role of drug preference. N Engl J Med. 1979;301:1310–4.

673. Verdoux H, Mury M, Besancon G, Bourgeois M. Comparative study of substance dependence comorbidity in bipolar, schizophrenic and schizoaffective disorders. Encéphale. 1996;22(2):95–101.

674. Brown ES, Jeffress J, Liggin JD, Garza M, Beard L. Switching outpatients with bipolar or schizoaffective disorders and substance abuse from their current antipsychotic to aripiprazole. J Clin Psychiatry. 2005;66(6):756–60.

675. Zimmett SV, Strous RD, Burgess ES, Kohnstamm S, Green AL. Effects of clozapine on substance use in patients with schizophrenia and schizoaffective disorder: a retrospective survey. J Clin Pharmacol. 2000;20(1):94–8.

676. Dixon L. Dual diagnosis of substance abuse in schizophrenia: prevalence and impact on outcome. Schizophr Res. 1999;35(S):93–100.

677. Mueser KT, Bennett M, Kushner MG. Epidemiology of substance use disorder among persons with chronic mental illness. In: Lehman AF, Dixon LB, editors. Double jeopardy: chronic mental illness and substance use disorder. Bern: Harwood Academic Publisher; 1995. p. 9–26.

678. Buckley P, Thompson P, Way L, Melzer HY. Substance abuse among patients with treatment resistant schizophrenia: characteristics and implications for clozapine therapy. Am J Psychiatry. 1994;151(3):385–9.

679. Dixon L, Haas G, Weiden PJ, Sweeney J, Frances AJ. Acute effects of drug abuse in schizophrenic patients: clinical observations and patients' self report. Schizophr Bull. 1990;16:69–79.

680. Kane J. What Can we achieve by implementing a compliance-improvement program? Int Clin Psychopharmacol. 1997;12(S):43–6.

681. Yovell Y, Opler LA. Clozapine reverses cocaine craving in a treatment resistant mentally ill chemical abuser: a case report and a hypothesis. J Nerv Ment Dis. 1994;182:591–2.

682. Woolverton RH, Johnson P. Neurobiology of cocaine abuse. Trends Pharmacol Sci. 1992;13:193–200.

683. Mueser KT, Yarnold PR, Levinson DF, Singh H, Bellack AS, Kee K, Morrison RL, Yadalam KG. Prevalence of substance abuse in schizophrenia: demographic and clinical correlates. Schizophr Bull. 1990;16:31–56.

684. Kristal JH, D'souza DC, Madonick S, Petrakis IL. Toward rational pharmacotherapy of comorbid substance abuse in schizophrenic patients. Schizophr Res. 1999;35(S):35–9.

685. Brady K, Anton R, Ballenger JC, Lydiard RB, Adinoff B, Selander J. Cocaine abuse among schizophrenic patients. Am J Psychiatry. 1990;147:1164–7.

686. Karper LP, Freeman GK, Grillon C, Morgan CAR, Charney DS, Krystal JH. Preliminary evidence of an association between sensorimotor gating and distractibility Il psychosis. J Neuropsychiatry Clin Neurosci. 1996;8:60–6.

687. Lysaker P, Bell M, Beam-Goulet J, Milstein R. Relationship of positive and negative symptoms to cocaine abuse in schizophrenia. J Nerv Ment Dis. 1994;182:109–12.

688. Cloninger CR, Svrakic DM, Przybeck TR. A psychobiological model of temperament and character. Arch Gen Psychiatry. 1993;50:975–90.

689. Tsuang M, Simpson J, Kronfol Z. Subtypes of drug abuse with psychosis. Arch Gen Psychiatry. 1982;39:141–7.

690. Covey LS, Glassman AH, Stetner F. Major depression following smoking cessation. Am J Psychiatry. 1997;154:263–5.

691. Siris SG, Bermazohn PC, Mason SC, Shuwall MA. Antidepressants for substance abusing schizophrenic patients: a mini review. Prog Neuro-Psychopharmacol Biol Psychiatry. 1991;15:1–13.

692. Brady KT, Grice DE, Dustan L, Randall C. Gender differences in substance use disorders. Am J Psychiatry. 1993;150(11):1707–11.

693. Siris SG, Kane JM, Frechen K, Sellew AP, Mandeli J, Fasano-Dube B. Histories of substance abuse in patients with postpsychotic depression. Compr Psychiatry. 1988;29:550–7.

694. Calabrese JR, Kimmel SE, Woyshville MJ, Rapport DJ, Faust CJ, Thompson PA, Meltzer HY. Clozapine for treatment refractory mania. Am J Psychiatry. 1996;153:759–64.
695. Siris SG. Pharmacological treatment of substance-abusing schizophrenic patients. Schizophr Bull. 1990;16(1):111–22.
696. Schneier FR, Siris SG. A review of psychoactive substance use and abuse in shizophrenia: patterns of drug choice. J Nerv Ment Dis. 1987;175:641–50.
697. Mueser KT, Nishith P, Tracy JI, Di Girolamo J, Molinaro M. Expectation and motives for substance use in schizophrenia. Schizophr Bull. 1995;21:367–78.
698. Mueser KT, Bellack AS, Blanchard JJ. Comorbidity of schizophrenia and substance abuse: implications for treatment. J Consult Clin Psychol. 1992;60:845–56.
699. Dixon L, Haas G, Weiden PJ, Sweeney J, Frances AJ. Acute effects of drug abuse in schizophrenic patients: clinical correlates and reasons for use. Am J Psychiatry. 1991;148:224–30.
700. Brenner LM, Karper LP, Krystal JH. Short term use of disulfiram with clozapine. J Clin Pharmacol. 1994;14:213–5.
701. Regier DA, Farmer ME, Rae DS, Locke BZ, Keith SJ, Judd LL, Goodwin FK. Comorbidity of mental disorders with alchool and other drug abuse. JAMA. 1990;19(264):2511–8.
702. Maremmani AGI, Bacciardi S, Rovai L, Rugani F, Dell'Osso L, Maremmani I. Natural history of addiction in psychotic heroin addicted patients at their first agonist opioid treatment. Addict Disord Their Treat. 2013;12(1):31–9.
703. Maremmani I, Pani PP, Pacini M, Perugi G. Substance use and quality of life over 12 months among buprenorphine maintenance-treated and methadone maintenance-treated heroin-addicted patients. J Subst Abus Treat. 2007;33(1):91–8.
704. Maremmani I, Pacini M, Lovrecic M, Lubrano S, Perugi G. Maintenance therapy with opioid agonist for heroin addicted patients. Usefulness in the treatment of comorbid psychiatric diseases. In: Waal H, Haga E, editors. Maintenance treatment of heroin addiction. Evidence at the crossroads. Oslo: Cappelen Akademisk Forlag; 2003. p. 221–33.
705. Tenore PL. Psychotherapeutic benefits of opioid agonist therapy. J Addict Dis. 2008;27(3):49–65.
706. Pani PP, Maremmani I, Pacini M, Lamanna F, Maremmani AGI, Dell'Osso L. Effect of psychiatric severity on the outcome of methadone maintenance treatment. Eur Addict Res. 2011;17(2):80–9.
707. Maremmani I, Pani PP, Popovic D, Pacini M, Deltito J, Perugi G. Improvement of quality of life in heroin addicts: differences between methadone and buprenorphine treatment. Heroin Addict Relat Clin Probl. 2008;10(1):41–8.
708. Pani PP, Maremmani I, Pirastu R, Tagliamonte A, Gessa GL. Buprenorphine: a controlled clinical trial in the treatment of opioid dependence. Drug Alcohol Depend. 2000;60(1):39–50.
709. Pani PP, Trogu E, Carboni G, Palla P, Loi A. Psychiatric severity and treatment response in methadone maintenance treatment programmes: new evidence. Heroin Addict Relat Clin Probl. 2003;5(3):22–36.
710. Kessler RC, Nelson CB, McGonagle KA, Edlund MJ, Frank RG, Leaf PJ. The epidemiology of co-occurring addictive and mental disorders: implications for prevention and service utilization. Am J Orthopsychiatry. 1996;66(1):17–31.
711. Grant BF, Stinson FS, Dawson DA, Chou SP, Dufour MC, Compton W, Pickering RP, Kaplan K. Prevalence and co-occurrence of substance use disorders and independent mood and anxiety disorders: results from the National Epidemiologic Survey on alcohol and related conditions. Arch Gen Psychiatry. 2004;61(8):807–16.
712. Merikangas KR, Mehta RL, Molnar BE, Walters EE, Swendsen JD, Aguilar-Gaziola S, Bijl R, Borges G, Caraveo-Anduaga JJ, DeWit DJ, Kolody B, Vega WA, Wittchen HU, Kessler RC. Comorbidity of substance use disorders with mood and anxiety disorders: results of the international consortium in psychiatric epidemiology. Addict Behav. 1998;23(6):893–907.
713. Lahmeyer HW, Channon RA, Schlemmer FJ. Psychoactive substance abuse. In: Flaherty JA, Channon RA, Devis JM, editors. Psychiatry. Diagnosis & terapy. San Mateo, CA: Appleton & Lange; 1988. p. 182–99.

714. Dyer K, White J, Foster D, Bochner F, Menelaou A, Somogyi A. The relationship between mood state and plasma methadone concentration in maintenance patients. J Clin Psychopharmacol. 2001;21(1):78–84.

715. Angst J. The bipolar spectrum. Br J Psychiatry. 2007;190:189–91.

716. Kessler RC, Aguilar-Gaxiola S, Bijl R, Borges G, Caraveo-Anduaga JJ. Cross-national comparison of comorbidities between substance use disorders and mental disorders. Results Fron the international consortium in psychiatric epidemiology. In: Bukoski WJ, Sloboda Z, editors. Handbook for drug abuse prevention. Theory, science and practice. New York: Plenum Publisher; 2003. p. 448–71.

717. Wittchen HU, Perkonigg A, Reed V. Comorbidity of mental disorders and substance use disorders. Eur Addict Res. 1996;2:36–47.

718. Cruickshank CC, Dyer KR. A review of the clinical pharmacology of methamphetamine. Addiction. 2009;104(7):1085–99.

719. Caton CL, Drake RE, Hasin DS, Dominguez B, Shrout PE, Samet S, Schanzer B. Differences between early phase primary psychotic disorders with concurrent substance. Arch Gen Psychiatry. 2005;62(2):137–45.

720. Schuckit MA, Saunders JB. The empirical basis of substance use disorders diagnosis: research recommendations for the diagnostic and statistical manual of mental disorders, fifth edition (DSM-V). Addiction. 2006;101(Suppl 1):170–3.

721. Brady K, Casto S, Lydiand RB, Malcolm R, Arana G. Substance abuse in an inpatient psychiatric sample. Am J Drug Alcohol Abuse. 1991;17:389–97.

722. Bartlett E, Hallin A, Chapman B, Angrist B. Selective sensitization to the psychosis-inducing effects of cocaine: a possible marker for addiction relapse vulnerability? Neuropsychopharmacology. 1997;16(1):77–82.

723. Griffith JD. Experimental psychosis induced by the administration of D-amphetamine. In: Costa E, Garattini S, editors. Amphetamine and related compounds. New York: Raven Press; 1970. p. 876–904.

724. Angrist BM, Gershon S. The phenomenology of experimentally induced amphetamine psychosis. Preliminary observations. Biol Psychiatry. 1970;2:95–107.

725. Bell DS. The experimental reproduction of amphetamine psychosis. Arch Gen Psychiatry. 1973;29:35–40.

726. Janowsky DS, Risch C. Amphetamine psychosis and psychotic symptoms. Psychopharmacology. 1979;65:73–7.

727. Angrist B. Amphetamine psychosis: clinical variations of the syndrome. In: Cho AK, Segal DS, editors. Amphetamine and its analogs. New York: Academic Press; 1995. p. 387–414.

728. Kalayasiri R, Sughondhabirom A, Gueorguieva R, Coric V, Lynch WJ, Morgan PT, Cubells JF, Malison RT. Self-reported paranoia during laboratory "binge" cocaine self administration in humans. Pharmacol Biochem Behav. 2006;83:249–56.

729. Lucas AR, Weiss M. Methylphenidate hallucinosis. JAMA. 1971;217:1079–81.

730. Gelperin K, Phelan K. Psychiatric adverse events associated with drug treatment of ADHD: review of Postmarketing safety data. FDA report PID D050243. US Food and Drug Administration. 2006. https://www.fda.gov/ohrms/dockets/ac/06/briefing/2006-4210b_11_01_AdverseEvents.pdf. Accessed 18 March 2009.

731. Mosholder A. Psychiatric adverse events in clinical trials of drugs for ADHD. FDA Report PID D060163. US Food and Drug Administration. 2006). http://www.fda.gov/ohrms/dockets/ac/06/briefing/2006-4210b_10_01_Mosholder.pdf. Accessed 3 March 2010.

732. Phelan K. Summary of psychiatric and neurological adverse events from June 2005 1-year post pediatric exclusivity reviews of concerta and other methylphenidate products. US Food and Drug Administration. 2006. https://www.fda.gov/ohrms/dockets/ac/06/briefing/2006-4210b_09_01_Methsummary.pdf. Accessed 18 March 2009.

733. Phelan KM. One year post-pediatric exclusivity postmarketing adverse event review: Adderall XR. FDA report PID D040761. US Food and Drug Administration. 2006. https://www.fda.gov/ohrms/dockets/ac/06/briefing/20064210b_05_02_AdderallSafetyreview.Pdf. Accessed 18 March 2009.

734. Reichart CG, Nolen WA. Earlier onset of bipolar disorder in children by antidepressants or stimulants? An hypothesis. J Affect Disord. 2004;78:81–4.

735. Ross RG. Psychotic and manic-like symptoms during stimulant treatment of attention deficit hyperactivity disorder. Am J Psychiatry. 2006;163(7):1149–52.

736. Thomas H. A community survey of adverse effects of cannabis use. Drug Alcohol Depend. 1996;42(3):201–7.

737. Chaudry HR, Moss HB, Bashir A, Suliman T. Cannabis psychosis following bhang ingestion. Br J Addict. 1991;86:1075–81.

738. Solomons K, Neppe VM, Kuyl JM. Toxic cannabis psychosis is a valid entity. S Afr Med J. 1990;78:476–81.

739. Wylie AS, Scott RTA, Burnett SJ. Psychosis due to 'skunk'. BMJ. 1995;311:125.

740. Zammit S, Allebeck P, Andreasson S, Lundberg I, Lewis G. Self reported cannabis use as risk factor for schizophrenia in Swedish conscript of 1969: historical cohort study. Br Med J. 2002;325:1195.

741. Andreasen S, Allebeck P, Engstrom A, Rydberg U. Cannabis and schizophrenia. A longitudinal study of Swedish conscripts. Lancet. 1987;2:1483–6.

742. Van Os J, Bak M, Hansenn M, Bijl RV, De Graaf R, Verdoux H. Cannabis use and psychosis: a longitudinal population-based study. Am J Epidemiol. 2002;156(3):19–27.

743. Arseneault L, Cannon M, Poulton R, Murray R, Caspi A, Moffit TE. Cannabis use in adolescence and risk for adult psychosis: longitudinal study. Br Med J. 2002;325(11):1212–3.

744. Degenhardt L, Hall W, Lynskey M. Testing hypotheses about the relationship between cannabis use and psychosis. Drug Alcohol Depend. 2003;71:37–48.

745. Khantzian EJ. The ego, the self and opiate addiction: theoretical and treatment considerations. In: Blaine JD, Julius EA, editors. Psychodinamics of drug dependence, NIDA Research Monograph No. 12; HEW Pub No. 101–116. Washington, DC: U.S. Government Printing Office; 1977.

746. Khantzian EJ. Self-regulation and self-medication factors in alcoholism and the addictions: similarities and differences. Recent Dev Alcohol. 1990;8:255–71.

747. Rauch L. The poet syndrome: opiates, psychosis and creativity. J Psychoactive Drugs. 2000;32(3):343–9.

748. Berger PA, Watson SJ, Akil H, Elliot GR, Rubin RT, Pfefferbaum A. Betaendorphin and schizophrenia. Arch Gen Psychiatry. 1980;37:635–40.

749. Wurmser L. Psychoanalytic considerations of the etiology of compulsive drug use. J Am Psychoanal Assoc. 1974;22(4):820–43.

750. Khantzian EJ. An ego/self theory of substance dependence: a contemporary psychoanalitic perspective. NIDA Res Monogr. 1980;30:29–33.

751. McKenna GJ. The use of methadone as a psychotropic agent. Nat Conf Methadone Treat Proc. 1973;5:1317–24.

752. Woody GE, McLellan AT, Luborsky L. Sociopathy and psychotherapy outcome. Arch Gen Psychiatry. 1985;42:1081–6.

753. Gandhi DH, Bogrov MU, Osher FC, Myers CP. A comparison of the patterns of drug use among patients with and without severe mental illness. Am J Addict. 2003;12(5):424–31.

754. Tournier M, Sorbara F, Gindre C, Swendsenm JD, Verdoux H. Cannabis use and anxiety in daily life: a naturalistic investigation in a non-clinical population. Psychiatry Res. 2003;118(1):1–8.

755. Ogborne AC, Smart RG, Weber T, Birchmore-Timney C. Who is using cannabis as a medicine and why: an exploratory study. J Psychoactive Drugs. 2000;32(4):435–43.

756. Aharonovich E, Nguyen HT, Nunes EV. Anger and depressive states among treatment-seeking drug abusers: testing the psychopharmacological specificity hypothesis. Am J Addict. 2001;10(4):327–34.

757. Perugi G, Frare F, Madaro D, Maremmani I, Akiskal HS. Alcohol abuse in social phobic patients: is there a bipolar connection? J Affect Disord. 2002;68(1):33–9.

758. Schuckit MA, Tipp JE, Bucholz KK, Nurnberger JI, Hesselbrock Crowe RR, Kramer J. The life-time rates of three major mood disorders and four major anxiety disorders in alcoholics and controls. Addiction. 1997;92(10):1289–304.

759. Gilder DA, Wall TL, Ehlers CL. Comorbidity of select anxiety and affective disorders with alcohol dependence in Southwest California Indians. Alcohol Clin Exp Res. 2004;28:1805–13.

760. Hesselbrock MN, Hesselbrock VM, Segal B, Schuckit MA, Bucholz K. Ethnicity and psychiatric comorbidity among alcohol-dependent persons who receive inpatient. Alcohol Clin Exp Res. 2003;27(8):1368–73.

761. Brown SA, Schuckit MA. Changes in depression among abstinent alcoholics. J Stud Alcohol. 1988;49:312–7.

762. Mueller TI, Lavori PW, Keller MB, Swartz A, Warshaw M, Hasin D. Prognostic effect of the variable course of alcoholism on the 10-year course of depression. Am J Psychiatry. 1994;151:701–6.

763. Conner KR, Sörensen S, Leonard KE. Initial depression and subsequent drinking during alcoholism treatment. J Stud Alcohol. 2005;66:401–6.

764. Birnbaum I, Taylor T, Parker E. Alcohol and sober mood state in female social drinkers. Alcohol Clin Exp Res. 1983;7:362–8.

765. Strakowski SM, McElroy SL, Keck PEJ, West SA. The effects of antecedent substance abuse on the development of first-episode psychotic mania. J Psychiatr Res. 1996;30(1):59–68.

766. Strakowski SM, Sax KW, McElroy SL, Keck PEJ, Hawkins JM, West SA. Course of psychiatric and substance abuse syndromes co-occurring with bipolar disorder after a first psychiatric hospitalization. J Clin Psychiatry. 1998;59(9):465–71.

767. Strakowski SM, DelBello MP, Fleck DE, Alder CM, Anthenelli RM, Keck PE, Arnold LM, Amicone J. Effects of co-occurring alcohol abuse on the course of bipolar disorder following a first hospitalization for mania. Arch Gen Psychiatry. 2000;62(8):851–8.

768. Favazza AR. Bodies under siege self-mutilation and body modification in culture and psychiatry. Baltimore, MD: The Johns Hopkins University Press; 1996.

769. Whitlock J, Knox KL. The relationship between self-injurious behavior and suicide in a young adult population. Arch Pediatr Adolesc Med. 2007;161(7):634–40.

770. White Kress VE. Self-injurious behaviors: assessment and diagnosis. J Couns Dev. 2003;81(4):490–6.

771. Gratz KL. Measurement of deliberate self-harm: preliminary data on the deliberate self-harm inventory. J Psychopathol Behav Assess. 2001;23:253–63.

772. Evren C, Evren B. Self-mutilation in substance-dependent patients and relationship with childhood abuse and neglect, alexithymia and temperament and character dimensions of personality. Drug Alcohol Depend. 2005;80(1):15–22.

773. Muehlenkamp JJ, Gutierrez PM. An investigation of differences between self-injurious behavior and suicide attempts in a sample of adolescents. Suicide Life Threat Behav. 2004;34(1):12–23.

774. Sansone RA, Levitt JL. Self-harm behaviors among those with eating disorders: an overview. Eat Disord. 2002;10(3):205–13.

775. Grossman R, Siever L. Impulsive self-injurious behaviors: phenomenology, neurobiology and treatment. In: Simeon D, Hollander E, editors. Self-injurious behaviors. American Psychiatric Publishing: Washington, DC; 2001. p. 117–48.

776. Faye P. Addictive characteristics of the behavior of self-mutilation. J Psychosoc Nurs Ment Health Serv. 1995;33(6):36–9.

777. Washburn JJ, Juzwin KR, Styer DM, Aldridge D. Measuring the urge to self-injure: preliminary data from a clinical sample. Psychiatry Res. 2010;178(3):540–4.

778. Nixon MK, Cloutier PF, Aggarwal S. Affect regulation and addictive aspects of repetitive self-injury in hospitalized adolescents. J Am Acad Child Adolesc Psychiatry. 2002;41(11):1333–41.

779. Victor SE, Glenn CR, Klonsky ED. Is non-suicidal self-injury an "addiction"? A comparison of craving in substance use and non-suicidal self-injury. Psychiatry Res. 2012;197(1–2):73–7.

780. Sher L, Stanley BH. The role of endogenous opioids in the pathophysiology of self-injurious and suicidal behavior. Arch Suicide Res. 2008;12(4):299–308.
781. Kitanaka J, Kitanaka N, Hall FS, Uhl GR, Fukushima Y, Sawai T, Watabe K, Kubo H, Takahashi H, Tanaka K, Nishiyama N, Tatsuta T, Morita Y, Takemura M. The selective mu opioid receptor antagonist beta-funaltrexamine attenuates methamphetamine-induced stereotypical biting in mice. Brain Res. 2013;1522:88–98.
782. Kempf DJ, Baker KC, Gilbert MH, Blanchard JL, Dean RL, Deaver DR, Bohm RP Jr. Effects of extended-release injectable naltrexone on self-injurious behavior in rhesus macaques (Macaca Mulatta). Comp Med. 2012;62(3):209–17.
783. Symons FJ, Tapp J, Wulfsberg A, Sutton KA, Heeth WL, Bodfish JW. Sequential analysis of the effects of naltrexone on the environmental mediation of self-injurious behavior. Exp Clin Psychopharmacol. 2001;9(3):269–76.
784. Modesto-Lowe V, Van Kirk J. Clinical uses of naltrexone: a review of the evidence. Exp Clin Psychopharmacol. 2002;10(3):213–27.
785. Odlaug BL, Grant JE. Pathologic skin picking. Am J Drug Alcohol Abuse. 2010;36(5):296–303.
786. Roth AS, Ostroff RB, Hoffman RE. Naltrexone as a treatment for repetitive self-injurious behaviour:an open-label trial. J Clin Psychiatry. 1996;57(6):233–7.
787. Sandman CA, Hetrick W, Taylor DV, Marion SD, Touchette P, Barron JL, Martinezzi V, Steinberg RM, Crinella FM. Long-term effects of naltrexone on self-injurious behavior. Am J Ment Retard. 2000;105(2):103–17.
788. Thompson T, Hackenberg T, Cerutti D, Baker D, Axtell S. Opioid antagonist effects on self-injury in adults with mental retardation: response form and location as determinants of medication effects. Am J Ment Retard. 1994;99(1):85–102.
789. Gratz KL. Risk factors for and functions of deliberate self-harm: an empirical and conceptual review. Clin Psychol (New York). 2003;10(2):192–205.
790. Winchel RM, Stanley M. Self-injurious behavior: a review of the behavior and biology of self-mutilation. Am J Psychiatry. 1991;148(3):306–17.
791. Fong T. Self-mutilation: impulsive traits suggest new drug therapies. Curr Psychiat. 2003;2:1–8.
792. Nishida A, Sasaki T, Nishimura Y, Tanii H, Hara N, Inoue K, Yamada T, Takami T, Shimodera S, Itokawa M, Asukai N, Okazaki Y. Psychotic-like experiences are associated with suicidal feelings and deliberate self-harm behaviors in adolescents aged 12–15 years. Acta Psychiatr Scand. 2010;121(4):301–7.
793. Pluck G, Lekka NP, Sarkar S, Lee KH, Bath PA, Sharif O, Woodruff PW. Clinical and neuropsychological aspects of non-fatal self-harm in schizophrenia. Eur Psychiatry. 2013;28(6):344–8.
794. Hafner H, Loffler W, Maurer K, Hambrecht M, an der Heiden W. Depression, negative symptoms, social stagnation and social decline in the early course of schizophrenia. Acta Psychiatr Scand. 1999;100(2):105–18.
795. Milak MS, Aniskin DB, Eisenberg DP, Prikhojan A, Cohen LJ, Yard SS, Galynker II. The negative syndrome as a dimension: factor analyses of PANSS in major depressive disorder and organic brain disease compared with negative syndrome structures found in the schizophrenia literature. Cogn Behav Neurol. 2007;20(2):113–20.
796. Winograd-Gurvich C, Fitzgerald PB, Georgiou-Karistianis N, Bradshaw JL, White OB. Negative symptoms: a review of schizophrenia, melancholic depression and Parkinson's disease. Brain Res Bull. 2006;70(4–6):312–21.
797. Tamminga CA, Buchanan RW, Gold JM. The role of negative symptoms and cognitive dysfunction in schizophrenia outcome. Int Clin Psychopharmacol. 1998;13(Suppl 3):S21–6.
798. O'Leary DS, Flaum M, Kesler ML, Flashman LA, Arndt S, Andreasen NC. Cognitive correlates of the negative, disorganized, and psychotic symptom dimensions of schizophrenia. J Neuropsychiatry Clin Neurosci. 2000;12(1):4–15.
799. Sax KW, Strakowski SM, Keck PE Jr, Upadhyaya VH, West SA, McElroy SL. Relationships among negative, positive, and depressive symptoms in schizophrenia and psychotic depression. Br J Psychiatry. 1996;168(1):68–71.

800. Gerbaldo H, Fickinger MP, Wetzel H, Helisch A, Philipp M, Benkert O. Primary enduring negative symptoms in schizophrenia and major depression. J Psychiatr Res. 1995;29(4):297–302.
801. Toomey R, Faraone SV, Simpson JC, Tsuang MT. Negative, positive, and disorganized symptom dimensions in schizophrenia, major depression, and bipolar disorder. J Nerv Ment Dis. 1998;186(8):470–6.
802. Maziade M, Roy MA, Martinez M, Cliche D, Fournier JP, Garneau Y, Nicole L, Montgrain N, Dion C, Ponton AM. Negative, psychoticism, and disorganized dimensions in patients with familial schizophrenia or bipolar disorder: continuity and discontinuity between the major psychoses. Am J Psychiatry. 1995;152(10):1458–63.
803. Lewine RR. A discriminant validity study of negative symptoms with a special focus on depression and antipsychotic medication. Am J Psychiatry. 1990;147(11):1463–6.
804. Chaturvedi SK, Sarmukaddam SB. Prediction of outcome in depression by negative symptoms. Acta Psychiatr Scand. 1986;74(2):183–6.
805. Bonanno GA, Neria Y, Mancini A, Coifman KG, Litz B, Insel B. Is there more to complicated grief than depression and posttraumatic stress disorder? A test of incremental validity. J Abnorm Psychol. 2007;116(2):342–51.
806. Shear K, Shair H. Attachment, loss, and complicated grief. Dev Psychobiol. 2005;47(3):253–67.
807. Shear K, Monk T, Houck P, Melhem N, Frank E, Reynolds C, Sillowash R. An attachment-based model of complicated grief including the role of avoidance. Eur Arch Psychiatry Clin Neurosci. 2007;257(8):453–61.
808. Stroebe M, Boelen PA, van den Hout M, Stroebe W, Salemink E, van den Bout J. Ruminative coping as avoidance: a reinterpretation of its function in adjustment to bereavement. Eur Arch Psychiatry Clin Neurosci. 2007;257(8):462–72.
809. Prigerson HG, Frank E, Kasl SV, Reynolds CF 3rd, Anderson B, Zubenko GS, Houck PR, George CJ, Kupfer DJ. Complicated grief and bereavement-related depression as distinct disorders: preliminary empirical validation in elderly bereaved spouses. Am J Psychiatry. 1995;152(1):22–30.
810. Boelen PA, Huntjens RJ, van Deursen DS, van den Hout MA. Autobiographical memory specificity and symptoms of complicated grief, depression, and posttraumatic stress disorder following loss. J Behav Ther Exp Psychiatry. 2010;41(4):331–7.
811. Olley A, Malhi G, Sachdev P. Memory and executive functioning in obsessive-compulsive disorder: a selective review. J Affect Disord. 2007;104(1–3):15–23.
812. Kuelz AK, Hohagen F, Voderholzer U. Neuropsychological performance in obsessive-compulsive disorder: a critical review. Biol Psychol. 2004;65(3):185–236.
813. Lynskey M, Hall W. The effects of adolescent cannabis use on educational attainment: a review. Addiction. 2000;95(11):1621–30.
814. French ED, Dillon K, Wu X. Cannabinoids excite dopamine neurons in the ventral tegmentum and substantia Nigra. Neuroreport. 1997;8(3):649–52.
815. Gardner EL, Vorel SR. Cannabinoid transmission and reward-related events. Neurobiol Dis. 1998;5(6 Pt B):502–33.
816. Tanda G, Goldberg SR. Cannabinoids: reward, dependence, and underlying neurochemical mechanisms—a review of recent preclinical data. Psychopharmacology. 2003;169(2):115–34.
817. Bossong MG, van Berckel BN, Boellaard R, Zuurman L, Schuit RC, Windhorst AD, van Gerven JM, Ramsey NF, Lammertsma AA, Kahn RS. Delta 9-tetrahydrocannabinol induces dopamine release in the human striatum. Neuropsychopharmacology. 2009;34(3):759–66.
818. Filbey FM, Schacht JP, Myers US, Chavez RS, Hutchison KE. Marijuana craving in the brain. Proc Natl Acad Sci U S A. 2009;106(31):13016–21.
819. Devane WA, Dysarz FA 3rd, Johnson MR, Melvin LS, Howlett AC. Determination and characterization of a cannabinoid receptor in rat brain. Mol Pharmacol. 1988;34(5):605–13.
820. Munro S, Thomas KL, Abu-Shaar M. Molecular characterization of a peripheral receptor for cannabinoids. Nature. 1993;365:61–5.
821. Gardner EL. Addictive potential of cannabinoids: the underlying neurobiology. Chem Phys Lipids. 2002;121(1–2):267–90.

822. Wise RA. Neurobiology of addiction. Curr Opin Neurobiol. 1996;6:243–51.
823. van Hell HH, Vink M, Ossewaarde L, Jager G, Kahn RS, Ramsey NF. Chronic effects of cannabis use on the human reward system: an FMRI study. Eur Neuropsychopharmacol. 2010;20(3):153–63.
824. Howlett AC, Breivogel CS, Childers SR, Deadwyler SA, Hampson RE, Porrino LJ. Cannabinoid physiology and pharmacology: 30 years of progress. Neuropharmacology. 2004;47(Suppl 1):345–58.
825. Sim-Selley LJ. Regulation of cannabinoid CB1 receptors in the central nervous system by chronic cannabinoids. Crit Rev Neurobiol. 2003;15(2):91–119.
826. Bovasso GB. Cannabis abuse as a risk factor for depressive symptoms. Am J Psychiatry. 2001;158(12):2033–7.
827. Janiri L, Martinotti G, Dario T, Reina D, Paparello F, Pozzi G, Addolorato G, Di Giannantonio M, De Risio S. Anhedonia and substance-related symptoms in detoxified substance-dependent subjects: a correlation study. Neuropsychobiology. 2005;52(1):37–44.
828. Tanda G, Pontieri FE, Di Chiara G. Cannabinoid and heroin activation of mesolimbic dopamine transmission by a common M1 opioid receptor mechanism. Science. 1997;276:2048–50.
829. Tanda G, Loddo P, Di Chiara G. Dependence of mesolimbic dopamine transmission on Delta9-tetrahydrocannabinol. Eur J Pharmacol. 1999;376(1–2):23–6.
830. Ledent C, Valverde O, Cossu G, Petitet F, Aubert JF, Beslot F, Boheme GA, Imperato A, Pedrazzini T, Roques BP, Vassart G, Fratta W, Parmentier M. Unresponsiveness to cannabinoid and reduced addictive effects of opiates in CBI receptor knockout mice. Science. 1999;283:401–4.
831. Navarro M, Carrera MR, Fratta W, Valverde O, Cossu G, Fattore L, Chowen JA, Gomez R, del Arco I, Villanua MA, Maldonado R, Koob GF, Rodriguez de Fonseca F. Functional interaction between opioid and cannabinoid receptors in drug self-administration. J Neurosci. 2001;21(14):5344–50.
832. Zimmer A, Valjent E, Konig M, Zimmer AM, Robledo P, Hahn H, Valverde O, Maldonado R. Absence of delta −9-tetrahydrocannabinol dysphoric effects in dynorphin-deficient mice. J Neurosci. 2001;21(23):9499–505.
833. Ghozland S, Matthes HW, Simonin F, Filliol D, Kieffer BL, Maldonado R. Motivational effects of cannabinoids are mediated by mu-opioid and kappa-opioid receptors. J Neurosci. 2002;22(3):1146–54.
834. Maremmani I, Castrogiovanni P. Disturbi Da Uso Di Sostanze. Disturbi Da Oppiacei Ed Analgesici. In: Cassano GB, D'Errico A, Pancheri P, Pavan L, Pazzagli A, Ravizza L, Rossi R, Smeraldi E, Volterra V, editors. Trattato Italiano Di Psichiatria. Milano: Masson; 1992. p. 1148–61.
835. Bozarth MA, Wise R. Heroin reward is dependent on a dopaminergic substrate. Life Sci. 1981;29:1881–6.
836. Karler R, Calder L, Thai L, Bedingfield B. A dopaminergic-glutamatergic basis for the action of amphetamine and cocine. Brain Res. 1994;658:8–14.
837. Roberts DC, Ranaldi R. Effect of dopaminergic drugs on cocaine reinforcement. Clin Neuropharmacol. 1995;18:S84–95.
838. Di Chiara G, Imperato A. Drugs abused by humans preferentially increase synaptic dopamine concentrations in the mesolimbic system of freely moving rats. Proc Natl Acad Sci U S A. 1988;85(14):5274–378.
839. Pontieri FE, Tanda G, Di Chiara G. Intravenous cocaine, morphine, and amphetamine preferentially increase extracellular dopamine in the "shell" as compared with the "core" of the rat nucleus accumbens. Proc Natl Acad Sci U S A. 1995;92(26):12304–8.
840. Drevets WC, Gautier C, Price JC, Kupfer DJ, Kinahan PE, Grace AA, Price JL, Mathis CA. Amphetamine-induced dopamine release in human ventral striatum correlates with euphoria. Biol Psychiatry. 2001;49(2):81–96.
841. Kelley AE, Berridge KC. The neuroscience of natural rewards: relevance to addictive drugs. J Neurosci. 2002;22:3306–11.

842. Berridge KC. The debate over dopamine's role in reward: the case for incentive salience. Psychopharmacology. 2007;191(3):391–431.

843. Hyman SE. Addiction: a disease of learning and memory. Am J Psychiatry. 2005;162:1414–22.

844. Pierce RC, Kalivas PW. A circuitry model of the expression of behavioral sensitization to amphetamine-like psychostimulants. Brain Res. 1997;25(2):192–216.

845. Robinson TE, Berridge KC. Incentive-sensitization and addiction. Addiction. 2001;96(1):103–14.

846. Carlezon WAJ, Nestler EJ. Elevated levels of GluR1 in the midbrain: a trigger for sensitization to drugs of abuse? Trends Neurosci. 2002;25(12):610–5.

847. Vezina P. Sensitization of midbrain dopamine neuron reactivity and the self-administration of psychomotor stimulant drugs. Neurosci Biobehav Rev. 2004;27(8):827–39.

848. Nestler EJ. Common molecular and cellular substrates of addiction and memory. Neurobiol Learn Mem. 2002;78(3):637–47.

849. Bolaños CA, Nestler EJ. Neurotrophic mechanisms in drug addiction. NeuroMolecular Med. 2004;5(1):69–83.

850. Volkow ND, Fowler JS, Wang GJ, Goldstein RZ. Role of dopamine, the frontal cortex and memory circuits in drug addiction: insight from imaging studies. Neurobiol Learn Mem. 2002;78(3):610–24.

851. Robbins TW, Everitt BJ. Limbic-striatal memory systems and drug addiction. Neurobiol Learn Mem. 2002;8(3):625–36.

852. Childress AR, Mozley PD, McElgin W, Fitzgerald J, Reivich M, O'Brien CP. Limbic activation during cue-induced cocaine craving. Am J Psychiatry. 1999;156:11–8.

853. Garavan H, Pankiewicz J, Bloom A, Cho JK, Sperry L, Ross TJ, Salmeron BJ, Risinger R, Kelley D, Stein EA. Cue-induced cocaine craving: neuroanatomical specificity for drug users and drug stimuli. Am J Psychiatry. 2000;157(11):1789–98.

854. Wexler BE, Gottschalk CH, Fulbright RK, Prohovnik I, Lacadie CM, Rounsaville BJ, Gore JC. Functional magnetic resonance imaging of cocaine craving. Am J Psychiatry. 2001;158:86–95.

855. Wang GJ, Volkow ND, Fowler JS, Cervany P, Hitzemann RJ, Pappas NR, Wong CT, Felder C. Regional brain metabolic activation during craving elicited by recall of previous drug experiences. Life Sci. 1999;64:775–84.

856. Grant S, London ED, Newlin DB, Villemagne VL, Liu X, Contoreggi C, Phillips RL, Kimes AS, Margolin A. Activation of memory circuits during cue-elicited cocaine craving. Proc Natl Acad Sci U S A. 1996;93(21):12040–5.

857. Maas LC, Lukas SE, Kaufman MJ, Weiss RD, Daniels SL, Rogers VW, Kukes TJ, Renshaw PF. Functional magnetic resonance imaging of human brain activation during cue-induced cocaine craving. Am J Psychiatry. 1998;155:124–6.

858. Breiter HC, Gollub RL, Weisskoff RM, Kennedy DN, Makris N, Berke JD, Goodman JM, Kantor HL, Gastfriend DR, Riorden JP, Mathew RT, Rosen BR, Hyman SE. Acute effects of cocaine on human brain activity and emotion. Neuron. 1997;19(3):591–611.

859. Volkow ND, Wang GJ, Fowler JS, Hitzemann R, Angrist B, Gatley SJ, Logan J, Ding YS, Pappas N. Association of Methylphenidate-Induced Craving with changes in right striato-orbitofrontal metabolism in cocaine abusers: implications in addiction. Am J Psychiatry. 1999;156:19–26.

860. Volkow ND, Wang GJ, Ma Y, Fowler JS, Zhu W, Maynard L, Telang R, Vaska P, Ding YS, Wong C, Swanson JM. Expectation enhances the regional brain metabolic and the reinforcing effects of stimulants in cocaine abusers. J Neurosci. 2003;23:11461–8.

861. Volkow ND, Hitzemann R, Wang GJ, Fowler JS, Wolf AP, Dewey SL, Handlesman L. Long-term frontal brain metabolic changes in cocaine abusers. Synapse. 1992;11:184–90.

862. Volkow ND, Hitzemann R, Wang GJ, Fowler JS, Burr G, Pascani K, Dewey SL, Wolf AP. Decreased brain metabolism in neurologically intact healthy alcoholics. Am J Psychiatry. 1992;149:1016–22.

863. Volkow ND, Wang GJ, Hitzemann R, Fowler JS, Overall JE, Burr G, Wolf AP. Recovery of brain glucose metabolism in detoxified alcoholics. Am J Psychiatry. 1994;151:178–83.

864. Volkow ND, Wang GJ, Overall JE, Hitzemann R, Fowler JS, Pappas N, Frecska E, Piscani K. Regional brain metabolic response to lorazepam in alcoholics during early and late alcohol detoxification. Alcohol Clin Exp Res. 1997;21:1278–84.

865. Catafau AM, Etcheberrigaray A, Perez de los Cobos J, Estorch M, Guardia J, Flotats A, Berna L, Mari C, Casas M, Carrio I. Regional cerebral blood flow changes in chronic alcoholic patients induced by naltrexone challenge during detoxification. J Nucl Med. 1999;40:19–24.

866. Kaufman JN, Ross TJ, Stein EA, Garavan H. Cingulate hypoactivity in cocaine users during a GO-NOGO task as revealed by event-related functional magnetic resonance imaging. J Neurosci. 2003;23:7839–43.

867. Forman SD, Dougherty GG, Casey BJ, Siegle GJ, Braver TS, Barch DM, Stenger VA, Wick-Hull C, Pisarov LA, Lorensen E. Opiate addicts lack error-dependent activation of rostral anterior cingulate. Biol Psychiatry. 2004;55:531–7.

868. Volkow ND, Fowler JS, Wolf AP, Schlyer D, Shiue CY, Alpert R, Dewey SL, Logan J, Bendriem B, Christman D. Effects of chronic cocaine abuse on postsynaptic dopamine receptors. Am J Psychiatry. 1990;147(6):719–24.

869. Volkow ND, Fowler JS, Wang GJ, Hitzemann R, Logan J, Schlyer D, Dewey S, Wolf AP. Decreased dopamine D2 receptor availability is associated with reduced frontal metabolism in cocaine abusers. Synapse. 1993;14:169–77.

870. Wang GJ, Volkow ND, Fowler JS, Logan J, Abumrad NN, Hitzemann RJ, Pappas NS, Pascani K. Dopamine D2 receptor availability in opiate-dependent subjects before and after naloxone-precipitated withdrawal. Neuropsychopharmacology. 1997;16:174–82.

871. Volkow ND, Chang L, Wang GJ, Fowler JS, Leonido-Yee M, Franceschi D, Sedler MJ, Gatley SJ, Hitzemann R, Ding YS, Logan J, Wong C, Miller EN. Association of dopamine transporter reduction with psychomotor impairment in methamphetamine abusers. Am J Psychiatry. 2001;158:377–82.

872. Volkow ND, Wang GJ, Telang F, Fowler JS, Logan J, Jayne M, Ma Y, Pradhan K, Wong C. Profound decreases in dopamine release in striatum in detoxified alcoholics: possible orbitofrontal involvement. J Neurosci. 2007;27(46):12700–6.

873. Piazza PV, Le Moal M. The role of stress in drug self-administration. Trends Pharmacol Sci. 1998;19:67–74.

874. Goeders NE. The impact of stress on addiction. Eur Neuropsychopharmacol. 2003;13:435–41.

875. Richter R, Weiss F. In vivo CRF release in rat amygdala is increased during cocaine withdrawal in self-administration rats. Synapse. 1999;32:254–61.

876. Maj M, Turchan J, Smialowska M, Przewlocka B. Morphine and cocaine influence on CRF biosynthesis in the rat central nucleus of amygdala. Neuropeptides. 2003;37:105–10.

877. Cador M, Cole BJ, Koob GF, Stinus L, Le Moal M. Central administration of corticotropin releasing factor induces long-term sensitization to D-amphetamine. Brain Res. 1993;606:181–6.

878. Merlo Pich E, Lorang M, Yeganeh M, Rodriguez de Fonseca F, Raber J, Koob GF, Weiss FI. Increase of extracellular corticotrophin releasing factor-like immunoreactivity levels in the amygdala of awake rats during restraint stress and ethanol withdrawal as measured by microdialysis. J Neurosci. 1995;15:5439–47.

879. Koob GF. Stress, corticotropin-releasing factor, and drug addiction. Ann N Y Acad Sci. 1999;897:27–45.

880. Koob GF. Neuroadaptive mechanisms of addiction: studies on the extended amygdala. Eur Neuropsychopharmacol. 2003;13(6):442–52.

881. Prado-Alcala R, Wise RA. Brain stimulation reward and dopamine terminal fields. I. Caudate-putamen, nucleus accumbens and amygdala. Brain Res. 1984;297(2):265–73.

882. Imperato A, Di Chiara G. Preferential stimulation of dopamine release in the nucleus accumbens of freely-moving rats by ethanol. J Pharmacol Exp Ther. 1986;239:219–38.

883. Damsma G, Day J, Fibiger HC. Lack of tolerance to nicotine-induced dopamine release in the nucleus accumbens. Eur J Pharmacol. 1989;168(3):363–8.

884. Kuczenski R, Segal DS, Aizenstein ML. Amphetamine, cocaine, and fencamfamine: relationship between locomotor and stereotypy response profiles and caudate and accumbens dopamine dynamics. J Neurosci. 1991;11(9):2703–12.

885. Chang JY, Sawyer SF, Lee RS, Woodward DJ. Electrophysiological and pharmacological evidence for the role of the nucleus accumbens in cocaine self-administration in freely moving rats. J Neurosci. 1994;14(3 Pt 1):1224–44.

886. Pontieri FE, Tanda G, Orzi F, Di Chiara G. Effects of nicotine on the nucleus accumbens and similarity to those of addictive drugs. Nature. 1996;382(6588):255–7.

887. Benwell ME, Balfour DJ. The effects of acute and repeated nicotine treatment on nucleus accumbens dopamine and locomotor activity. Br J Pharmacol. 1992;105(4):849–56.

888. Perez MF, Ford KA, Goussakov I, Stutzmann GE, Hu XT. Repeated cocaine exposure decreases dopamine D(2)-like receptor modulation of Ca(2+) homeostasis in rat nucleus accumbens neurons. Synapse. 2011;65(2):168–80.

889. Bowirrat A, Oscar-Berman M. Relationship between dopaminergic neurotransmission, alcoholism, and reward deficiency syndrome. Am J Med Genet B Neuropsychiatr Genet. 2005;132B(1):29–37.

890. Blum K, Noble EP. Allelic association of human dopamine D2 receptor gene in alcoholism. JAMA. 1994;263:2055–60.

891. Blum K, Wood RC, Braverman ER, Chen TJ, Sheridan PJ. The D2 dopamine receptor gene as a predictor of compulsive disease: Bayes' theorem. Funct Neurol. 1995;10(1):37–44.

892. Crunelle CL, Miller ML, Booij J, van den Brink W. The nicotinic acetylcholine receptor partial agonist varenicline and the treatment of drug dependence: a review. Eur Neuropsychopharmacol. 2010;20(2):69–79.

893. Palmatier MI, Levin ME, Mays KL, Donny EC, Caggiula AR, Sved AF. Bupropion and nicotine enhance responding for nondrug reinforcers via dissociable pharmacological mechanisms in rats. Psychopharmacology. 2009;207(3):381–90.

894. Grieder TE, Sellings LH, Vargas-Perez H, Ting AKR, Siu EC, Tyndale RF, van der Kooy D. Dopaminergic signaling mediates the motivational response underlying the opponent process to chronic but not acute nicotine. Neuropsychopharmacology. 2010;35(4):943–54.

895. Danna CL, Elmer GI. Disruption of conditioned reward association by typical and atypical antipsychotics. Pharmacol Biochem Behav. 2010;96(1):40–7.

896. Kapur S, Seeman P. Does fast dissociation from the dopamine D(2) receptor explain the action of atypical antipsychotics? A new hypothesis. Am J Psychiatry. 2001;158(3):360–9.

897. Pancheri P. La Ricerca Di Nuove Terapie Antipsicotiche: I Neuropeptidi. In: Reda GC, Pancheri P, editors. Terapia Della Schizofrenia. Il Pensiero Scientifico Ed: Roma; 1985.

898. Feinberg DT, Hartman N. Methadone and schizophrenia. Am J Psychiatry. 1991;148(12):1750–1.

899. Resnick RB, Fink M, Freedmann AM. A cyclazocine typology in opiate dependence. Am J Psychiatry. 1970;126:1256–60.

900. McLellan AT. "Psychiatric severity" as a predictor of outcome from substance abuse treatments. In: Meyer RE, editor. Psychopathology and addictive disorders. New York: Guilford Press; 1986. p. 97–139.

901. Rounsaville BJ, Kleber HD. Psychiatric disorders in opiate addicts: preliminary findings on the cause and interaction with program type. In: Meyer RE, editor. Psychopathology and addictive disorders. New York: Guilford Press; 1986. p. 140–68.

902. Bowers MBJ, Mazure CM, Nelson JC, Jatlow PI. Psychotogenic drug use and neuroleptic response. Schizophr Bull. 1990;16:81–5.

903. Buchley PF. Substance abuse in schizophrenia. A review. J Clin Psychiatry. 1998;59(S3):26–30.

904. McEvoy J, Freudenreich O, Levin E, Rose GE. Haloperidol increases smoking in patients with schizophrenia. Psychopharmacology. 1995;119:124–6.

905. McEvoy J, Freudenreich O, McGee M, VanderZwaag C, Levin E, Rose J. Clozapine decrease smoking in patients with chronic schizophrenia. Biol Psychiatry. 1995;37:550–2.

906. Meltzer HY. The mechanism of action of novel antipsychotic drugs. Schizophr Bull. 1991;17:263–87.

907. Albanese MJ, Khantzian EJ, Murphy SL, Green AI. Decreased substance use in chronically psychotic patients treated with clozapine. Am J Psychiatry. 1994;151:5.
908. Buckley PF, Thompson P, Way L, Meltzer HY. Substance abuse and clozapine treatment. J Clin Psychiatry. 1994;55:114–6.
909. Franckenbourg FR. Experience with clozapine in refractory psychotic illness. In: Standards of care in schizophrenia. Sandoz Pharmaceutical Corporation; Basel, 1994. p. 3–19.
910. Franckenbourg FR, Baldessarrini RJ. Clozapine: a novel antipsychotic agent. N Engl J Med. 1991;324(11):746–54.
911. Marcus P, Snyder R. Reduction of comorbid substance abuse with clozapine. Am J Psychiatry. 1995;152:959.
912. Ciccone PE, O'Brien CP, Manoochehr K. Psychotropic agents in opiate addiction: a brief review. Int J Addict. 1980;15:449–513.
913. Kleber HD, Gold MS. Use of psychotropic drugs in treatment of methadone maintained narcotic addicts. Ann N Y Acad Sci. 1978;311:81–98.
914. Stoops WW, Bennett JA, Lile JA, Sevak RJ, Rush CR. Influence of Aripiprazole pretreatment on the reinforcing effects of methamphetamine in humans. Prog Neuro-Psychopharmacol Biol Psychiatry. 2013;47:111–7.
915. Stoops WW. Aripiprazole as a potential pharmacotherapy for stimulant dependence: human laboratory studies with D-amphetamine. Exp Clin Psychopharmacol. 2006;14(4):413–21.
916. Sevak RJ, Vansickel AR, Stoops WW, Glaser PE, Hays LR, Rush CR. Discriminative-stimulus, subject-rated, and physiological effects of methamphetamine in humans pretreated with aripiprazole. J Clin Psychopharmacol. 2011;31(4):470–80.
917. Newton TF, Reid MS, De La Garza R, Mahoney JJ, Abad A, Condos R, Palamar J, Halkitis PN, Mojisak J, Anderson A, Li SH, Elkashef A. Evaluation of subjective effects of aripiprazole and methamphetamine in methamphetamine-dependent volunteers. Int J Neuropsychopharmacol. 2008;11(8):1037–45.
918. Lile JA, Stoops WW, Glaser PE, Hays LR, Rush CR. Discriminative stimulus, subject-rated and cardiovascular effects of cocaine alone and in combination with aripiprazole in humans. J Psychopharmacol. 2011;25(11):1469–79.
919. Moran LM, Phillips KA, Kowalczyk WJ, Ghitza UE, Agage DA, Epstein DH, Preston KL. Aripiprazole for cocaine abstinence: a randomized-controlled trial with ecological momentary assessment. Behav Pharmacol. 2017;28(1):63–73.
920. Haney M, Rubin E, Foltin RW. Aripiprazole maintenance increases smoked cocaine self-administration in humans. Psychopharmacology. 2011;216(3):379–87.
921. Stoops WW, Tindall MS, Havens JR, Oser CB, Webster JM, Mateyoke-Scrivner A, Wright PB, Booth BM, Leukefeld CG. Kentucky rural stimulant use: a comparison of methamphetamine and other stimulant users. J Psychoactive Drugs. 2007;Suppl 4:407–17.
922. Tiihonen J, Kuoppasalmi K, Fohr J, Tuomola P, Kuikanmaki O, Vorma H, Sokero P, Haukka J, Meririnne E. A comparison of Aripiprazole, methylphenidate, and placebo for amphetamine dependence. Am J Psychiatry. 2007;164(1):160–2.
923. Meini M, Moncini M, Cecconi D, Cellesi V, Biasci L, Simoni G, Ameglio M, Pellegrini M, Forgione RN, Rucci P. Aripiprazole and ropinirole treatment for cocaine dependence: evidence from a pilot study. Curr Pharm Des. 2011;17(14):1376–83.
924. Coffin PO, Santos GM, Das M, Santos DM, Huffaker S, Matheson T, Gasper J, Vittinghoff E, Colfax GN. Aripiprazole for the treatment of methamphetamine dependence: a randomized, double-blind, placebo-controlled trial. Addiction. 2013;108(4):751–61.
925. Kranzler HR, Covault J, Pierucci-Lagha A, Chan G, Douglas K, Arias AJ, Oncken C. Effects of aripiprazole on subjective and physiological responses to alcohol. Alcohol Clin Exp Res. 2008;32(4):573–9.
926. Haass-Koffler CL, Goodyear K, Zywiak WH, Leggio L, Kenna GA, Swift RM. Comparing and combining topiramate and aripiprazole on alcohol-related outcomes in a human laboratory study. Alcohol Alcohol. 2018;53(3):268–76.

927. Voronin K, Randall P, Myrick H, Anton R. Aripiprazole effects on alcohol consumption and subjective reports in a clinical laboratory paradigm—possible influence of self-control. Alcohol Clin Exp Res. 2008;32(11):1954–61.

928. Anton RF, Kranzler H, Breder C, Marcus RN, Carson WH, Han J. A randomized, multi-center, double-blind, placebo-controlled study of the efficacy and safety of aripiprazole for the treatment of alcohol dependence. J Clin Psychopharmacol. 2008;28(1):5–12.

929. Martinotti G, Di Nicola M, Di Giannantonio M, Janiri L. Aripiprazole in the treatment of patients with alcohol dependence: a double-blind, comparison trial vs. naltrexone. J Psychopharmacol. 2009;23(2):123–9.

930. Beresford TP. Medications for alcohol use disorders. JAMA. 2014;312(13):1350.

931. Beresford T, Buchanan J, Thumm EB, Emrick C, Weitzenkamp D, Ronan PJ. Late reduction of cocaine cravings in a randomized, double-blind trial of aripiprazole vs perphenazine in schizophrenia and comorbid cocaine dependence. J Clin Psychopharmacol. 2017;37(6):657–63.

932. Sulaiman AH, Gill JS, Said MA, Zainal NZ, Hussein HM, Guan NC. A randomized, placebo-controlled trial of aripiprazole for the treatment of methamphetamine dependence and associated psychosis. Int J Psychiatry Clin Pract. 2013;17(2):131–8.

933. Szerman N, Basurte-Villamor I, Vega P, Martinez-Raga J, Parro-Torres C, Cambra Almerge J, Grau-Lopez L, De Matteis M, Arias F. Once-monthly long-acting injectable aripiprazole for the treatment of patients with schizophrenia and co-occurring substance use disorders: a multicentre, observational study. Drugs Real World Outcomes. 2020;7(1):75–83.

934. Han DH, Kim SM, Choi JE, Min KJ, Renshaw PF. Adjunctive aripiprazole therapy with escitalopram in patients with co-morbid major depressive disorder and alcohol dependence: clinical and neuroimaging evidence. J Psychopharmacol. 2013;27(3):282–91.

935. Sepede G, Di Iorio G, Lupi M, Sarchione F, Acciavatti T, Fiori F, Santacroce R, Martinotti G, Gambi F, Di Giannantonio M. Bupropion as an add-on therapy in depressed bipolar disorder type I patients with comorbid cocaine dependence. Clin Neuropharmacol. 2014;37(1):17–21.

936. Bruno A, Romeo VM, Pandolfo G, Scimeca G, Zoccali RA, Muscatello MR. Aripiprazole plus topiramate in opioid-dependent patients with schizoaffective disorder: an 8-week, open-label, uncontrolled, preliminary study. Subst Abus. 2014;35(2):119–21.

937. Cassano GB, Lattanzi L, Litta A, Lombardi V, Tatulli A, Benedetti A, Longobardi A, Maremmani I. Is aripriprazole useful to refrain from cocaine use after detoxification (avoiding relapses)? Addict Disord Their Treat. 2009;8(4):161–6.

938. Petrakis IL, Carroll KM, Nich C, Gordon LT, McCance-Katz EF, Frankforter T, Rounsaville BJ. Disulfiram treatment for cocaine dependence in methadone-maintained opioid addicts. Addiction. 2000;95(2):219–28.

939. Grabowski J. Cocaine: pharmacology, effects and treatment of abuse, NIDA Research Monograph Series No. 50. Rockville, MD: NIDA; 1984.

940. Tims FM, Leukefeld CG. Cocaine treatment: research and clinical perspectives, NIDA Research Monograph Series No. 135. Rockville, MD: NIDA; 1993.

941. Roncero C, Barral C, Rodriguez-Cintas L, Perez-Pazos J, Martinez-Luna N, Casas M, Torrens M, Grau-Lopez L. Psychiatric comorbidities in opioid-dependent patients undergoing a replacement therapy programme in Spain: the Proteus study. Psychiatry Res. 2016;243:174–81.

942. Maremmani I, Pacini M. The issues of dosage. In: Maremmani I, editor. The principles and practice of methadone treatment. Pisa: Pacini Editore Medicina; 2009. p. 97–102.

943. Clark CB, Hendricks PS, Brown A, Cropsey KL. Anxiety and suicidal ideation predict successful completion of substance abuse treatment in a criminal justice sample. Subst Use Misuse. 2014;49(7):836–41.

944. Ros-Cucurull E, Miquel L, Franco MQ, Casas M. Reduction of psychotic symptoms during the use of exogenous opiates. Heroin Addict Relat Clin Probl. 2012;14(2):57–8.

945. Walby FA, Borg P, Eikeseth PH, Neegaard E, Kjerpeseth K, Bruvik S, Waal H. Use of methadone in the treatment of psychotic patients with heroin dependence. Tidsskr Nor Laegeforen. 2000;120(2):195–8.

946. Parvaresh N, Masoudi A, Majidi S, Mazhari S. The correlation between methadone dosage and comorbid psychiatric disorders in patients on methadone maintenance treatment. Addict Health. 2012;4(1–2):1–8.

947. Deglon JJ, Wark E. Methadone: a fast and powerful anti-anxiety, anti-depressant and anti-psychotic treatment. Heroin Addict Relat Clin Probl. 2008;10(1):49–56.

948. Darke S, Mills K, Teesson M, Ross J, Williamson A, Havard A. Patterns of major depression and drug-related problems amongst heroin users across 36 months. Psychiatry Res. 2009;166(1):7–14.

949. Friedmann PD, Lemon SC, Anderson BJ, Stein MD. Predictors of follow-up health status in the drug abuse treatment outcome study (Datos). Drug Alcohol Depend. 2003;69(3):243–51.

950. Fernandez Miranda J, Gonzalez Garcia-Portilla M, Saiz Martinez P, Gutierrez Cienfuegos E, Bobes Garcia J. Influence of psychiatric disorders in the effectiveness of a long-term methadone maintenance treatment. Actas Luso Esp Neurol Psiquiatr Cienc Afines. 2001;29(4):228–32.

951. Maremmani I, Canoniero S, Pacini M. Psycho(Patho)logy of "addiction" interpretative hypothesis. Ann Ist Super Sanita. 2002;38(3):241–57.

952. Pani PP, Agus A, Gessa GL. Methadone as a mood stabilizer [letter]. Heroin Addict Relat Clin Probl. 1999;1(1):43–4.

953. Eiden C, Leglise Y, Clarivet B, Blayac JP, Peyriere H. Psychiatric disorders associated with high-dose methadone (>100 mg/d): a retrospective analysis of treated patients. Therapie. 2012;67(3):223–30.

954. Herrero MJ, Domingo-Salvany A, Brugal MT, Torrens M, Itinere I. Incidence of psychopathology in a cohort of young heroin and/or cocaine users. J Subst Abus Treat. 2011;41(1):55–63.

955. Freud S. Beyond the pleasure principle. London: The International Psycho-Analytical Press; 1922.

956. Klein M. The psychoanalysis of children. New York: Grove Press; 1960.

957. Adler A. Understanding human nature. New York: Greenberg; 1927.

958. Fromm E. The anatomy of human destructiveness. London: Cape; 1974.

959. Storr H. Human aggression. London: Penguin; 1995.

960. Lorenz K. On aggression. New York: Harcourt, Brace & World; 1966.

961. Dollard J, Doob LW, Miller NE, Mowrer OH, Sears RR, Ford CS, Hovland CI, Sollenberger RT. Frustration and aggression. New Haven: Yale University Press; 1939.

962. Berkowitz L. The frustration-aggression hypothesis revisited. In: Berkowitz L, editor. Roots of aggression. New York: Atherton Press; 1969. p. 1–28.

963. Bandura A. Aggression: a social learning analysis. Englewood Cliffs: Prentice Hall; 1973.

964. Buss AH, Durkee A. An inventory for assessing different kinds of hostility. J Consult Clin Psychol. 1957;21:343–9.

965. Derogatis LR, Lipman RS, Covi L. SCL-90: an outpatient psychiatric rating scale. Preliminary report. Psychopharmacol Bull. 1973;9(1):13–28.

966. Castrogiovanni P, Andreani MF, Maremmani I, Nannini-Innocenti MA. Per Una Valutazione Dell'aggressività Nell'uomo: contributo Alla Validazione Di un Questionario per La Tipizzazione Del Comportamento Aggressivo. Riv Psichiatr. 1982;17:276–95.

967. Maremmani I, Massimetti G, Bozzi G, Carlucci P, Castrogiovanni P. Un Questionario per La Tipizzazione Del Comportamento Aggressivo Dal Possibile Impiego in Psicosomatica. Prima Standardizzazione Nella Popolazione Italiana. Bollettino Società Medico Chirurgica di Pisa. 1988;LIV:37–43.

968. Derogatis LR, Lipman RS, Rickels K. The Hopkins symptom checklist (HSCL). A self report symptom inventory. Behav Sci. 1974;19:1–16.

969. Maremmani I, Maremmani AGI, Pani PP. Psicopatologia Del Disturbo Da Uso Di Sostanze. Pisa: Pacini Editore Medicina & AU-CNS; 2016.

970. Bacciardi S, Maremmani AGI, Rovai L, Rugani F, Pacini M, Lamanna F, Dell'Osso L, Maremmani I. Aggressive behaviour in heroin dependent subjects at treatment entry. Heroin Addict Relat Clin Probl. 2013;15(1):5–13.

971. Gerra LM, Gerra G, Mercolini L, Manfredini M, Somaini L, Pieri CM, Antonioni M, Protti M, Ossola P, Marchesi C. Increased oxytocin levels among abstinent heroin addicts: association with aggressiveness, psychiatric symptoms and perceived childhood neglect. Prog Neuropsychopharmacol Biol Psychiatry. 2017;75:70–6.

972. Conversano C, Belcari I, Marchi L, Maremmani AGI, Maremmani I. Personality profiles and aggressive behaviour of heroin use disorder patients compared with non-substance-use peers. Heroin Addict Relat Clin Probl. 2018;20(4):45–54.

973. Gerra G, Zaimovic A, Raggi MA, Giusti F, Delsignore R, Bertacca S, Brambilla F. Aggressive responding of male heroin addicts under methadone treatment: psychometric and neuroendocrine correlates. Drug Alcohol Depend. 2001;65(1):85–95.

974. Gerra G, Zaimovic A, Raggi MA, Moi G, Branchi B, Moroni M, Brambilla F. Experimentally induced aggressiveness in heroin-dependent patients treated with buprenorphine: comparison of patients receiving methadone and healthy subjects. Psychiatry Res. 2007;149(1–3):201–13.

975. Tremeau F, Darreye A, Staner L, Correa H, Weibel H, Khidichian F, Macher JP. Suicidality in opioid-dependent subjects. Am J Addict. 2008;17(3):187–94.

976. Kazour F, Soufia M, Rohayem J, Richa S. Suicide risk of heroin dependent subjects in Lebanon. Community Ment Health J. 2016;52(5):589–96.

977. Lovrecic M, Lovrecic B, Maremmani I, Maremmani AGI. Excess suicide mortality in heroin use disorder patients seeking opioid agonist treatment in Slovenia and risk factors for suicide. Heroin Addict Relat Clin Probl. 2018;20(2):35–40.

978. Zhong BL, Xu YM, Zhu JH, Liu XJ. Non-suicidal self-injury in Chinese heroin-dependent patients receiving methadone maintenance treatment: prevalence and associated factors. Drug Alcohol Depend. 2018;189:161–5.

979. Maremmani AGI, Maiello M, Carbone MG, Pallucchini A, Brizi F, Belcari I, Conversano C, Perugi G, Maremmani I. Towards a psychopathology specific to substance use disorder: should emotional responses to life events be included? Compr Psychiatry. 2018;80:132–9.

980. Carbone MG, Tagliarini C, Ricci M, Lupi AM, Sarandrea L, Ceban A, Casella P, Maremmani I. Ethnicity and specific psychopathology of addiction. Comparison between migrant and Italian heroin use disorder patients. Heroin Addict Relat Clin Probl. 2019;21(5):61–6.

981. Maremmani AGI, Lovrecic M, Lovrecic B, Maremmani I. Ethnicity and specific psychopathology of addiction. Comparison between Slovenian and Italian heroin use disorder patients. Heroin Addict Relat Clin Probl. 2019;21(4):35–9.

982. Maremmani AGI, Rovai L, Bacciardi S, Massimetti E, Gazzarrini D, Rugani F, Pallucchini A, Piz L, Maremmani I. An inventory for assessing the behavioural covariates of craving in heroin substance use disorder. Development, theoretical description, reliability, exploratory factor analysis and preliminary construct validity. Heroin Addict Relat Clin Probl. 2015;17(5):51–60.

983. Turgeon SM, Pollack AE, Fink JS. Enhanced CREB phosphorylation and changes in c-FOS and FRA expression in striatum accompany amphetamine sensitization. Brain Res. 1997;749(1):120–6.

984. Maremmani I, Pacini M, Perugi G, Akiskal HS. Addiction and bipolar spectrum: dual diagnosis with a common substrate? Addict Disord Their Treat. 2004;3(4):156–64.

985. Maremmani AGI, Cerniglia L, Cimino S, Bacciardi S, Rovai L, Pallucchini A, Spera V, Perugi G, Maremmani I. Further evidence of a specific psychopathology of addiction. differentiation from other psychiatric psychopathological dimensions (such as obesity). Int J Environ Res Public Health. 2017;14:943.

986. Maremmani AGI, Gazzarrini D, Fiorin A, Cingano V, Bellio G, Perugi G, Maremmani I. Psychopathology of addiction: is the SCL90-based five dimensional structure applicable to a non-substance-related addictive disorder such as gambling disorder? Ann General Psychiatry. 2018;17(3):1–9.

987. Rugani F, Paganin W, Maremmani AGI, Perugi G, Maremmani I. Towards a specific psychopathology of heroin addiction. Comparison between heroin use disorder and chronic psychotic patients. Heroin Addict Relat Clin Probl. 2019;21(3):53–9.

988. Michelazzi A, Vecchiet F, Leprini R, Popovic D, Deltito J, Maremmani I. GPS' office based metadone maintenance treatment in Trieste, Italy. Therapeutic efficacy and predictors of clinical response. Heroin Addict Relat Clin Probl. 2008;10(2):27–38.

989. Gerra G, Zaimovic A, Moi G, Bussandri M, Bubici C, Mossini M, Raggi MA, Brambilla F. Aggressive responding in abstinent heroin addicts: neuroendocrine and personality correlates. Prog Neuro-Psychopharmacol Biol Psychiatry. 2004;28(1):129–39.

990. Gerra G, Di Petta G, D'Amore A, Iannotta P, Bardicchia F, Falorni F, Coacci A, Strepparola G, Campione G, Lucchini A, Vedda G, Serio G, Manzato E, Antonioni M, Bertacca S, Moi G, Zaimovic A. Effects of olanzapine on aggressiveness in heroin dependent patients. Prog Neuro-Psychopharmacol Biol Psychiatry. 2006;30(7):1291–8.

991. Zarghami M, Sheikhmoonesi F, Ala S, Yazdani J, Farnia S. A comparative study of beneficial effects of olanzapine and sodium valproate on aggressive behavior of patients who are on methadone maintenance therapy: a randomized triple blind clinical trial. Eur Rev Med Pharmacol Sci. 2013;17(8):1073–81.

992. Evren C, Yilmaz A, Can Y, Bozkurt M, Evren B, Umut G. Severity of impulsivity and aggression at 12-month follow-up among male heroin dependent patients. Bull Clin Psychopharmacol. 2014;24(2):158–67. https://doi.org/10.5455/bcp.20131218094342.

993. Shaikh MB, Dalsass M, Siegel A. Opioidergic mechanisms mediating aggressive behavior in the cat. Aggress Behav. 1990;16:191–206.

994. Khantzian EJ. Psychological (structural) vulnerabilities and the specific appeal of narcotics. Ann N Y Acad Sci. 1982;398:24–32.

995. Pichot P. La Nosologie des États Depréssifs. Bases Éthiologiques. Geigy: Acte Psychosom Doc; 1960.

996. Walker PW. Zum Krankheitsbild Der Lavierten Endogenen depression. Wien Med Wschr Suppl. 1963;98:111.

997. Ball JC, Corty E, Petroski SP, Bond H, Tommasello A, Graff H. Medical services provided to 2394 patients at methadone programs in three states. J Subst Abus Treat. 1986;3:203–9.

998. Barr HL, Cohen A. The problem drinking drug addiction. In: National Drug/Alcohol Collaborative Project: issues in multiple substance abuse. Washington, DC: U.S. Government Printing Office; 1980. p. 78–0.

999. Barr HL, Cohen A. Abusers of alcohol and narcotics: who are they? Int J Addict. 1987;22:525–32.

1000. Chambers CD. Characteristics of combined opiate and alcohol abusers. In: Gardner SE, editor. Drug and alcohol abuse: implication for treatment, NIDA treatment research monograph Series. Rockville, MD: U.S. Department of Health and Human Services; 1972. p. 1131–40.

1001. Green J, Jaffe JH, Carlisi J, Zaks A. Alcohol use in the opiate use cycle of the heroin addict. Int J Addict. 1978;13:1415–6.

1002. Hunt DE, Strud DL, Goldsmith DS. Alcohol use and abuse: heavy drinking among methadone clients. Am J Drug Alcohol Abuse. 1986;12:147–0.

1003. Kosten TR, Rounsaville J, Kleber HD. Parental alcoholism in opioid addicts. J Nerv Ment Dis. 1985;173:461–9.

1004. Rounsaville BJ, Weissman MM, Kleber HB. The significance of alcoholism in treated opiate addicts. J Nerv Ment Dis. 1982;170:479–88.

1005. Wixon HN, Hunt WA. Effect of acute and chronic ethanol treatment on gamma amino butyric acid levels and on Aminooxyacetic acid-induced gaba accumulation. Subst Alcohol Ab/Mis. 1980;1:481–91.

1006. Hudolin V. Manuale di alcologia. Trento: Edizioni Centro Studi Erikson; 1991.

1007. Gerston A, Cohen MJ, Stimmel B. Alcoholism, heroin dependency, and methadone maintenance: alternatives and aids to conventional methods of therapy. Am J Drug Alcohol Abuse. 1977;4:517–31.

1008. Charuvastra CV, Pannell J, Hopper M, Erhmann M, Blakis M, Ling W. The medical safety of the combined usage of disulfiram and methadone (pharmacological treatment for alcoholic heroin addicts). Arch Gen Psychiatry. 1976;33:391–3.

1009. Ling W, Weiss DG, Charuvastra VC, O'Brien CP. Use of disulfiram for alcoholics in methadone maintenance programs. A veterans administration cooperative study. Arch Gen Psychiatry. 1983;40:851–4.
1010. Tong TG, Benowitz NL, Kreek MJ. Methadone-disulfiram interaction during methadone maintenance. J Clin Pharmacol. 1980;20:506–13.
1011. Mamelak M. Gamma-hydroxybutyrate: an endogenous regulator of energy metabolism. Neurosci Biobehav Rev. 1989;13:187–98.
1012. Snead OCR, Liu CC. Gamma-Hydroxybutyric acid binding sites in rat and human brain Synaptosomal membranes. Biochem Pharmacol. 1984;33(16):2587–90.
1013. Tunnicliff G. Significance of gamma-hydroxybutyric acid in the brain. Gen Pharmacol. 1992;23:1028–34.
1014. Diana M, Rossetti ZL, Gessa GL. Central dopaminergic mechanism of alcohol and opiate withdrawal syndromes. In: Tagliamonte A, Maremmani I, editors. Drug addiction and related clinical problems. Wien: Springer-Verlag; 1995. p. 18–26.
1015. Gessa GL, Agabio R, Carai MAM, Lobina C, Pani M, Reali R, Colombo G. Mecchanism of antialcohol effect of gammahydroxybutyric acid. Alcohol. 2000;20:271–6.
1016. Gessa GL, Crabai F, Yargiu L, Spano PF. Selective increase of brain dopamine induced by gamma-hydroxybutyrate: study of the mechanism of action. J Neurochem. 1968;15(5):377–81.
1017. Addolorato G, Stefanini GF, Gasbarrini G. Manageability and tollerability of gamma-hidroxybutyric acid in the medium-term outpatient treatment of alcoholism. Alcohol Clin Exp Res. 1997;21(2):380.
1018. Ferrara SD, Zotti S, Tedeschi L, Frison G, Castagna F, Gallimberti L, Gessa GL, Palatini P. Pharmacokinetics of gamma-hydroxybutyric acid in alcohol dependent patients after single and repeated oral doses. Br J Clin Pharmacol. 1992;34(3):231–5.
1019. Maremmani I, Balestri C, Lamanna F, Tagliamonte A. Efficacy of split doses of GHB used as anticraving in the treatment of alcohol dependence. Preliminary results. Alcoholism. 1998;34(1–2):73–80.
1020. Palatini P, Tedeschi L, Frison G, Padrini R, Zordan R, Orlando R, Gallimberti L, Gessa GL, Ferrara SD. Dose-dependent absorption and elimination of gamma-hydroxybutyric acid in healthy volunteers. Eur J Clin Pharmacol. 1993;45(4):353–6.
1021. Levy MI, Davis BM, Mohs RC, Trigos GC, Mathe AA, Davis KL. Gamma-hydroxybutyrate in the treatment of schizophrenia. Psychiatry Res. 1983;9:1–8.
1022. Schulz SC, van Kammen DP, Buchsbaum MS, Roth RH, Alexander P, Bunney WE Jr. Gamma-hydroxybutyrate treatment of schizophrenia: a pilot study. Pharmacopsychiatria. 1981;14(4):129–34.
1023. Poldrugo F, Addolorato G. The role of gamma-hydroxybutyric acid in the treatment of alcoholism: from animal to clinical studies. Alcohol Alcohol. 1999;34(1):15–24.
1024. Gessa GL, Colombo G. L'acido gamma-idrossibutirrico (GHB): un neurotrasmettitore, una medicina, una sostanza D'abuso. Boll Farmacodip Alcol. 1998;21(Suppl 1):43–6.
1025. Di Bello MG, Gambassi F, Mignai L, Masini E, Mannaioni PF. Gammahydroxy-butyrric acid induced suppression and prevention of alcohol withdrawal syndrome and relief of craving in alcohol dependent patients. Alcologia. 1995;VII(2):9–16.
1026. Gallimberti L, Gentile N, Cibin M, Fadda F, Canton G, Ferri M, Ferrara SD, Gessa GL. Gamma-hydroxybutyric acid for treatment of alcohol withdrawal syndrome. Lancet. 1989;2(8666):787–9.
1027. Addolorato G, Balducci G, Capristo E, Attilia ML, Taggi F, Gasbarrini G, Ceccanti M. Gammahydroxybutyric acid (GHB) in the treatment of alcohol withdrawal syndrome: a randomized comparative study versus benzodiazepine. Alcohol Clin Exp Res. 1992;23:1596–604.
1028. Lenzenhuber E, Muller C, Rommelspacher H, Spies C. Gamma-hydroxybutyrate for treatment of alcohol withdrawal syndrome in intensive care patients. A comparison between with two symptom-oriented therapeutic concepts. Anaesthesist. 1999;48(2):89–96.

1029. Nimmerrichter AA, Walter H, Gutierrez-Lobos KE, Lesch OM. Double-blind controlled trial of gamma-hydroxybutyrate and clomethiazole in the treatment of alcohol withdrawal. Alcohol Alcohol. 2002;37(1):67–73.
1030. Addolorato G, Castelli E, Stefanini GF, Casella G, Caputo F, Marsigli L, Bernardi M, Gasbarrini G. An open multicentric study evaluating 4-hydroxybutyric acid sodium salt in the medium-term treatment of 179 alcohol dependent subjects. GHB study group. Alcohol Alcohol. 1996;31(4):341–5.
1031. Addolorato G, Cibin M, Caputo F, Capristo E, Gessa GL, Stefanini GF, Gasbarrini G. Gamma-hydroxybutyric acid in the treatment of alcoholism: dosage fractioning utility in non-responder alcoholic patients. Drug Alcohol Depend. 1998;53(1):7–10.
1032. Maremmani I, Lamanna F, Tagliamonte A. Long-term therapy using GHB (sodium gamma hydroxybutyrate) for treatment-resistant chronic alcoholics. J Psychoactive Drugs. 2001;33(2):135–42.
1033. Maremmani AGI, Pani PP, Rovai L, Pacini M, Dell'Osso L, Maremmani I. Long-term Γ-hydroxybutyric acid (GHB) and disulfiram combination therapy in GHB treatment-resistant chronic alcoholics. Int J Environ Res Public Health. 2011;8(7):2816–27.
1034. Addolorato G, Lesch O-M, Maremmani I, Walter H, Nava F, Raffaillac Q, Caputo F. Post-marketing and clinical safety experience with sodium oxybate for the treatment of alcohol withdrawal syndrome and maintenance of abstinence in alcohol-dependent subjects. Expert Opin Pharmacother. 2020;19(2):159–66. https://doi.org/10.1080/14740338.2020.1709821.
1035. van den Brink W, Addolorato G, Aubin H-J, Benyamina A, Caputo F, Dematteis M, Gual A, Lesch O-M, Mann K, Maremmani I, Nutt D, Paille F, Perney P, Rehm J, Reynaud M, Simon N, Söderpalm B, Sommer W, Walter H, Spanagel R. Efficacy and safety of sodium oxybate in alcohol dependent patients with a very high drinking risk level. Addict Biol. 2018;23:969–86.
1036. Gallimberti L, Cibin M, Pagnin P, Sabbion R, Pani PP, Pirastu R, Ferrara SD, Gessa GL. Gamma-hydroxybutyric acid for treatment of opiate withdrawal syndrome. Neuropsychopharmacology. 1993;9(1):77–81.
1037. US Xyrem® Multi-Center Study Group. The abrupt cessation of therapeutically administered sodium oxybate (GHB) does not cause withdrawal symptoms. Toxicol Clin Toxicol. 2003;41(2):131–5.
1038. Craig K, Gomez HF, McManus JL, Bania TC. Severe gamma-hydroxybutyrate withdrawal: a case report and literature review. J Emerg Med. 2000;18:65–70.
1039. Dyer JE, Roth B, Hyma BA. Gamma-hydroxybutyrate withdrawal syndrome. Ann Emerg Med. 2001;37:147–53.
1040. Galloway GP, Frederick SL, Staggers FE Jr, Gonzales M, Stalcup S, Smith D. Gamma-hydroxybutyrate: an emerging drug of abuse that causes physical dependence. Addiction. 1997;92:89–96.
1041. McDaniel CH, Miotto KA. Gamma hydroxybutyrate (GHB) and gamma butyrolactone (GBL) withdrawal: five case studies. J Psychoactive Drugs. 2001;33(2):143–9.
1042. Rosenberg MH, Deerfield LJ, Baruch EM. Two cases of severe gamma-hydroxybutyrate withdrawal delirium on a psychiatric unit: recommendations for management. Am J Drug Alcohol Abuse. 2003;29(2):487–96.
1043. Tarabar AF, Nelson LS. The gamma-hydroxybutyrate withdrawal syndrome. Toxicol Rev. 2004;23(1):45–9.
1044. Addolorato G, Caputo F, Capristo E, Gasbarrini G. Diazepam in the treatment of GHB dependence. Br J Psychiatry. 2001;178:183.
1045. Rosen MI, Pearsall HR, Woods SW, Kosten TR. Effects of gamma-hydroxybutyric acid (GHB) in opioid-dependent patients. J Subst Abus Treat. 1997;14(2):149–54.
1046. Hernandez M, McDaniel CH, Costanza CD, Hernandez OJ. GHB-induced delirium: a case report and review of the literature of gamma hydroxybutyric acid. Am J Drug Alcohol Abuse. 1998;24:179–83.
1047. Miotto K, Darakjian J, Basch J, Murray S, Zogg J, Rawson R. Gamma-hydroxybutyric acid: patterns of use, effects and withdrawal. Am J Addict. 2001;10(3):232–41.

1048. Friedman J, Westlake R, Furman M. Grievous bodily harm: gamma hydroxybutyrate abuse leading to a Wernicke-Korsakoff syndrome. Neurology. 1996;46:469–71.

1049. Caputo F, Addolorato G, Stoppo M, Francini S, Vignoli T, Lorenzini F, Del Re A, Comaschi C, Andreone P, Trevisani F, Bernardi M. Comparing and combining gamma-hydroxybutyric acid (GHB) and naltrexone in maintaining abstinence from alcohol: an open randomised comparative study. Eur Neuropsychopharmacol. 2007;17(12):781–9.

1050. Gallimberti L, Schifano F, Forza G, Miconi L, Ferrara SD. Clinical efficacy of gamma-hydroxybutyric acid in treatment of opiate withdrawal. Eur Arch Psychiatry Clin Neurosci. 1994;244(3):113–4.

1051. Feigenbaum JJ, Simantov R. Lack of effect of gamma-hydroxybutyrate on mu, delta and kappa opioid receptor binding. Neurosci Lett. 1996;212(1):5–8.

1052. Maremmani I, Lamanna F. Clinica E Terapia Dell'alcolismo Nei Tossicodipendenti. In: Maremmani I, Canoniero S, Pacini M, editors. Manuale Di Neuropsicofarmacoterapia Psichiatrica E Dell'abuso Di Sostanze. Pisa: Pacini Editore Medicina & AUC-CNS Onlus; 2001. p. 413–8.

1053. Dineeva NR. Adolescent narcotism in Russia. Heroin Addict Relat Clin Probl. 1999;1(2):27–34.

1054. Coppel A, Bloch-Laine JF, Charpak Y, Spira R. Evaluation survey of a methadone treatment share care programme between a specialized clinic and a network of GPS. Heroin Addict Relat Clin Probl. 2001;3(2):21–8.

1055. Lubrano S, Pacini M, Giuntoli G, Maremmani I. Is craving for heroin and alcohol related to low methadone dosages in methadone maintened patients. Heroin Addict Relat Clin Probl. 2002;4(2):11–7.

1056. Maremmani I, Pacini M. Use of sodium gamma-hydroxybutyrate (GHB) in alcoholic heroin addicts and polydrug-abusers. Heroin Addict Relat Clin Probl. 2007;9(1):55–76.

1057. Caputo F, Addolorato G, Domenicali M, Mosti A, Viaggi M, Trevisani F, Gasbarrini G, Bernardi M, Stefanini G. Services for addiction treatment. Short-term methadone administration reduces alcohol consumption in non-alcoholic heroin addicts. Alcohol Alcohol. 2002;37(2):164–8.

1058. Maxwell S, Shinderman MS. Optimizing response to methadone maintenance treatment: use of higher-dose methadone. J Psychoactive Drugs. 1999;31(2):95–102.

1059. Lamanna F, Maremmani I. Il trattamento degli eroinomani alcolisti. 5 casi clinici. Heroin addict Relat Clin Probl Suppl. 2006;XI:25–7.